AF760985

Current Clinical Pathology

Series Editor

Antonio Giordano MD PhD
Philadelphia, PA, USA

More information about this series at http://www.springer.com/series/7632

Vincenzo Canzonieri
Antonio Giordano
Editors

Gastric Cancer In The Precision Medicine Era

Diagnosis and Therapy

Humana Press

Editors
Vincenzo Canzonieri
Pathology Unit and Biobank
CRO-Aviano, IRCCS,
National Cancer Institute
Aviano
Italy

University of Trieste
Trieste TS
Italy

Department of Biology
Temple University
Philadelphia, PA
USA

Antonio Giordano
Sbarro Institute for Cancer
Research and Molecular Medicine
Department of Biology
Temple University
Philadelphia, PA
USA

Department of Medicine
Surgery and Neuroscience
University of Siena
Siena
Italy

ISSN 2197-781X ISSN 2197-7828 (electronic)
Current Clinical Pathology
ISBN 978-3-030-04860-0 ISBN 978-3-030-04861-7 (eBook)
https://doi.org/10.1007/978-3-030-04861-7

Library of Congress Control Number: 2018962131

© Springer Nature Switzerland AG 2019
This work is subject to copyright. All rights are reserved by the Publisher, whether the whole or part of the material is concerned, specifically the rights of translation, reprinting, reuse of illustrations, recitation, broadcasting, reproduction on microfilms or in any other physical way, and transmission or information storage and retrieval, electronic adaptation, computer software, or by similar or dissimilar methodology now known or hereafter developed.
The use of general descriptive names, registered names, trademarks, service marks, etc. in this publication does not imply, even in the absence of a specific statement, that such names are exempt from the relevant protective laws and regulations and therefore free for general use.
The publisher, the authors, and the editors are safe to assume that the advice and information in this book are believed to be true and accurate at the date of publication. Neither the publisher nor the authors or the editors give a warranty, express or implied, with respect to the material contained herein or for any errors or omissions that may have been made. The publisher remains neutral with regard to jurisdictional claims in published maps and institutional affiliations.

This Humana Press imprint is published by the registered company Springer Nature Switzerland AG
The registered company address is: Gewerbestrasse 11, 6330 Cham, Switzerland

Preface

Gastric cancer is an aggressive disease that represents a serious problem and has a daunting impact on global health. Despite an appreciable decrease in incidence over the last several decades, gastric cancer remains one of the most common types of cancer in the world. In recent years, a great progress has been made in understanding the pathogenesis of gastric cancer, especially regarding the importance of *Helicobacter pylori* and its associated inflammatory response. Furthermore, for early and advanced gastric cancers, appropriate treatments have been implemented to maximize curative results, as in the setting of adjuvant oncologic therapies of proven benefit for advanced cases, in addition to surgery.

Our purpose through this book is to provide a general overview of the different aspects of gastric cancer.

The first part aims to clarify the main aspects of tumorigenesis, such as the role of inflammation linked to the presence of *H. pylori* infection, and the genetic and epigenetic mechanisms so far known.

The second part includes the pathological and clinical features and contains information regarding the most recent tissue and serological biomarkers in these neoplasms.

The three successive parts are intended to provide the "state of art" of multimodal treatment approaches to gastric cancer, i.e., standard and novel surgical aspects, common and innovative chemo and radio protocols, and modern targeted therapies. Novel molecular classifications are under consideration to improve diagnostic and prognostic definitions and to prospect future treatments based on the use of immunotherapies and innovative molecules such as noncoding RNA and nanoparticles.

Aviano, Italy — Vincenzo Canzonieri
Philadelphia, PA, USA — Antonio Giordano

Contents

Introduction

About 90–95% of gastric cancers (GC) or stomach cancers are adenocarcinomas. These cancers develop within the cells of the mucosa, the innermost lining of the stomach. Other GC histotypes are lymphoma, gastrointestinal stromal tumors (GISTs), carcinoid tumors, and other rare tumors.

Gastric adenocarcinoma (GAC) is the fourth most common type of cancer and the second most common cause of cancer-related deaths in the world; this is determined, in part, by the late appearance of symptoms, usually associated with disease's advanced stages. In the last decades, the incidence of GAC is declining due to improved nutrition, food preservation, increase in hygiene standards, better prevention, earlier diagnosis and treatment, and *Helicobacter pylori* (*H. pylori*) eradication.

The incidence of GAC varies geographically: more than 50% of new cases of GAC occur in developing countries. The high-risk areas are Eastern Europe, East Asia, and Central and South America; the low-risk areas are North and East Africa, Southern Asia, North America, New Zealand, and Australia [1, 2].

Like other carcinomas, also GAC results from a combination of genetic alterations and environmental factors. Prevention is always the best way to avoid the disease and includes anti-*H. pylori* therapies, healthy diet, chemoprevention, and screening for early cancer detection. Infection with *H. pylori* bacteria seems to be a major cause of stomach cancer, especially cancers in the lower (distal) part of the stomach. Infections caused by this long-lasting germ can cause inflammation (chronic atrophic gastritis) and precancerous alterations of the inner lining of the stomach. An increased risk of stomach cancer is seen in people with diets that have large amounts of smoked foods, salted fish and meat, pickled vegetables, and alcohol drinking abuse. Healthy dietary habits rich in high fresh fruits and vegetables can also lower stomach cancer risk. Furthermore, many studies have confirmed that tobacco smoke increases stomach cancer risk, particularly for cancers of the upper portion of the stomach near the esophagus. Accordingly, the rate of stomach cancer is about doubled in smokers [3, 4].

Only a small percentage of stomach cancers are known to be caused by hereditary diffuse gastric cancer syndrome or by another hereditary cancer syndrome called Lynch syndrome.

From the pathological point of view, GAC mainly consists of two pathological variants, intestinal type and diffuse type. The intestinal type is the end result of an inflammatory process that progresses from chronic gastritis to atrophic gastritis and finally to intestinal metaplasia and dysplasia. While the intestinal type of gastric cancer is often related to environmental factors such as *Helicobacter pylori* infection, diet, and lifestyle, and it is more common in elderly men, the diffuse type is more often associated with genetic abnormalities [5], and it is more prevalent among women and in individuals under the age of 50. Furthermore, the diffuse type is associated with an unfavorable prognosis because the diagnosis is carried out mainly in advanced stages.

Depending on the site and extent of cancer, surgery is the only potentially curative treatment for all T1b-T4 GACs, and extended lymphadenectomy should be recommended as standard of care in resectable tumors. Endoscopic submucosal resection is the preferred option for early-stage cancer. Furthermore, a survival benefit for postoperative chemotherapy, chemoradiotherapy, and perioperative chemotherapy in case of pathologic $T > 2$ and/or node-positive gastric cancer patients has been established, and chemotherapy should contain 5-fluorouracil and cisplatin or their analogs capecitabine and oxaliplatin. Finally, in select metastatic gastric cancer patients, chemotherapy is better than best supportive care only, with cisplatin-5-fluorouracil or capecitabine as the most widely used drugs. In patients that show HER2 overexpression, the addition of anti-HER2 antibody trastuzumab to first-line chemotherapy is advisable. For HER2-negative patients, two or three combinations, including irinotecan, docetaxel, oxaliplatin, or 5FU prodrugs, are valid treatments. Furthermore, the addition of the anti-VEGFR-2 antibody ramucirumab in second line improves overall survival and progression-free survival when compared to chemotherapy only [6]. The following sections report different aspects related to GC, such as tumorigenesis mechanisms, clinical-pathological features and new molecular classifications, and multimodal treatments ranging from surgical strategies to chemo- and radiotherapy, up to the most recent approaches of precision medicine and the most innovative treatments that involve the use of noncoding RNA, immunotherapy, and nanotechnologies.

Aviano, Italy Vincenzo Canzonieri
Philadelphia, PA, USA Antonio Giordano

References

1. Sitarz R, Skierucha M, Mielko J, Offerhaus GJ, Maciejewski R, Polkowski WP. Gastric cancer: epidemiology, prevention, classification, and treatment. Cancer Manag Res. 2018;10:239–48. https://doi.org/10.2147/CMAR.S149619.
2. Jemal A, Bray F, Center MM, Ferlay J, Ward E, Forman D. Global cancer statistics. CA Cancer J Clin. 2011;61(2):69–90. https://doi.org/10.3322/caac.20107. Epub 2011 Feb 4.
3. The American Cancer Society medical and editorial content team, Last Revised: December 14, 2017. Available on: https://www.cancer.org/cancer/stomach-cancer/causes-risks-prevention/risk-factors.html#written_by.

4. Karimi P, Islami F, Kamangar F. Gastric cancer: descriptive epidemiology, risk factors, screening, and prevention. Cancer Epidemiol Biomark Prev. 2014;23(5):700–13. https://doi.org/10.1158/1055-9965.EPI-13-1057.
5. Carcas LP. Gastric cancer review. J Carcinog. 2014;13:14. https://doi.org/10.4103/1477-3163.146506.
6. Orditura M, Galizia G, Sforza V, Gambardella V, Fabozzi A, Laterza MM, Andreozzi F, Ventriglia J, Savastano B, Mabilia A, Lieto E, Ciardiello F, De Vita F. Treatment of gastric cancer. World J Gastroenterol. 2014;20(7):1635–49. https://doi.org/10.3748/wjg.v20.i7.1635.

Contributors

Lara Alessandrini Pathology Department, IRCCS, CRO Aviano, National Cancer Institute, Aviano, PN, Italy

Department of Medicine (DIMED), Surgical Pathology & Cytopathology Unit, University Hospital of Padova, Padova, Italy

Danilo Antona Surgical Oncology Department, IRCCS, CRO Aviano, National Cancer Institute, Aviano, PN, Italy

Claudio Belluco Surgical Oncology Department, IRCCS, CRO Aviano, National Cancer Institute, Aviano, PN, Italy

Massimiliano Berretta Medical Oncology Department, IRCCS, CRO Aviano, National Cancer Institute, Aviano, PN, Italy

Giulio Bertola Surgical Oncology Department, IRCCS, CRO Aviano, National Cancer Institute, Aviano, PN, Italy

Angela Buonadonna Medical Oncology Department, IRCCS, CRO Aviano, National Cancer Institute, Aviano, Italy

Isabella Caligiuri Pathology Unit, Department of Translational Research, IRCCS, CRO Aviano, National Cancer Institute, Aviano, PN, Italy

Renato Cannizzaro Oncological Gastroenterology Department, IRCCS, CRO Aviano, National Cancer Institute, Aviano, Italy

Vincenzo Canzonieri Pathology Department, IRCCS, CRO Aviano, National Cancer Institute, Aviano, Italy

Department of Medical, Surgical and Health Sciences, University of Trieste, Trieste, TS, Italy

CRO Biobank, IRCCS, CRO Aviano, National Cancer Institute, Aviano, PN, Italy

Department of Biology, Temple University, Philadelphia, PA, USA

Mariateresa Casarotto Immunopathology and Cancer Biomarkers, IRCCS, CRO Aviano, National Cancer Institute, Aviano, PN, Italy

Silvia Cervo Immunopathology and Cancer Biomarkers, IRCCS, CRO Aviano, National Cancer Institute, Aviano, PN, Italy

CRO-Biobank, IRCCS, CRO Aviano, National Cancer Institute, Aviano, PN, Italy

Antonino De Paoli Radiation Oncology Department, IRCCS, CRO Aviano, National Cancer Institute, Aviano, PN, Italy

Paolo De Paoli IRCCS, CRO Aviano, National Cancer Institute, Aviano, PN, Italy

Valli De Re Immunopathology and Biomarker Unit/Bio-proteomics Facility, Department of Research and Advanced Tumor Diagnostics, IRCCS, CRO Aviano, National Cancer Institute, Aviano, PN, Italy

Riccardo Dolcetti Immunopathology and Biomarker Unit/Bio-proteomics Facility, Department of Research and Advanced Tumor Diagnostics, Aviano, PN, Italy

Translational Research Institute, University of Queensland Diamantina Institute, Brisbane, QLD, Australia

Maguie El Boustani Pathology Unit, Department of Translational Research, IRCCS, CRO Aviano, National Cancer Institute, Aviano, PN, Italy

Valentina Fanotto Medical Oncology, IRCCS, CRO Aviano, National Cancer Institute, Aviano, PN, Italy

Department of Clinical Oncology, IRCCS, CRO Aviano, National Cancer Institute, Aviano, PN, Italy

Department of Medicine (DAME), University of Udine, Udine, UD, Italy

Mara Fornasarig Oncological Gastroenterology Department, IRCCS, CRO Aviano, National Cancer Institute, Aviano, PN, Italy

Antonio Giordano Sbarro Institute for Cancer Research and Molecular Medicine, Department of Biology, Temple University, Philadelphia, PA, USA

Department of Medicine, Surgery and Neuroscience, Anatomic Pathology Section, University of Siena, Siena, Italy

Michela Guardascione Medical Oncology Department, IRCCS, CRO Aviano, National Cancer Institute, Aviano, PN, Italy

Roberto Innocente Radiation Oncology Department, IRCCS, CRO Aviano, National Cancer Institute, Aviano, PN, Italy

Fabrizio Italia Oncopath Lab, Floridia, SR, Italy

Andrea Lauretta Surgical Oncology Department, IRCCS, CRO Aviano, National Cancer Institute, Aviano, PN, Italy

Raffaella Magris Oncological Gastroenterology Department, IRCCS, CRO Aviano, National Cancer Institute, Aviano, PN, Italy

Stefania Maiero Oncological Gastroenterology Department, IRCCS, CRO Aviano, National Cancer Institute, Aviano, PN, Italy

Melissa Manchi Pathology Department, IRCCS, CRO Aviano, National Cancer Institute, Aviano, PN, Italy

Gian Maria Miolo Medical Oncology Department, IRCCS, CRO Aviano, National Cancer Institute, Aviano, PN, Italy

Nayla Mouawad Pathology Unit, Department of Translational Research, IRCCS, CRO Aviano, National Cancer Institute, Aviano, PN, Italy

Federico Navarria Radiation Oncology Department, IRCCS, CRO Aviano, National Cancer Institute, Aviano, PN, Italy

Matteo Olivieri Surgical Oncology Department, IRCCS, CRO Aviano, National Cancer Institute, Aviano, PN, Italy

Elisa Palazzari Radiation Oncology Department, IRCCS, CRO Aviano, National Cancer Institute, Aviano, PN, Italy

Tiziana Perin Pathology Department, IRCCS, CRO Aviano, National Cancer Institute, Aviano, PN, Italy

CRO Biobank, IRCCS, CRO Aviano, National Cancer Institute, Aviano, PN, Italy

Chiara Pratesi Immunopathology and Cancer Biomarkers, IRCCS, CRO Aviano, National Cancer Institute, Aviano, PN, Italy

Fabio Puglisi Department of Clinical Oncology, IRCCS, CRO Aviano, National Cancer Institute, Aviano, PN, Italy

Department of Medicine (DAME), University of Udine, Udine, UD, Italy

Federica Rao Pathology Department, IRCCS, CRO Aviano, National Cancer Institute, Aviano, PN, Italy

Clara Rizzardi Department of Medical, Surgical and Health Sciences, University of Trieste, Trieste, Italy

Flavio Rizzolio Pathology Department, IRCCS, CRO Aviano, National Cancer Institute, Aviano, PN, Italy

Department of Molecular Sciences and Nanosystems, Ca' Foscari University, Venice-Mestre, VE, Italy

Department of Biology, Temple University, Philadelphia, PA, USA

Rossella Rotondo Pathology Department, IRCCS, CRO Aviano, National Cancer Institute, Aviano, PN, Italy

Paola Spessotto Molecular Oncology Unit, IRCCS, CRO Aviano, National Cancer Institute, Aviano, PN, Italy

Agostino Steffan Immunopathology and Cancer Biomarkers, IRCCS, CRO Aviano, National Cancer Institute, Aviano, PN, Italy

CRO-Biobank, IRCCS, CRO Aviano, National Cancer Institute, Aviano, PN, Italy

Fabrizio Zanconati Department of Medical, Surgical and Health Sciences, University of Trieste, Trieste, Italy

Stefania Zanussi Immunopathology and Cancer Biomarkers, IRCCS, CRO Aviano, National Cancer Institute, Aviano, PN, Italy

Part I

Gastric Tumorigenesis

1 Gastric Tumorigenesis: Role of Inflammation and *Helicobacter pylori*

Stefania Zanussi, Mariateresa Casarotto, Chiara Pratesi, and Paolo De Paoli

Introduction

Great improvements in molecular and cellular technologies and decades of in-depth studies were needed so that inflammation was added to the hallmarks of cancer, and pioneering observations of Virchow and Coley became widely accepted perspectives to be pursued for translation in cancer cures [1–3]. Inflammation is a coordinated response following infection or tissue damage by exogenous or endogenous agents, which involves innate and adaptive immune system cells and soluble factors. Macrophages, neutrophils, eosinophils, mast cells, dendritic cells (DCs), and natural killer (NK) cells represent the antigen-independent first line of immunological defense against homeostatic perturbation of tissue microenvironment. These cell subsets initiate inflammatory response by sensing pathogen-associated molecular patterns, which are present during microbial infections, and danger-associated molecular patterns, which are components of the host cells released during cell damage or death. At early stages of inflammation, tissue antigens are processed and transported to lymphoid organs by specialized antigen-presenting cells, which allow the activation and expansion of B and T lymphocyte-specific immune responses. In this scenario, intracellular regulatory pathways are activated, which ultimately lead to the secretion of reactive oxygen and reactive nitrogen species (ROS and RNS), of diffusible growth factors, of inflammatory cytokines, and of matrix-remodeling enzymes. These elements induce mobilization and infiltration of additional leucocytes in the affected field and magnify the inflammatory reaction until the resolution of the injury or infection.

The tumorigenic fate of the immune response largely depends on the physiological state of the epithelial, stromal, and vascular microenvironment and on the immune cell profile that are part of it, hence from the signals conveyed toward autophagy/death, differentiation, proliferation, and angiogenetic circuits and from the cross talk between them. The duration of the inflammation is another key feature affecting the outcome of the immune responses. This is strictly linked to the presence of host immunogenetic predisposition and/or ongoing chemical, physical, or biological irritation. In the case of gastric mucosa, infection with persistent microorganisms bearing oncogenic potential such as Epstein-Barr virus

S. Zanussi (✉) · M. Casarotto · C. Pratesi
Immunopathology and Cancer Biomarkers, IRCCS, CRO Aviano, National Cancer Institute, Aviano, PN, Italy
e-mail: szanussi@cro.it; mtcasarotto@cro.it; cpratesi@cro.it

P. De Paoli
IRCCS, CRO Aviano, National Cancer Institute, Aviano, PN, Italy
e-mail: pdepaoli@cro.it

© Springer Nature Switzerland AG 2019

V. Canzonieri, A. Giordano (eds.), *Gastric Cancer In The Precision Medicine Era*, Current Clinical Pathology, https://doi.org/10.1007/978-3-030-04861-7_1

and *Helicobacter pylori* (*H. pylori*) can initiate local inflammation and, after elusion of immune clearance mechanisms, may cause chronic inflammation. Specific or non-specific viral and bacterial virulence factors in conjunction with immunity defects can cause aberrant interactions between microbes and gastric epithelial cells. This condition can drive premalignancy, implementing the inflammatory response with the accumulation of new genetic and epigenetic modifications in epithelial cells, actually favoring the establishment of a gastric cancerized field.

Helicobacter and Inflammation: The Two Facet Janus

H. pylori is a Gram-negative, spiral-shaped, microaerophilic bacterium colonizing the human stomach. From a biological and evolutionary point of view, *H. pylori* has coevolved with humans for at least 50,000 years to be transmitted from person to person and become a commensal of the stomach [4, 5]. An homeostatic equilibrium between bacterial effectors and host responses allows microbial persistence, but also confers the risk of gastric neoplasia. In 1994 *H. pylori* was classified as a class I human carcinogen by the International Agency for Research on Cancer working group for its association with an increased risk for gastric cancer, in particular non-cardia gastric cancer, and mucosa-associated lymphoid tissue (MALT) lymphoma [6]. Since that time, *H. pylori* infection is considered the primary cause of gastric neoplasms [7], although the etiology is multifactorial. One of the first mechanisms by which *H. pylori* may express its pathogenetic potential is inflammation-related and refers to the production of autoreactive immunoglobulins; these may cause complement-dependent cell lysis and small immune complexes formation that may promote local damage [8]. Autoantibodies originate through molecular mimicry of host epitopes by lipopolysaccharide (LPS) structures of *H. pylori* [9]. These observations prompt to evaluate the inflammation-related carcinogenic potential of the structural components of a broad range of microbial populations colonizing the gastric environment.

Both the undifferentiated and the differentiated gastric cancer types (named diffuse-type carcinoma and intestinal-type adenocarcinoma, respectively) are associated with *H. pylori*. However, only the pathogenesis of the intestinal cancer seems to significantly involve the chronic inflammation, which directs the abnormal differentiation of the normal gastric mucosa toward the precancerous gastric lesions. This can be done according to the cascade model hypothesized by Correa, which involves the evolution of the forms of non-atrophic gastritis, toward multifocal atrophic gastritis without intestinal metaplasia, intestinal metaplasia, dysplasia, and finally cancer [10]. All these lesions occur in a setting of inflammation and in a complex milieu of diffusible factors. Despite the variable, but significant, prevalence of *H. pylori* infection in various countries [11], it is estimated that 1–3% of infected people will develop non-cardia gastric cancer and lymphoma [12, 13]. Indeed, besides the environmental factors, such as smoking and diet, and the commensal microbes, the clinical outcome of the infection is conditioned by virulence factors of *H. pylori*, by its high phenotypic and genomic heterogeneity within the gastric niche [14] as well as by genetic susceptibility and immune profile of the host [15].

Each host is not colonized by a single type of *H. pylori*, but by a multitude of genetically closely related microorganisms similar to quasispecies, which interfere with signaling pathways influencing host cell growth and death [16, 17]. From an ecological and teleological point of view, the diversity is originated by the bacterium in an attempt to persist in the microenvironment, notwithstanding the oxidative stress directly caused by *H. pylori* virulence factors and indirectly by inflammatory response. Pro-inflammatory cytokines, such as tumor necrosis factor (TNF)-α, interleukin (IL)1-β and IL-8, sustain inflammation in gastric mucosa, but anti-inflammatory cytokines, such as IL-10, tend to turn it off. They are released by several components of the immune system as well as by cells immersed in the stromal microenvironment, such as fibroblasts, epithelial, and endothelial cells. They can accomplish pleiotropic effects on a wide range of cell types, including immune and epithelial cells. Since variations in genotypes heightening cytokine levels have been associated with an increased risk of gastric cancer [18–22], cytokines are believed to enhance overall rather than attenuate the pathogenicity of the bacterium. However, it's elemental to highlight that the cellular composition of the microenvironment might deeply influence the cancer risk; the own different CD4$^+$ T cell subsets can secrete different cytokine and chemokine types, which in turn can stimulate different signal transduction pathways and activation of transcription factors, leading to pro-inflammatory reactive or anti-inflammatory suppressive responses.

Helicobacter pylori-Specific Determinants Affecting Inflammation and Tumorigenesis

A plenty of virulence factors have been described in *H. pylori* infection. Some of them are highly studied and specifically involved in inflammatory response after infection. Moreover, they cooperate to the inflammation-related tumorigenic process. Among the most mentioned virulence determinants for their relevance in colonization, persistence, and oxidative stress induction, there are the *H. pylori* neutrophil-activating protein (HP-NAP), the γ-glutamyl-transpeptidase (GGT), the cytotoxin-associated gene pathogenicity island (*Cag*PAI), and the vacuolating cytotoxin A (VacA).

While GGT and HP-NAP are constitutively expressed and show little genetic variability among *H. pylori* isolates, perhaps indicating a structural function or a lack of immune selection for diversification [23], on the other hand, *vacA* and *Cag*PAI show plasticity, being apt to genetic modifications which modulate their virulence [24–26]. The characteristics and modalities of action of these different virulence factors are summarized in the following paragraphs.

H. pylori Neutrophil-Activating Protein

H. pylori neutrophil-activating protein (HP-NAP) has probably evolved as a pro-inflammatory molecule to sustain the production of reactive oxygen intermediates by human neutrophils, functional to the release of nutrients, which can speed *H. pylori* growth [27]. It has been described that HP-NAP can trigger inflammation in conjunction with other bacterial and host-derived factors [28], but also as an only molecule. Indeed, several studies sustain a model in which HP-NAP represents a critical element in initiating the inflammatory process. HP-NAP is probably released after cell lysis in the infected mucosa of the stomach, and, after its transfer through gastric epithelial lining, it activates subepithelial resident mast cells and macrophages [29]. Consequently, these innate immune components release biochemical mediators and, in particular, the pleiotropic cytokine TNF-α. Overall, soluble factors attract and stimulate the adhesion and extravasation of polymorphonucleates (PMN) and lympho-monocytes through the endothelium lining the vessels, as suggested by the TNF-α-induced upregulation of adhesion molecules V-CAM and I-CAM on the surface of endothelial cells and by *in vitro* and *in vivo* experiments on animal models [30, 31]. PMN and monocytes produce and secrete ROS through the HP-NAP-induced increase of cytoplasmic Ca^{2+} and phosphorylation of proteins, leading to assembly of nicotinamide adenine dinucleotide phosphate (NADPH) oxidase on plasma membrane. Moreover, PMN and monocytes are activated to secrete cytokines and chemokines which amplify the inflammatory state. Among these, IL-12 and IL-23 contribute to differentiate the monocytes into a mature dendritic phenotype and the T- lymphocytic response toward a cytotoxic T- helper type 1 (Th1) phenotype producing interferon-γ (IFN-γ), TNF-β, IL-12, IL-18, IL-17, and TNF-α [32]. Preclinical studies demonstrate that HP-NAP inhibits the differentiation of Th0 into Th2 profile [23].

γ-Glutamyl-Transpeptidase

γ-Glutamyl-transpeptidase (GGT) is a virulence factor virtually associated with all wild-type *H. pylori* strains, although strain-to-strain variations in GGT expression among clinical isolates from patients with different disease statuses have been observed. GGT is related to ROS production from the epithelium and to oxidation of DNA and membrane lipids by using the body's master antioxidant glutathione (GSH), which is catabolized by GGT itself. Besides pro-apoptotic and necrotic effects evoked by ROS compounds and potentially sustained by other virulence factors such as VacA, GGT shows anti-apoptotic activities by activation of p38 mitogen-activated protein kinases (MAPKs), protein kinase B (AKT), and nuclear factor k-light-chain-enhancer of activated B cell (NF-kB) signaling pathways; the subsequent production of inducible nitric oxide synthase (iNOS), DNA damage, IL-8, and prostaglandin synthase cyclooxygenase-2 (COX-2) enhances the inflammatory reaction and induces epithelial cell proliferation [33]. Additionally, GGT suppresses T cell proliferation by inducing cell cycle arrest through the disruption of the Ras signaling pathway [34]. *In vitro* and *in vivo* studies suggest that GGT contributes to DC tolerization and directs the T cell response toward a regulatory immunosuppressive phenotype [35]. A suppressive milieu inhibits lymphocyte activation and favors *H. pylori* escape and persistent infection.

Cytotoxin-Associated Gene A Pathogenicity Island and Vacuolating Cytotoxin A

Cytotoxin-associated gene A pathogenicity island (*Cag*PAI) is a 40,000 base pairs sequence containing coding regions for virulence determinants and several proteins participating to the assembly of a specialized syringe machinery called type IV secretion system. Through this structure, *H. pylori* is able to inject into cells inflammation- and tumorigenesis-related bacterial components, such as the cytotoxin-associated gene A (CagA), peptidoglycans, and methyltransferases. Proteins encoded by *Cag*PAI genes induce inflammation by using the host signaling pathways essential for maintenance of the normal gastric mucosa homeostasis [36]. In the case of CagA, after translocation into epithelial cells, it acts through direct interaction with intracellular receptors in a phosphorylation-dependent or phosphorylation-independent manner. In the first case, CagA becomes phosphorylated by members of the Src and Abl family kinases at specific amino acidic motifs in the C-terminus of the protein (Glu-Pro-Ile-Tyr-Ala, EPIYA). This phosphorylation allows CagA binding to SH2 domain-containing proteins, such as SHP2 tyrosine phosphatase, causing its activation and subsequent induction of the extracellular signal-regulated kinases (ERK)-MAPK pathway, which leads to mitogenic response and cellular migration [37]. In the second case, CagA is translocated, but not phosphorylated, and it determines altered activation of β-catenin, disruption of apical junctional complexes, and loss of cellular polarity. Moreover, non-phosphorylated CagA targets a series of adhesion, enzymatic, and transducer molecules, which leads to mitogenic and pro-inflammatory responses [38–41]. CagA also interacts with tumor suppressor proteins, such as Runt-related transcription factor 3 (RUNX3) and protein 53 (p53) leading to their proteasomal degradation [37]. It has been reported that translocated CagA into the host cell is degraded by oxidative stress-dependent autophagy and, hence, short-lived, except when it enters CD44v9^{+} gastric cancer stem-like cells, that show oxidative stress resistance due to their high GSH content [42]. The expression of the CD44 homing receptor can be induced upon chronic inflammation [43], is involved in the upregulation of GSH synthesis, contributes to the progression of precancerous gastric lesions in patients with *H. pylori* infection, and correlates positively with recurrence of gastric cancer [44–46]. These observations suggest that the accumulation of alterations due to ROS and the cell survival through protection against ROS may play a considerable role for the generation of cancer cells in the infected gastric mucosa.

CagPAI-codified type IV secretion system can also deliver peptidoglycans into host cells, where they are recognized by the nucleotide-binding oligomerization domain-containing protein 1 (NOD1). The subsequent activation of NF-kB, p38, and extracellular ERK signaling induces the production of pro-inflammatory cytokines macrophage inflammatory protein (MIP)-2, β-defensins, and IL-8. Additionally, the interaction between NOD1 and post-translational-modified peptidoglycans modulates the production of type I interferons which are involved in the activation of DCs and of T cell cytotoxic effector functions [47–49].

CagA and other *H. pylori* molecules can be injected not only into gastric epithelial cells, but also into B lymphoid cells and DCs. As a consequence, host's immune responses can be suppressed through the reduction in the secretion of pro-inflammatory cytokines, such as IL-12p40, and the increase in the expression of suppressive cytokines, such as IL-10 [50]. This highlights the existence of pro-inflammatory and anti-inflammatory effects produced by the same virulence component in dependence on the cellular metabolic status and composition of the microenvironment.

VacA is a pore-forming protein which is secreted by *H. pylori* through a type V autotransport secretion system. It exerts multiple effects on epithelial and immune cells in synergy with other virulence determinants. VacA can be internalized into the host cells by endocytosis; afterward it accumulates in different cellular compartments inducing apoptosis. In parallel, it contributes to the successful colonization of the gastric niche disrupting epithelial cell tight connections and allowing the access of bacterial molecules and *H. pylori* to the lamina propria. This function is shared with CagA that is able to bind and inhibit PAR1b, a protein essential for the establishment and maintenance of cell polarity. Once in the innermost layers of the gastric mucosa, VacA encounters granulocytes and T cells recruited to the sites of infection by the triggered inflammation program. Herein, VacA is capable of inducing an influx of Ca^{2+}, probably NF-kB activation, and consequent inflammation through generation of oxidative stress and IL-8 secretion [51, 52]. On the other hand, it modulates the inflammatory response restricting T lymphocytes proliferation and effector functions [53]. *In vitro* and *in vivo* experiments demonstrate that VacA, in cooperation with GGT, contributes critically and non-redundantly to *H. pylori* tolerizing effects on murine DCs allowing persistence of the bacterium [35, 54].

Helicobacter pylori Affects Early Phases of Inflammation

Several evidences point to an involvement of *H. pylori* in the first phases of the carcinogenesis while long lasting molecular changes in epithelial cells, which result from the initial infection with virulent *H. pylori* strains, contribute to tissue damage progression [55, 56]. Indeed, the reversibility of oxidative and nitrosative stress processes, one of the crucial initial steps of the inflammatory reaction contributing to carcinogenesis in gastric mucosa, has been documented after *H. pylori* eradication [57]. Moreover, prospective studies show that *H. pylori* eradication by antibiotics reduces the incidence of precancerous lesions, and it is effective in reversing atrophic gastritis, but not intestinal metaplasia [58, 59]. Finally, *H. pylori* eradication does not decrease the risk of gastric cancer in patients with more advanced metaplastic or dysplastic mucosal lesions [60].

Inflammation and *H. pylori*-Mediated Oxidative and Nitrosative Stresses

RNS are produced mainly by neutrophils and macrophages, but also by gastric epithelial cells through the action of the nitric oxide synthase (NOS) and, especially, of iNOS. Nitric oxide (NO) is sufficiently long-lived to diffuse through the extracellular matrix and enter the nucleus of epithelial cells infected by *H. pylori* and those surrounding them within the gastric pit. ROS, such as superoxide (O_2^-), is active in this biochemical pathway. The source of effective ROS is the epithelial cell itself, since ROS generated by neutrophils and macrophages are not sufficiently long-lived to diffuse through extracellular matrix and penetrate epithelial cell membranes. Here, NO and O_2^- react to form peroxynitrite ($ONOO^-$), which causes DNA damage through guanine nitration and, finally, mutations, impairment of DNA repair enzymes and genomic instability [61–63]. Changes in lipid and protein expression consequent to oxidative stress have been observed [64, 65]. Last but not least, induced NO production interferes with transcriptional modulation by promoting DNA hyper-methylation both in noncoding and coding sequences for clincher proteins of the carcinogenetic intracellular pathways, such as p53, the cyclin-dependent kinase inhibitors (CDKN2A/CDKN2B), the epithelial cadherin-1 (CDH1) or mutL homolog 1 (MLH1), and many others. It's worth noting that passenger genes, namely, genes that are not directly causally involved in gastric carcinogenesis, are even significantly subjected to silencing by aberrant methylation in the cancerized field [55, 66, 67]. These observations point to methylation rather than silencing of genes by mutation as the main mechanism for inactivation of driver and passenger tumor suppressor genes, indicating that gastric cancer is an epigenetic disease [56].

ROS accumulation in differentiated and stem gastric cells can be directly and indirectly induced by *H. pylori*. Due to its poor immunogenicity, LPS helps the bacteria to develop a chronic infection and, following activation of epithelial Toll-like receptor (TLR) 4 signaling, contributes to epithelial cell ROS production [68, 69]. Moreover, especially highly virulent $CagA^+$ *H. pylori* strains can cause pro-oxidant activities through induction of NADPH oxidase or spermidine oxidase activity in host gastric cells [70–72]. ROS generation is indirectly induced by *H. pylori* infection through interaction of TNF-α-receptor on mucosal cell surface with TNF-α released by inflammatory cells in response to the infection. Epigenetic modifications can be directly induced by *H. pylori* possessing a functional type IV secretion system [36]. Indeed, through this structure, specific methyltransferases encoded by *H. pylori* may be injected into the host cell [73]. However, studies in gerbil-based models of carcinogenesis evidenced a major role of *H. pylori*-induced inflammation rather than a unique direct role of *H. pylori*-specific virulence factors in DNA methylation modulation. Indeed, increases of iNOS, IL1-β, TNF-α, and CXCL2 transcription, which are consequent to and synergistic with *H. pylori* infection immunopathologic effects, were shown to parallel the DNA methylation levels in gastric mucosa [74, 75]. Further experiments in animal models suggest that infiltrating mucosa monocytes are central components for *H. pylori*-dependent methylation induction and that the specificity of aberrant gene methylation in target cells is conditioned from their genomic architecture and from epigenetic elements already present in the cells where methylation is activated [56].

Inflammation and *H. pylori*-Mediated Alteration of DNA Repair Mechanisms

H. pylori may affect activation-induced cytidine deaminase (AID), which is an inducible enzyme, physiologically responsible for editing the human genome, e.g., for generating genomic diversity within the variable regions of immunoglobulin genes in activated B lymphocytes through somatic hypermutation and class switch recombination. AID is not expressed in normal gastric mucosa, but it is overexpressed in a proportion of *H. pylori*-infected gastric epithelium and in gastric cancer tissues, especially in the presence of mononuclear cell infiltration and intestinal metaplasia [76]. Most importantly, AID expression decreases after *H. pylori* eradication, suggesting a cause-effect link with the bacterium [77]. *Cag*PAI^+, but not *cag*PAI^- *H. pylori* isolates, are able to stimulate aberrant AID expression in epithelial cell lines, causing chromosomal aberrations and somatic point mutations in tumor suppressor genes such as the aforementioned *p53* and *CDKN2A/CDKN2B* [76, 78]. Moreover, also pro-inflammatory cytokines, such as TNF-α, indirectly increase the expression of AID through NF-kB intracellular pathway activation [55].

In vitro experiments on infected gastric epithelial cells demonstrate *H. pylori*-induced downregulation of proteins that are sequentially involved in the mechanism of base excision repair (BER) and which mediate the removal of incorrect single base residues [79]. Also the proteins of the DNA base mismatch repair are downregulated by *H. pylori* infection in gastric epithelial cells as well as in a *H. pylori*-infected mouse model and in *H. pylori*-positive patients with chronic gastritis [80, 81].

In gastric cell lines and primary gastric epithelial cells, it has been demonstrated that *H. pylori* infection prompts downregulation of several components engaged in double-strand DNA break (DSB) repair pathway, which generate carcinogenetic lesions if they are not appropriately restored [61]. Indeed, DNA damage affecting chromosomal ends resulting in telomere shortening and chromosomal instability has been reported [61]. Even if the precise mechanisms by which these events occur are not completely understood and elucidated, *ex vivo* and *in vitro* studies demonstrate that *H. pylori* infection is associated with alteration in DNA repair by direct host-pathogen contact, and prolonged infection may result in unrepaired breaks [82]. A genome-wide screening in gastric epithelial cell lines suggests an involvement of a type IV secretion system-dependent injection of XPF/XPG endonucleases together with NF-kB activation in DSB induction [83].

Toward Cellular Autophagy or Death

The molecular damage in gastric epithelial and immune cells, consequent to the activation of oxidative stress pathways by *H. pylori*-induced inflammation, stimulates caspase-mediated autophagy or apoptosis, with a raise in cell turnover during the initial steps of the infection [84, 85]. Autophagy is an intrinsic cytoprotective mechanism by self-eating and recycling of cellular components. Hence, autophagy can suppress tumor initiation by preserving normal cells and inhibiting inflammation. However, it can promote proliferation of damaged cells with precancerous characteristics by favoring inflammatory cell growth and providing sufficient oxygen and nutrients [86]. Hence, an increase in cell survival and proliferation may be induced in infected and in neighboring cells, adding on the possibility of malignant characteristics acquirement thanks to accumulation of mutagenic DNA lesions, altered methylation, and block of the DNA repair machinery [87]. VacA is important in autophagy induction through the formation of autophagosome, a double membrane structure encapsulating intracellular and pathogen-derived damaged organelles and proteins, among them VacA itself and CagA, whose activities are modulated [84, 88]. As the chronic infection establishes and progresses, DNA damage may determine aberrations in autophagy-associated proteins, such as the oncoprotein p62/SQSTM1, which is overexpressed in gastric lesions and has been found to promote tumorigenesis through the NF-kB signaling transduction pathway [89, 90].

In vitro studies demonstrate that autophagy and apoptosis are molecular mechanisms which could cross talk between them and may control the cell fate in autonomous or cooperative ways [91, 92]. The selected pathway seems to be dependent on the cellular surface receptor status, such as the presence of TRAIL or CD95, on Bcl-2 as a central regulator of autophagy and apoptosis, and on the intracellular signaling milieu [93–95]. A key intracellular component driving death and autophagy is the inflammasome, a cytosolic multiprotein oligomer containing caspases, whose exact composition depends on the activator which initiates inflammasome assembly. Inflammasome has dual opposite roles in the oncogenesis: one in the anti-tumor inflammatory response by eliminating precancerous precursors through apoptosis and, on the other hand, a pro-tumorigenic effect by stimulating production of trophic factors for precancerous cells and stroma [96]. Anti-tumorigenic and pro-tumorigenic properties are largely determined by the types of cells, tissues, and organs involved [97]. For instance, some cells with DNA damage elicited by $CagA^+$ *H. pylori* strains are less likely to undergo apoptosis, and thus they are at high risk of malignant transformation [72]. This highlights that the interplay between the host and different *H. pylori* strains with differentially expressed virulence determinants is complex and may strongly influence the progression of the disease.

The Progression of *H. pylori*-Induced Precancerous Lesions: A Continuous Tolerizing Relationship

Beyond the biochemical, genetic, and molecular mechanisms triggered in the early phases of *H. pylori* infection and of inflammation, cellular and soluble factors deeply influence the relationships between *H. pylori* and the gastric microenvironment, sustaining bacterial persistence and survival of those cells altered from inflammation and that are shaped toward a precancerous lesion. Pro-inflammatory factors derived from damaged cells, such as IL-1β, and from activated T lymphocytes, such as IFN-γ, IL-4, IL-10, and IL-12, trigger immunosuppressive pathways from myeloid cells [98]. In addition, $CD4^+$ T cells recruited in the inflamed microenvironment secrete pleiotropic chemokines and cytokines, which play a fundamental role in the final clinical outcome of the infection and of the cancerized field, through the activation of many pathways, such as those leading to epithelial-to-mesenchymal transition or development of gastric cancer stem cells [99–103].

Mechanisms of *H. pylori* Attenuation and Evasion from Immune Surveillance

Despite the activation of a strong immune response, *H. pylori* is able to sustain the infection for several years or throughout lifetime. *H. pylori* survives oxidative stress by the production of enzyme oxidase and superoxide catalase, thus determining its persistence in the gastric mucosa and the further enhancement of the oxidative burst. Strains with high virulence levels and carriers of bacterial determinants with toxic activity seem to account for a high risk of gastric cancer development [26, 104]. However, the *H. pylori* gastric niche harbors bacterial strains with differential virulence acquired by genetic recombination as a strategy for survival and persistence in the site of infection. Indeed, DNA damage induced by inflammation in epithelial and stromal cells can involve not only the host genetic background, but also the *H. pylori* genome. Homologous recombination can act as a repair pathway of DNA breaks, prompting antigenic variation in *H. pylori* [105]; for instance, rearrangements in the genes encoding post-translational modifying enzymes, such as alpha-fucosyltransferases or peptidoglycan deacetylases, can determine changes in their activity with modulation of bacterial cell wall antigenic specificity [106, 107].

Molecular biology studies suggest functional relationships between different genomic traits of *H. pylori*. In particular, the composition of the *Cag*PAI greatly affects bacterial motility, survival capacity in different gastric microenvironments, production of pro-inflammatory cytokines, and antimicrobial susceptibility [108–112]. It has been highlighted that a single infective *H. pylori* strain may include variable proportions of subtypes with different *Cag*PAI genotypes, a phenomenon consistent with host-induced adaptive changes of the bacterial population infecting the stomach [113, 114]. Indeed, heterogeneous genomic and proteomic profiles of *H. pylori* strains and subtypes have been described showing a tendency to an association with different precancerous or pathologic conditions [26, 115–117]. Deletions of *Cag*PAI genes are more frequently detected among individuals with metaplasia and atrophic gastritis than non-atrophic gastritis or duodenal ulcers [118, 119]. These mechanisms entail virulence attenuation favoring colonization and persistence, but also modify the interaction capacity of the bacterium favoring the escape from the immunosurveillance.

Myeloid and Lymphoid Cellular and Soluble Factors Affecting the Clinical Outcome of *H. pylori* Infection

The secretion of inflammatory cytokines from healthy and damaged cells can be promoted by interaction of bacterial LPS, flagellins, toxins, and cellular products with membrane receptors, such as TLRs, or cytosolic components, such as inflammasomes. A paradigmatic example of membrane receptor is TLR4. It is expressed in immune as well as epithelial and stromal cells, where it can activate MyD88-dependent pathways, with the transcription of genes encoding for pro-inflammatory cytokines and chemokines (TNF, IL-1β, IL-18), immunosuppressive cytokines (IL-10 and transforming growth factor (TGF)-β), and angiogenic mediators (vascular endothelial growth factor (VEGF), epidermal growth factor (EGF)). In addition, TLR4 has been detected in tumoral cells, where it is capable of activating mitogen-activated protein kinases (MAPK) and NF-kB, suggesting its direct role in apoptosis inhibition and proliferation stimulation [120]. Inflammasomes are predominantly expressed in macrophages and can promote cytokine and chemokine production as well, especially IL-18 and IL-1β. The *Cag*PAI-encoded type IV secretion system, LPS, VacA, and bacterial urease B subunit seem to play a role in inflammasome activation. Recent studies highlight that the *H. pylori*-induced inflammasome activation and consequent IL-18 and IL-1β secretion need the coordinated cooperation between TLR-2, Nod-like receptor family pyrin domain-containing 3 (NLRP3) and caspase-1 [121].

IL-18 is a multifactorial chemokine, which intervenes directly activating $CD8^+$ cytotoxic T lymphocytes and $CD4^+$ naïve T cells that acquire a Th1-IFN-γ-secreting phenotype under the synergic action of IL-12 [99, 122]. Besides this anti-inflammatory action, mucosa integrity protection, and anti-cancer effect, IL-18 manifests pro-cancer properties [123]. This effect seems to be related to an impaired NK cell function through a PD-1-dependent mechanism, as it has been evidenced by *in vitro* and murine models [124]. However, IL-18 role in gastric cancer is not clearly understood in the clinical settings [125]. Overexpression of IL-1β is involved in the pathogenesis of gastric cancer through an immune-tolerizing effect of the mucosal gastric microenvironment guided by the mobilization of myeloid-derived suppressor cells (MDSCs) to the stomach [126]. MDSCs are one of the representative immune suppressive cells having the capacity to increase T cell apoptosis and suppress T cell responses, directing the result of the infection toward evasion from immune system and pathology [127]. MDSC levels are significantly increased in cancer patients and correlate with cancer clinical stages and poor prognosis [128–130], to such an extent that they have been mentioned as possible prognostic biomarkers of gastric cancer together with macrophages, neutrophils, and DCs [131, 132]. Finally, IL-1β production by MDSCs may induce secretion of IL-17 by CD4+ T cells [102].

Th17

Th17 and Th1 are the predominant subsets during the inflammatory phases of *H. pylori* infection, with Th17 response involved at earlier stages of infection than Th1 response [133]. In particular, $CagA^+$ strains stimulate DCs to IL-1β and IL-23 production. In the presence of antigen presentation, DCs activate $CD4^+$ naïve T cells to differentiation toward a Th17 phenotype. At intracellular level, the process is controlled by signal transducers, such as Signal Transducer and Activator of Transcription-3 (STAT-3), and by the transcription factors retinoic acid receptor-Related Orphan Receptors (ROR) γt and α. TGF-β, BAFF, and IL-6 secreted by DCs may be additional important factors for Th17 differentiation. They act through STAT-3 and NF-kB pathways [134]. In particular, TGF-β induces the expression of both RORγt and of forkhead box P3 (FoxP3) in naïve T cells; the latter molecule is a transcription factor capable of suppressing the activation of RORγt by a physical interaction and of deviating the differentiation of naïve T cells toward an immunosuppressive T regulatory (Treg) signature [135]. IL-6 links the differentiative pathways of Th17 and Treg, by activating STAT-3 pathway and down-modulating FoxP3 expression, finally unbalancing the ratio between these two subsets in favor of Th17. IL-6 expression is high in *H. pylori*-infected subjects as well as in physiological aging, where this cytokine is involved in the maintenance of a low level of systemic and local chronic inflammation, that can unbalance immune system functions toward tolerance and senescence, with a high risk of morbidity [136, 137].

Th17 cell subsets are able to release several chemokines and cytokines, namely, IL-17A, IL-17F, IL-21, IL-22, IL-23, IL-26, TNF-α, CCL20, and GM-CSF, although not all are Th17 specific. Epithelial cells and fibroblasts are stimulated by Th17 cytokines/chemokines toward pro-inflammatory soluble factors secretion, further recalling infiltration of macrophages, activated monocytes, T cells, and DCs in the microenvironment. Functional for tissue remodeling, but of relevance for re-localization of cells with malignant or premalignant characteristics,

Th17 cells stimulate epithelial cells to produce matrix metalloproteinases (MMP) that disrupt microenvironment architecture. Although IL-17 responses are downregulated by immunosuppressive enzymes, such as indoleamine 2,3-dioxygenase (IDO), or by reduced expression of co-stimulatory receptors on the Th17 surface, the activity of this T cell subset continues also after disappearance of the bacterium thanks to the action of IL-1β, which levels remain elevated in the gastric mucosa [138].

Th1

Th1 cells are involved primarily in defense against intracellular pathogens and in the isotypic switch of immunoglobulins to isotypes with complement-activation properties. *H. pylori* colonization of gastric mucosa seems to be directly proportional to Th1 immune response, since an insufficiency in this lineage is associated with enhanced bacterial density [139]. Outer membrane proteins of *H. pylori* induce NK and DC activation and maturation with predominant production of IL-12, IL-18, and IFN-γ. The synergic action of DCs and NK cells and their soluble mediators induces the expression of the transcription factor T-box expressed in T cells (T-bet) in T cell receptor (TCR)-engaged naïve $CD4^+$ T cells, leading to their differentiation in Th1 secreting at least IL-2 and IFN-γ. Hence, through an autocrine mechanism, IFN-γ enforces the Th1 polarization operated by NK, while IL-2 stimulates the progression of target cells from G0 to G1 phase, initiating the process of clonal expansion of activated T, B, and NK cells. Moreover, the Th1 cytokines cause further recruitment of macrophages into the infection site [140], emphasizing Th1 hyperactivation and reinforcing gastric inflammation finalized to the decrease of bacterial density.

During the early phases of infection, T lymphocytes from the *H. pylori*-infected gastric mucosa are not able to secrete Th2 cytokines. Indeed, IL-4 from basophils and mast cells stimulates the expression of the Th2 cell-specific master transcription factor GATA-binding protein-3 (GATA-3) in TCR-engaged naïve T cells. GATA-3 have reciprocal antagonistic activity with T-bet, and both transcription factors are involved in attenuating the harmful effects of Th1 response to maintain an healthy homeostasis [141]. Moreover, *H. pylori*, through HP-NAP and other virulence determinants, plays a central role in inhibiting the pathway of Th2 differentiation, promoting IL-12 and IL-23 secretion by neutrophils and monocytes, which support the polarization of Th1 and Th17 against *H. pylori*, respectively. However, negative feedbacks down-modulating Th1 responses can be exerted by some *H. pylori* virulence factors and by components of the inflammatory milieu. For instance, bacterial molecules such as GGT or Lewis-antigens on LPS can activate tolerogenic DC subsets unable to foster a Th1 differentiation and response [142, 143]. In addition, IDO, high levels of COX-2 and prostaglandin-2 (PGE-2) modify the Th1/Th2 balance in favor of the Th2 response [144–146].

Th2

The Th2 cytokine profile includes IL-4, IL-5, and IL-13, which are involved in a paracrine and autocrine self-activation and self-maintenance circuit. These cell subsets are important for the production of *H. pylori*-specific IgG, IgM, and IgA, which intervene in systemic and local antibody-mediated protection against the bacterium. Especially IgA are relevant in inhibiting the bacterial colonization of the mucosa [147]. Th1 immune responses are more efficient than Th2 responses against bacteria [148], but, when mechanisms down-modulating Th1 expression occur, Th2 and Th17 seem to prevail, and an imbalance toward Th2 responses is shown. Patients with precancerous gastric lesions and gastric cancer express a predominant Th2 signature [149, 150]. One of the mechanisms which links Th2 profile to worse prognosis is represented by the ability of GATA-3 to down-modulate onco-suppressor genes [151].

T Regulatory (Treg)

Treg subsets, together with MDSCs, play a clincher role in *H. pylori* immune escape, since they can suppress DCs and effector T cells by cell to cell contact and production of TGF-β, IL-10, and IL-35, which limit the inflammatory responses. They are delegated to maintain self-tolerance and physiological conditions avoiding autoimmunity. Two kinds of Tregs have been described with different ontogeny but some common features: the natural Tregs (nTregs) and the induced Tregs (iTregs). While nTregs are generated within the thymus from lymphoid precursors, the naïve $CD4^+$ T cells residing in peripheral lymphoid organs and stimulated by the antigen can differentiate into iTregs in the presence of TGF-β and IL-2. Commonly both kinds of Tregs are defined by the intracytoplasmic expression of the transcription factor FoxP3.

Triggering of TLR-2 signaling pathway through *H. pylori* components LPS or HP-NAP is an important mechanism for Treg activation accompanied by Th1 inhibition. The Treg-induced onset of immunologically tolerant gastric microenvironment modulates the survival and persistence of *H. pylori* and directs the disease to a worse outcome [152, 153]. The increase in Tregs levels within gastric mucosa seems to be associated with increased expression of programmed death-ligand 1 (PD-L1) on epithelial cells in the site of infection. The binding of PD-L1 to inhibitory receptors present on the surface of $CD4^+$ T lymphocytes, such as PD-1 or B7.1, transmits inhibitory signals which reduce the effector capacity of these subsets [154]. Hence, globally, an immunological anergy is established in the field of infection and cancerization, favoring the immune evasion of the bacterium and transformed cells. It has been observed that *H. pylori*-induced DCs stimulate proliferation of Treg possessing a reduced suppressive function due to the *H. pylori*-dependent IL-1β secretion by DCs itself, suggesting an attempt to maintain or restore an inflammatory milieu with effector proprieties [155]. The transition to anergic or reactive immunity also depends on the balance between the signaling pathways conveyed toward Tregs or Th17 subset differentiation. In particular, the absence or the presence of IL-6, together with the activation of IL-6/STAT-3 axis in naïve CD4+ T cells, prompts or suppresses the expression of FoxP3, determining the fate toward the differentiation of suppressive or reactive T cells, respectively [156, 157].

Besides the essential immunological components described in this paragraph and their basic relationships participating to an evolving immune profile within the gastric precancerous lesion, other cellular subsets, such as Th9 and Th22, are strictly interrelated and committed in the progression/regression of the infection and of the field cancerization. They are elegantly reviewed elsewhere [102, 103]. Furthermore, host genetic factors related to immunological and regulatory elements composing the mucosal milieu and entangled in bacterial interactions may play a pivotal role in addressing the outcome of *H. pylori* infection.

Host Factors Affecting Inflammation and Its Clinical Outcome

Functional polymorphisms that influence the level or the quality of the expression of genes encoding for intracellular and extracellular receptors, enzymes, cytokines, and chemokines modulating the inflammatory response have been associated with increased risk of gastric cancer [158]. The clinical significance of these associations is dependent from ethnicity, which is an important confounding factor in epidemiological studies [159, 160]. Interestingly, a correlation between the presence of certain single nucleotide substitutions (SNPs) and a high proportion of highly virulent *H. pylori* strains has been found, suggesting the existence of a selective pressure exerted by the host on the microorganism subtypes. This possible synergistic interaction could lead to the progression or regression of precancerous lesions [20, 161]. Individual genetic predisposition to exacerbate or dampen the effects of *H. pylori* infection may concern several steps of the interplay between the bacterium and the host (Table 1.1).

Table 1.1 Some genetic polymorphisms involved in modulating host response during *Helicobacter pylori* infection

Host gene	Polymorphism	Associated clinical condition	Ethnicity	References
Mucosal invasion and damage				
PTPN11	rs2301756 A>G	Hp-related atrophic gastritis	Japanese; Japanese Brazilian	[162, 163]
	rs2301756 A>G	GC	Japanese	[164]
	rs12229892	GC and/or AG	Chinese	[165]
CDH1	rs16260 (−160 C>A)	GC	Caucasian	[166–172]
DNA repair				
PARP-1	rs1136410 T>C	Cardiac adenocarcinoma	Chinese	[173]
	rs1136410 T>C	High proportion of high virulence strains	Brazilian	[161]
DNMT	rs1550117 AA	GC	Chinese	[174]
Immune evasion and attenuation				
TLR1	rs4833095	Gastroduodenal diseases (including GC)	Malaysian	[175]
TLR4	rs4986790	Hp infection, AG, GC	Italian, Caucasian	[176, 177]
	rs4986791	Hp infection, AG, GC	Italian	[176, 178]
	rs4986790, −1	Digestive cancers	Caucasian	[179]
	rs11536889 G>C	Atrophy in Hp$^+$ pts	Japanese	[180]
TLR2	−196 to −174 del	GC; IGC, DGC	Brazilian; Japanese	[181, 182]
	−196 to −174 ins	Atrophy, IM	Japanese	[183]
TLR5	rs5744174 C	GC	Chinese	[184]
TLR10	rs10004195	Gastroduodenal diseases (including GC)	Malaysian	[175]
NOD1	rs2075820 AA	DU, atrophy, IM, Hp eradication failure	Hungarians; Turkish	[185, 186]
	rs2075820 AA	DGC	Chinese	[187]
	rs2075820 AA	Gastritis, ↑IL-8, and COX-2 mRNA	Korean	[188]
	rs2709800 GT	Gastric lesions; IM	Chinese	[189, 190]
	rs7789045 TT	GC	Chinese	[187]
NOD2	rs718226 G	Dysplasia	Chinese	[189]
	rs2111235 C	↑risk of disease progression in Hp$^+$ pts	Caucasian	[191]
	rs7205423 G	↑risk of disease progression in Hp$^+$ pts	Chinese	[187]
	rs7205423 GC	GC	Chinese	[187]
	rs2066842 (c.802CC>T)	GC	German, Polish	[192, 193]
	rs2066844 T	GC	Italian	[194]
	rs2066844 and rs2066845	↓autophagy and presentation to MHCII	Not specified	[195]
	rs2066847	↓bacterial clearance by monocytes	Italian	[196]
IL-1β	31C>T	GC, only in Hp$^+$ pts	Chinese	[197]
	511C/T	GC	Mixed; Caucasian	[19, 20, 198]
IL1-RN	IL1-RN*2 VNTR	GC	Non-Asian populations; Caucasian	[20, 199]

Table 1.1 (continued)

Host gene	Polymorphism	Associated clinical condition	Ethnicity	References
IL8	251 A/T	GC	Chinese; Asian	[200, 201]
IL10	1082 A/G	GC	Asian; Taiwanese	[199, 200, 202]
	819 C/T	GC	Taiwanese	[202]
TNF-α	308 G/A	GC	Caucasian	[203]
	238 G/A	GC	Asian	[204]

PTPN11 tyrosine-protein phosphatase non-receptor type 11, *Hp Helicobacter pylori*, *GC* gastric cancer, *AG* atrophic gastritis, *PARP-1* poly-ADP-ribose polymerase 1, *DNMT* DNA methyltransferase, *TLR* toll-like receptor, *pts* patients, *IGC* intestinal-type gastric cancer, *DGC* diffuse-type gastric cancer, *IM* intestinal metaplasia, *NOD* nucleotide-binding oligomerization domain-containing protein, *DU* duodenal ulcer, *IL* interleukin, *COX-2* cyclooxygenase-2, *MHCII* major histocompatibility complex II, *VNTR* variable number tandem repeat, *TNF-α* tumor necrosis factor α

Accumulation of DNA damage following oxidative stresses can be worsen by SNPs present in the host genes coding for DNA repair enzymes, which may unbalance the relationship between apoptosis and cellular proliferation. Poly-ADP-ribose polymerase 1 (PARP-1) is a component of the BER system whose polymorphisms have been mentioned to be associated with gastric cancer in some studies [161, 173]. However, some investigations report no relationship between worse prognosis and this mutated enzyme [205], while only combined effect of genetic and *H. pylori* profile covariates shows significant associations with gastric cancer in other studies [206].

One of the intracellular receptors which plays a pivotal role in the transformation of the infected cells is the tyrosine phosphatase Src homology region 2 domain-containing phosphatase-2 (SHP-2), which is first intercepted by the phosphorylated CagA and which was found to induce cell morphological and physiological modifications. SHP-2 is coded by the *PTPN11* gene, whose polymorphisms have been associated to increased risk of atrophic gastritis in Chinese population with, but not without, *H. pylori* infection. This effect is probably due to a different strength of signal transduction through the CagA-SHP-2 complex [165]. Although wide association studies focusing on hundreds of SNPs possibly involved in CagA interaction have identified new susceptibility loci for gastric cancer, the insufficient statistical power of these studies does not allow to assess the exact relationship between the selected SNPs and gastric cancer risk, providing only clues on the mechanisms entailing CagA function [207, 208].

Among polymorphisms concerning TLRs, two SNPs within *TLR4* coding gene have been linked with susceptibility to chronic infection, atrophic gastritis, and gastric cancer in Caucasian population by more than one study [176–178]; moreover, an alteration in the ligand-binding receptor site with proven diminished LPS responsiveness has been underlined [209, 210].

In addition to TLR, NLRs are important in the recognition of *H. pylori*. Polymorphisms of NOD1 and NOD2 are the best characterized in manifold studies. Overall, they highlight that functional SNPs reducing NOD1-/NOD2-mediated immune response to *H. pylori* contribute to bacterial survival and persistence and that a subsequent over-activation of other inflammatory responses may result in inflammation-related carcinogenesis [211].

As already mentioned, IL-1β is an important pro-inflammatory cytokine and a powerful inhibitor of gastric acid secretion, hence an inducer of atrophy progression. Polymorphisms in the *IL1B* promoter region, together with those concerning the IL-1 receptor antagonist (IL1-RN), have been reported to modulate IL-1β levels and action and be associated with an increased risk of gastric cancer [19]. These associations have been partially confirmed for Caucasian subjects by meta-analyses [212, 213], even if slightly contrasting results have emerged due to different grouping of subjects with different allelic frequencies or different genetic models of analyses [214]. A meta-analysis including 36 studies to evaluate the effect of TNFA on genetic susceptibility to gastritis and gastric cancer has shown that the TNFA -308G>A polymorphism is a risk factor for developing gastric tumors in different ethnic groups, with significant results found in Caucasians, but no significant associations among East Asians or other ethnicities [159]. A meta-analysis on a total of 203 studies assessing associations between gastric cancers and 225 polymorphisms in 95 genes showed ambiguous effects for several gene polymorphisms between Asian and Caucasian populations. However, this study was able to confirm, through gene clusters, two panels of polymorphisms that were significantly associated with the risk of gastric cancer and able to specifically distinguish these two different ethnic groups [160].

The results of association studies between genetic determinants and *H. pylori*-related gastric carcinogenesis may suffer from bias linked not only to the selection of the analyzed subjects but also to the population sample size, to the interactions between several covariates that can have an impact on this system and cannot be all eligible or valuable, and to the intrinsic limitations of the statistical methods applied in these complex contexts. However, they may help in personalization of the surveillance if they are directed to specific patient populations.

Conclusions

Gastric tumorigenesis is a multifactorial process involving complex interactions between gastric microenvironment, inflammation, and colonizing microorganisms, with *H. pylori* being the most studied and well-known cancer determinant. In dependence on its genetic and phenotypic heterogeneity, *H. pylori* triggers a number of innate and adaptive immune responses entangled in tumor formation process. *Cag*A^{+} strains present an increased risk of gastric cancer, and elevated levels of inflammatory cytokines have been observed in *H. pylori*-infected individuals. Through these mediators, several kinds of immune cells are stimulated to cooperate in the modulation of the oncogenic and anti-suppressive pathway activity. Methylation of tumor suppressor genes increases the risk of adenocarcinoma in the stomach. Autophagy and apoptosis processes may be hijacked toward cell growth and differentiation.

New technologies allow to discover additional elements, which can inflame the progression of the precancerous gastric lesions occurring in achlorhydria and atrophy settings. However, functional and mechanistic studies are needed to elucidate their specific activities within the evolution and dynamics of inflammation and their correlations with the pathogenesis of gastric cancer. Understanding of the mechanisms that regulate cancer-associated inflammation could open the way to new biomarkers able to distinguish patients with precancerous lesions that will remain indolent from those that will evolve, and to unexplored treatment opportunities influencing prevention and prognosis of therapeutic options.

References

1. Reese DM. Fundamentals-Rudolf Virchow and modern medicine. West J Med. 1998;169(2):105–8.
2. Orange M, Reuter U, Hobohm U. Coley's lessons remembered: augmenting mistletoe therapy. Integr Cancer Ther. 2016;15(4):502–11.
3. Hanahan D, Weinberg RA. Hallmarks of cancer: the next generation. Cell. 2011;144(5):646–74.
4. Blaser MJ, Atherton JC. Helicobacter pylori persistence: biology and disease. J Clin Invest. 2004;113(3):321–33.
5. Atherton JC, Blaser MJ. Coadaptation of Helicobacter pylori and humans: ancient history, modern implications. J Clin Invest. 2009;119(9):2475–87.
6. International Agency for Research on Cancer. IARC monographs on the evaluation of carcinogenic risks to humans. Schistosomes, liver flukes and helicobacter pylori, vol. 61. Lyon: International Agency for Research on Cancer; 1994. p. 177.
7. Parkin DM. The global health burden of infection-associated cancers in the year 2002. Int J Cancer. 2006;118(12):3030–44.
8. Chmiela M, Wadstrom T, Folkesson H, et al. Anti-Lewis X antibody and Lewis X-anti-Lewis X immune complexes in Helicobacter pylori infection. Immunol Lett. 1998;61(2–3):119–25.
9. Chmiela M, Gonciarz W. Molecular mimicry in Helicobacter pylori infections. World J Gastroenterol. 2017;23(22):3964–77.
10. Correa P, Piazuelo MB. The gastric precancerous cascade. J Dig Dis. 2012;13(1):2–9.

11. Burucoa C, Axon A. Epidemiology of Helicobacter pylori infection. Helicobacter. 2017;22 Suppl 1:1–5.
12. Peek RM Jr, Blaser MJ. Helicobacter pylori and gastrointestinal tract adenocarcinomas. Nat Rev Cancer. 2002;2(1):28–37.
13. Wroblewski LE, Peek RM Jr, Wilson KT. Helicobacter pylori and gastric cancer: factors that modulate disease risk. Clin Microbiol Rev. 2010;23:713–39.
14. Suerbaum S, Josenhans C. Helicobacter pylori evolution and phenotypic diversification in a changing host. Nat Rev Microbiol. 2007;5:441–52.
15. Atherton JC. The pathogenesis of Helicobacter pylori-induced gastro-duodenal diseases. Annu Rev Pathol. 2006;1:63–96.
16. Saberi S, Douraghi M, Azadmanesh K, et al. A potential association between Helicobacter pylori CagA EPIYA and multimerization motifs with cytokeratin 18 cleavage rate during early apoptosis. Helicobacter. 2012;17(5):350–7.
17. Greenfield LK, Jones NL. Modulation of autophagy by Helicobacter pylori and its role in gastric carcinogenesis. Trends Microbiol. 2013;21(11):602–12.
18. El-Omar EM, Rabkin CS, Gammon MD, et al. Increased risk of noncardia gastric cancer associated with proinflammatory cytokine gene polymorphisms. Gastroenterology. 2003;124(5):1193–201.
19. El-Omar EM, Carrington M, Chow WH, et al. Interleukin-1 polymorphisms associated with increased risk of gastric cancer. Nature. 2000;404(6776):398–402. Erratum in: Nature 2001 Jul 5;412(6842):99.
20. Machado JC, Pharoah P, Sousa S, et al. Interleukin 1B and interleukin 1RN polymorphisms are associated with increased risk of gastric carcinoma. Gastroenterology. 2001;121(4):823–9.
21. Lee WP, Tai DI, Lan KH, et al. The -251T allele of the interleukin-8 promoter is associated with increased risk of gastric carcinoma featuring diffuse-type histopathology in Chinese population. Clin Cancer Res. 2005;11(18):6431–41.
22. Taguchi A, Ohmiya N, Shirai K, et al. Interleukin-8 promoter polymorphism increases the risk of atrophic gastritis and gastric cancer in Japan. Cancer Epidemiol Biomark Prev. 2005;14(11 Pt 1): 2487–93.
23. De Bernard M, D'Elios MM. The immune modulating activity of the Helicobacter pylori HP-NAP: friend or foe? Toxicon. 2010;56(7):1186–92.
24. Palframan SL, Kwok T, Gabriel K. Vacuolating cytotoxin A (VacA), a key toxin for Helicobacter pylori pathogenesis. Front Cell Infect Microbiol. 2012;2:92.
25. Barrozo RM, Cooke CL, Hansen LM, et al. Functional plasticity in the type IV secretion system of Helicobacter pylori. PLoS Pathogens. 2013;9(2):e1003189.
26. Figura N, Marano L, Moretti E, et al. Helicobacter pylori infection and gastric carcinoma: not all the strains and patients are alike. World J Gastrointest Oncol. 2016;8(1):40–54.
27. Wang CA, Liu YC, Du SY, et al. Helicobacter pylori neutrophil-activating protein promotes myeloperoxidase release from human neutrophils. Biochem Biophys Res Commun. 2008;377(1):52–6.
28. Petersson C, Forsberg M, Aspholm M, et al. Helicobacter pylori SabA adhesin evokes a strong inflammatory response in human neutrophils which is down-regulated by the neutrophil-activating protein. Med Microbiol Immunol. 2006;195(4):195–206.
29. Montemurro P, Nishioka H, Dundon WG, et al. The neutrophil-activating protein (HP-NAP) of Helicobacter pylori is a potent stimulant of mast cells. Eur J Immunol. 2002;32(3):671–6.
30. Brisslert M, Enarsson K, Lundin S, et al. Helicobacter pylori induce neutrophil transendothelial migration: role of the bacterial HP-NAP. FEMS Microbiol Lett. 2005;249(1):95–103.
31. Polenghi A, Bossi F, Fischetti F, et al. The neutrophil-activating protein of Helicobacter pylori crosses endothelia to promote neutrophil adhesion in vivo. J Immunol. 2007;178(3):1312–20.
32. Amedei A, Cappon A, Codolo G, et al. The neutrophil-activating protein of Helicobacter pylori promotes Th1 immune responses. J Clin Invest. 2006;116(4):1092–101.
33. Ricci V, Giannouli M, Romano M, et al. Helicobacter pylori gamma-glutamyl transpeptidase and its pathogenic role. World J Gastroenterol. 2014;20(3):630–8.
34. Schmees C, Prinz C, Treptau T, et al. Inhibition of T-cell proliferation by Helicobacter pylori gamma-glutamyl transpeptidase. Gastroenterology. 2007;132(5):1820–33.
35. Oertli M, Noben M, Engler DB, et al. Helicobacter pylori γ-glutamyl transpeptidase and vacuolating cytotoxin promote gastric persistence and immune tolerance. Proc Natl Acad Sci U S A. 2013;110(8):3047–52.
36. Backert S, Tegtmeyer N, Fischer W. Composition, structure and function of the Helicobacter pylori cag pathogenicity island encoded type IV secretion system. Future Microbiol. 2015;10(6):955–65.
37. Hatakeyama M. Helicobacter pylori CagA and gastric cancer: a paradigm for hit-and-run carcinogenesis. Cell Host Microbe. 2014;15(3):306–16.
38. Churin Y, Al-Ghoul L, Kepp O, et al. Helicobacter pylori CagA protein targets the c-Met receptor and enhances the motogenic response. J Cell Biol. 2003;161(2):249–55.
39. Mimuro H, Suzuki T, Tanaka J, et al. Grb2 is a key mediator of helicobacter pylori CagA protein activities. Mol Cell. 2002;10(4):745–55.
40. Murata-Kamiya N, Kurashima Y, Teishikata Y, et al. Helicobacter pylori CagA interacts with E-cadherin and deregulates the beta-catenin signal that promotes intestinal transdifferentiation in gastric epithelial cells. Oncogene. 2007;26(32):4617–26.
41. Saadat I, Higashi H, Obuse C, et al. Helicobacter pylori CagA targets PAR1/MARK kinase to disrupt epithelial cell polarity. Nature. 2007;447(7142):330–3.
42. Tsugawa H, Suzuki H, Saya H, et al. Reactive oxygen species-induced autophagic degradation

of Helicobacter pylori CagA is specifically suppressed in cancer stem-like cells. Cell Host Microbe. 2012;12(6):764–77.
43. Ishimoto T, Oshima H, Oshima M, et al. CD44+ slow-cycling tumor cell expansion is triggered by cooperative actions of Wnt and prostaglandin E2 in gastric tumorigenesis. Cancer Sci. 2010;101(3):673–8.
44. Garay J, Piazuelo MB, Majumdar S, et al. The homing receptor CD44 is involved in the progression of precancerous gastric lesions in patients infected with Helicobacter pylori and in development of mucous metaplasia in mice. Cancer Lett. 2016;371(1):90–8.
45. Hirata K, Suzuki H, Imaeda H, et al. CD44 variant 9 expression in primary early gastric cancer as a predictive marker for recurrence. Br J Cancer. 2013;109(2):379–86.
46. Wakamatsu Y, Sakamoto N, Oo HZ, et al. Expression of cancer stem cell markers ALDH1, CD44 and CD133 in primary tumor and lymph node metastasis of gastric cancer. Pathol Int. 2012;62(2):112–9.
47. Watanabe T, Asano N, Fichtner-Feigl S, et al. NOD1 contributes to mouse host defense against Helicobacter pylori via induction of type I IFN and activation of the ISGF3 signaling pathway. J Clin Invest. 2010;120(5):1645–62.
48. Wang G, Lo LF, Forsberg LS, et al. Helicobacter pylori peptidoglycan modifications confer lysozyme resistance and contribute to survival in the host. MBio. 2012;3(6):e00409–12.
49. Wang G, Maier SE, Lo LF, et al. Peptidoglycan deacetylation in Helicobacter pylori contributes to bacterial survival by mitigating host immune responses. Infect Immun. 2010;78(11):4660–6.
50. Kalali B, Mejías-Luque R, Javaheri A, et al. H. pylori virulence factors: influence on immune system and pathology. Mediators Inflamm. 2014;2014:426309.
51. Kim JM, Kim JS, Lee JY, et al. Vacuolating cytotoxin in Helicobacter pylori water-soluble proteins upregulates chemokine expression in human eosinophils via Ca2+ influx, mitochondrial reactive oxygen intermediates, and NF-kappaB activation. Infect Immun. 2007;75(7):3373–81.
52. Takeshima E, Tomimori K, Takamatsu R, et al. Helicobacter pylori VacA activates NF-κB in T cells via the classical but not alternative pathway. Helicobacter. 2009;14(4):271–9.
53. Muller A, Oertli M, Arnold IC. H. pylori exploits and manipulates innate and adaptive immune cell signaling pathways to establish persistent infection. Cell Commun Signal. 2011;9(1):25.
54. Rizzuti D, Ang M, Sokollik C, et al. Helicobacter pylori inhibits dendritic cell maturation via interleukin-10-mediated activation of the signal transducer and activator of transcription 3 pathway. J Innate Immun. 2015;7(2):199–211.
55. Shimizu T, Chiba T, Marusawa H. Helicobacter pylori-mediated genetic instability and gastric carcinogenesis. Curr Top Microbiol Immunol. 2017;400:305–23.
56. Ushijima T, Hattori N. Molecular pathways: involvement of Helicobacter pylori-triggered inflammation in the formation of an epigenetic field defect, and its usefulness as cancer risk and exposure markers. Clin Cancer Res. 2012;18(4):923–9.
57. Pignatelli B, Bancel B, Plummer M, et al. Helicobacter pylori eradication attenuates oxidative stress in human gastric mucosa. Am J Gastroenterol. 2001;96(6):1758–66.
58. Mera R, Fontham ET, Bravo LE, et al. Long term follow up of patients treated for Helicobacter pylori infection. Gut. 2005;54(11):1536–40.
59. Massarrat S, Haj-Sheykholeslami A, Mohamadkhani A, et al. Precancerous conditions after H. pylori eradication: a randomized double blind study in first degree relatives of gastric cancer patients. Arch Iran Med. 2012;15(11):664–9.
60. Chen HN, Wang Z, Li X, Zhou ZG. Helicobacter pylori eradication cannot reduce the risk of gastric cancer in patients with intestinal metaplasia and dysplasia: evidence from a meta-analysis. Gastric Cancer. 2016;19(1):166–75.
61. Koeppel M, Garcia-Alcalde F, Glowinski F, et al. Helicobacter pylori infection causes characteristic DNA damage patterns in human cells. Cell Rep. 2015;11(11):1703–13.
62. Lee WP, Hou MC, Lan KH, et al. Helicobacter pylori-induced chronic inflammation causes telomere shortening of gastric mucosa by promoting PARP-1-mediated non-homologous end joining of DNA. Arch Biochem Biophys. 2016;606:90–8.
63. Kawanishi S, Ohnishi S, Ma N, et al. Crosstalk between DNA damage and inflammation in the multiple steps of carcinogenesis. Int J Mol Sci. 2017;18(8):E1808.
64. Baek HY, Lim JW, Kim H, et al. Oxidative-stress-related proteome changes in Helicobacter pylori-infected human gastric mucosa. Biochem J. 2004;379(Pt 2):291–9.
65. Huang FY, Chan AO, Rashid A, et al. Helicobacter pylori induces promoter methylation of E-cadherin via interleukin-1β activation of nitric oxide production in gastric cancer cells. Cancer. 2012;118(20):4969–80.
66. Hanada K, Uchida T, Tsukamoto Y, et al. Helicobacter pylori infection introduces DNA double-strand breaks in host cells. Infect Immun. 2014;82(10):4182–9.
67. Shimizu T, Marusawa H, Matsumoto Y, et al. Accumulation of somatic mutations in TP53 in gastric epithelium with Helicobacter pylori infection. Gastroenterology. 2014;147(2):407–17.e3.
68. Grivennikov SI, Greten FR, Karin M. Immunity, inflammation, and cancer. Cell. 2010;140(6):883–99.
69. Yuan X, Zhou Y, Wang W, et al. Activation of TLR4 signaling promotes gastric cancer progression by inducing mitochondrial ROS production. Cell Death Dis. 2013;4:e794.
70. Cha B, Lim JW, Kim KH, et al. HSP90beta interacts with Rac1 to activate NADPH oxidase in Helicobacter pylori-infected gastric epithelial cells. Int J Biochem Cell Biol. 2010;42(9):1455–61.

71. Handa O, Naito Y, Yoshikawa T. CagA protein of Helicobacter pylori: a hijacker of gastric epithelial cell signaling. Biochem Pharmacol. 2007;73(11):1697–702.
72. Chaturvedi R, Asim M, Romero-Gallo J, et al. Spermine oxidase mediates the gastric cancer risk associated with Helicobacter pylori CagA. Gastroenterology. 2011;141(5):1696–708. e1–2.
73. Vitkute J, Stankevicius K, Tamulaitiene G, et al. Specificities of eleven different DNA methyltransferases of Helicobacter pylori strain 26695. J Bacteriol. 2001;183(2):443–50.
74. Niwa T, Tsukamoto T, Toyoda T, et al. Inflammatory processes triggered by Helicobacter pylori infection cause aberrant DNA methylation in gastric epithelial cells. Cancer Res. 2010;70(4):1430–40.
75. Maeda M, Moro H, Ushijima T. Mechanisms for the induction of gastric cancer by Helicobacter pylori infection: aberrant DNA methylation pathway. Gastric Cancer. 2017;20(Suppl 1):8–15.
76. Matsumoto Y, Marusawa H, Kinoshita K, et al. Helicobacter pylori infection triggers aberrant expression of activation-induced cytidine deaminase in gastric epithelium. Nat Med. 2007;13(4):470–6.
77. Nagata N, Akiyama J, Marusawa H, et al. Enhanced expression of activation-induced cytidine deaminase in human gastric mucosa infected by Helicobacter pylori and its decrease following eradication. J Gastroenterol. 2014;49(3):427–35.
78. Matsumoto Y, Marusawa H, Kinoshita K, et al. Up-regulation of activation-induced cytidine deaminase causes genetic aberrations at the CDKN2b-CDKN2a in gastric cancer. Gastroenterology. 2010;139(6):1984–94.
79. Machado AM, Figueiredo C, Touati E, et al. Helicobacter pylori infection induces genetic instability of nuclear and mitochondrial DNA in gastric cells. Clin Cancer Res. 2009;15(9):2995–3002.
80. Kim JJ, Tao H, Carloni E, et al. Helicobacter pylori impairs DNA mismatch repair in gastric epithelial cells. Gastroenterology. 2002;123(2):542–53.
81. Park DI, Park SH, Kim SH, et al. Effect of Helicobacter pylori infection on the expression of DNA mismatch repair protein. Helicobacter. 2005;10(3):179–84.
82. Toller IM, Neelsen KJ, Steger M, et al. Carcinogenic bacterial pathogen Helicobacter pylori triggers DNA double-strand breaks and a DNA damage response in its host cells. Proc Natl Acad Sci U S A. 2011;108(36):14944–9.
83. Hartung ML, Gruber DC, Koch KN, et al. H. pylori-induced DNA Strand breaks are introduced by nucleotide excision repair endonucleases and promote NF-κB target gene expression. Cell Rep. 2015;13(1):70–9.
84. Terebiznik MR, Raju D, Vázquez CL, et al. Effect of Helicobacter pylori's vacuolating cytotoxin on the autophagy pathway in gastric epithelial cells. Autophagy. 2009;5(3):370–9.
85. Wang YH, Wu JJ, Lei HY. The autophagic induction in Helicobacter pylori-infected macrophage. Exp Biol Med (Maywood). 2009;234(2):171–80.
86. Yang X, Yu DD, Yan F, et al. The role of autophagy induced by tumor microenvironment in different cells and stages of cancer. Cell Biosci. 2015;5:14.
87. Polk DB, Peek RM Jr. Helicobacter pylori: gastric cancer and beyond. Nat Rev Cancer. 2010;10(6):403–14.
88. Raju D, Jones NL. Methods to monitor autophagy in H. pylori vacuolating cytotoxin A (VacA)-treated cells. Autophagy. 2010;6(1):138–43.
89. Mathew R, Karp CM, Beaudoin B, et al. Autophagy suppresses tumorigenesis through elimination of p62. Cell. 2009;137(6):1062–75.
90. Mohamed A, Ayman A, Deniece J, et al. P62/biquitin IHC expression correlated with clinicopathologic parameters and outcome in gastrointestinal carcinomas. Front Oncol. 2015;5:70.
91. Gump JM, Thorburn A. Autophagy and apoptosis: what is the connection? Trends Cell Biol. 2011;21(7):387–92.
92. Eisenberg-Lerner A, Bialik S, Simon HU, et al. Life and death partners: apoptosis, autophagy and the cross-talk between them. Cell Death Differ. 2009;16(7):966–75.
93. Xu MY, Lee DH, Joo EJ, et al. Akebia saponin PA induces autophagic and apoptotic cell death in AGS human gastric cancer cells. Food Chem Toxicol. 2013;59:703–8. https://doi.org/10.1016/j.fct.2013.06.059. Epub 2013 Jul 9.
94. Lim SC, Han SI. Ursodeoxycholic acid effectively kills drug-resistant gastric cancer cells through induction of autophagic death. Oncol Rep. 2015;34(3):1261–8.
95. Mukhopadhyay S, Panda PK, Sinha N, et al. Autophagy and apoptosis: where do they meet? Apoptosis. 2014;19(4):555–66.
96. Karki R, Man SM, Kanneganti TD. Inflammasomes and Cancer. Cancer Immunol Res. 2017;5(2):94–9.
97. Jorgensen I, Rayamajhi M, Miao EA. Programmed cell death as a defence against infection. Nat Rev Immunol. 2017;17(3):151–64.
98. Gabrilovich DI, Ostrand-Rosenberg S, Bronte V. Coordinated regulation of myeloid cells by tumours. Nat Rev Immunol. 2012;12(4):253–68.
99. O'Keeffe J, Moran AP. Conventional, regulatory, and unconventional T cells in the immunologic response to Helicobacter pylori. Helicobacter. 2008;13(1):1–19.
100. Choi YJ, Kim N, Chang H, et al. Helicobacter pylori-induced epithelial-mesenchymal transition, a potential role of gastric cancer initiation and an emergence of stem cells. Carcinogenesis. 2015;36(5):553–63.
101. Mesali H, Ajami A, Hussein-Nattaj H, et al. Regulatory T cells and myeloid-derived suppressor cells in patients with peptic ulcer and gastric cancer. Iran J Immunol. 2016;13(3):167–77.
102. Bockerstett KA, DiPaolo RJ. Regulation of gastric carcinogenesis by inflammatory cytokines. Cell Mol Gastroenterol Hepatol. 2017;4(1):47–53.

103. Jafarzadeh A, Larussa T, Nemati M, et al. T cell subsets play an important role in the determination of the clinical outcome of Helicobacter pylori infection. Microb Pathog. 2018. pii: S0882–4010(16)30548–4.
104. González CA, Figueiredo C, Lic CB, et al. Helicobacter pylori cagA and vacA genotypes as predictors of progression of gastric preneoplastic lesions: a long-term follow-up in a high-risk area in Spain. Am J Gastroenterol. 2011;106(5):867–74.
105. Hanada K, Yamaoka Y. Genetic battle between Helicobacter pylori and humans. The mechanism underlying homologous recombination in bacteria, which can infect human cells. Microbes Infect. 2014;16(10):833–9.
106. Rubin EJ, Trent MS. Colonize, evade, flourish: how glyco-conjugates promote virulence of Helicobacter pylori. Gut Microbes. 2013;4(6):439–53.
107. Ferreira JA, Magalhães A, Gomes J, et al. Protein glycosylation in gastric and colorectal cancers: toward cancer detection and targeted therapeutics. Cancer Lett. 2017;387:32–45.
108. Karita M, Blaser MJ. Acid-tolerance response in Helicobacter pylori and differences between cagA+ and cagA- strains. J Infect Dis. 1998;178:213–9.
109. Suerbaum S, Michetti P. Helicobacter pylori infection. N Engl J Med. 2002;347:1175–86.
110. Figura N, Trabalzini L, Mini R, et al. Inactivation of Helicobacter pylori cagA gene affects motility. Helicobacter. 2004;9:185–93.
111. Basaglia G, Sperandio P, Tomasini ML, et al. Analysis of antimicrobial susceptibility and virulence factors in Helicobacter pylori clinical isolates. J Chemother. 2004;16(5):504–6.
112. De Paoli P, Tomasini ML, Basaglia G. The predictive value of Helicobacter pylori in-vitro metronidazole resistance. Clin Microbiol Infect. 2004;10(12):1105–6.
113. Tomasini ML, Zanussi S, Sozzi M, et al. Heterogeneity of cag genotypes in Helicobacter pylori isolates from human biopsy specimens. J Clin Microbiol. 2003;41(3):976–80.
114. Sozzi M, Crosatti M, Kim SK, et al. Heterogeneity of Helicobacter pylori cag genotypes in experimentally infected mice. FEMS Microbiol Lett. 2001;203(1):109–14.
115. Figura N, Valassina M, Moretti E, et al. Histological variety of gastric carcinoma and Helicobacter pylori cagA and vacA polymorphism. Eur J Gastroenterol Hepatol. 2015;27(9):1017–21.
116. Repetto O, Zanussi S, Casarotto M, et al. Differential proteomics of Helicobacter pylori associated with autoimmune atrophic gastritis. Mol Med. 2014;20:57–71.
117. Bernardini G, Figura N, Ponzetto A, et al. Application of proteomics to the study of Helicobacter pylori and implications for the clinic. Expert Rev Proteomics. 2017;14(6):477–90.
118. Sozzi M, Valentini M, Figura N, et al. Atrophic gastritis and intestinal metaplasia in Helicobacter pylori infection: the role of CagA status. Am J Gastroenterol. 1998;93(3):375–9.
119. Sozzi M, Tomasini ML, Vindigni C, et al. Heterogeneity of cag genotypes and clinical outcome of Helicobacter pylori infection. J Lab Clin Med. 2005;146(5):262–70.
120. Korneev KV, Atretkhany KN, Drutskaya MS, et al. TLR-signaling and proinflammatory cytokines as drivers of tumorigenesis. Cytokine. 2017;89:127–35.
121. Pachathundikandi SK, Müller A, Backert S. Inflammasome activation by Helicobacter pylori and its implications for persistence and immunity. Curr Top Microbiol Immunol. 2016;397:117–31.
122. Kohyama M, Saijyo K, Hayasida M, et al. Direct activation of human CD8+ cytotoxic T lymphocytes by interleukin-18. Jpn J Cancer Res. 1998;89(10):1041–6.
123. Palma G, Barbieri A, Bimonte S, et al. Interleukin 18: friend or foe in cancer. Biochim Biophys Acta. 2013;1836(2):296–303.
124. Terme M, Ullrich E, Aymeric L, et al. IL-18 induces PD-1-dependent immunosuppression in cancer. Cancer Res. 2011;71(16):5393–9.
125. Yao J, Li ZH, Li YX, et al. Association between the −607 C > a polymorphism in interleukin-18 gene promoter with gastrointestinal cancer risk: a meta-analysis. Genet Mol Res. 2015;14(4):16880–7.
126. Tu S, Bhagat G, Cui G, et al. Overexpression of interleukin-1beta induces gastric inflammation and cancer and mobilizes myeloid-derived suppressor cells in mice. Cancer Cell. 2008;14(5):408–19.
127. Chen J, Ye Y, Liu P, et al. Suppression of T cells by myeloid-derived suppressor cells in cancer. Hum Immunol. 2017;78(2):113–9.
128. Diaz-Montero CM, Salem ML, Nishimura MI, et al. Increased circulating myeloid-derived suppressor cells correlate with clinical cancer stage, metastatic tumor burden, and doxorubicin-cyclophosphamide chemotherapy. Cancer Immunol Immunother. 2009;58(1):49–59.
129. Mantovani A. The growing diversity and spectrum of action of myeloid-derived suppressor cells. Eur J Immunol. 2010;40(12):3317–20.
130. Parker KH, Beury DW, Ostrand-Rosenberg S. Myeloid-derived suppressor cells: critical cells driving immune suppression in the tumor microenvironment. Adv Cancer Res. 2015;128:95–139.
131. Chang WJ, Du Y, Zhao X, et al. Inflammation-related factors predicting prognosis of gastric cancer. World J Gastroenterol. 2014;20(16):4586–96.
132. Shoji H, Tada K, Kitano S, et al. The peripheral immune status of granulocytic myeloid-derived suppressor cells correlates the survival in advanced gastric cancer patients receiving cisplatin-based chemotherapy. Oncotarget. 2017;8(56):95083–94.
133. Ricci V, Romano M, Boquet P. Molecular cross-talk between Helicobacter pylori and human gastric mucosa. World J Gastroenterol. 2011;17(11):1383–99.

134. Zhuang Y, Shi Y, Liu XF, et al. Helicobacter pylori infected macrophages induce Th17 cell differentiation. Immunobiology. 2011;216(1–2):200–7.
135. Ichiyama K, Yoshida H, Wakabayashi Y, et al. Foxp3 inhibits RORgammat-mediated IL-17A mRNA transcription through direct interaction with RORgammat. J Biol Chem. 2008;283(25):17003–8. https://doi.org/10.1074/jbc.M801286200. Epub 2008 Apr 23.
136. Caruso C, Lio D, Cavallone L, et al. Aging, longevity, inflammation, and cancer. Ann N Y Acad Sci. 2004;1028:1–13.
137. Zanussi S, Serraino D, Dolcetti R, et al. Cancer, aging and immune reconstitution. Anti Cancer Agents Med Chem. 2013;13(9):1310–24.
138. Serelli-Lee V, Ling KL, Ho C, et al. Persistent Helicobacter pylori specific Th17 responses in patients with past H. pylori infection are associated with elevated gastric mucosal IL-1beta. PLoS One. 2012;7(6):e39199.
139. Akhiani AA, Pappo J, Kabok Z, et al. Protection against Helicobacter pylori infection following immunization is IL-12-dependent and mediated by Th1 cells. J Immunol. 2002;169(12):6977–84.
140. Jager A, Kuchroo VK. Effector and regulatory T-cell subsets in autoimmunity and tissue inflammation. Scand J Immunol. 2010;72(3):173–84.
141. Zhang Y, Zhang Y, Gu W, et al. TH1/TH2 cell differentiation and molecular signals. Adv Exp Med Biol. 2014;841:15–44.
142. Kabisch R, Semper RP, Wustner S, et al. Helicobacter pylori gamma-glutamyltranspeptidase induces tolerogenic human dendritic cells by activation of glutamate receptors. J Immunol. 2016;196(10):4246–52.
143. Bergman MP, Engering A, Smits HH, et al. Helicobacter pylori modulates the T helper cell 1/T helper cell 2 balance through phase-variable interaction between lipopolysaccharide and DC-SIGN. J Exp Med. 2004;200(8):979–90.
144. Larussa T, Leone I, Suraci E, et al. Enhanced expression of indoleamine 2, 3-dioxygenase in Helicobacter pylori-infected human gastric mucosa modulates Th1/Th2 pathway and interleukin 17 production. Helicobacter. 2015;20(1):41–8.
145. Pellicanò A, Imeneo M, Leone I, et al. Enhanced activation of Cyclooxygenase-2 downregulates Th1 signaling pathway in Helicobacter pylori-infected human gastric mucosa. Helicobacter. 2007;12(3):193–9.
146. Toller IM, Hitzler I, Sayi A, et al. Prostaglandin E2 prevents Helicobacter-induced gastric preneoplasia and facilitates persistent infection in a mouse model. Gastroenterology. 2010;138(4):1455–67.
147. Forchielli ML, Walker WA. The role of gut-associated lymphoid tissues and mucosal defence. Br J Nutr. 2005;93(Suppl 1):S41–8.
148. Taylor JM, Ziman ME, Canfield DR, et al. Effects of a Th1-versus a Th2-biased immune response in protection against Helicobacter pylori challenge in mice. Microb Pathog. 2008;44(1):20–7.
149. Marotti B, Rocco A, De Colibus P, et al. Interleukin-13 mucosal production in Helicobacter pylori-related gastric diseases. Dig Liver Dis. 2008;40(4):240–7.
150. Yang P, Qiu G, Wang S, et al. The mutations of Th1 cell-specific T-box transcription factor may be associated with a predominant Th2 phenotype in gastric cancers. Int J Immunogenet. 2010;37(2):111–5.
151. Liu X, Cao K, Xu C, et al. GATA-3 augmentation down-regulates Connexin43 in Helicobacter Pylori associated gastric carcinogenesis. Cancer Biol Ther. 2015;16(6):987–96.
152. Sun X, Zhang M, El-Zataari M, et al. TLR2 mediates Helicobacter pylori-induced tolerogenic immune response in mice. PLoS One. 2013;8(9):e74595.
153. Nemati M, Larussa T, Khorramdelazad H, et al. Toll-like receptor 2: an important immunomodulatory molecule during Helicobacter pylori infection. Life Sci. 2017;178:17–29.
154. Das S, Suarez G, Beswick EJ, et al. Expression of B7-H1 on gastric epithelial cells: its potential role in regulating T cells during Helicobacter pylori infection. J Immunol. 2006;176(5):3000–9.
155. Mitchell P, Afzali B, Fazekasova H, et al. Helicobacter pylori induces in-vivo expansion of human regulatory T cells through stimulating interleukin-1β production by dendritic cells. Clin Exp Immunol. 2012;70(3):300–9.
156. Zhang C, Zhang X. ChenXH. Inhibition of the interleukin-6 signaling pathway: a strategy to induce immune tolerance. Clin. Rev. Allerg Immunol. 2014;47(2):163–73.
157. Zheng SG. Regulatory T cells vs Th17: differentiation of Th17 versus Treg, are they mutually exclusive? Afr J Clin Exp Immunol. 2013;2(1):94–106.
158. Hamajima N, Naito M, Kondo T, et al. Genetic factors involved in the development of Helicobacter pylori-related gastric cancer. Cancer Sci. 2006;97(11):1129–38.
159. Li M, Wang Y, Gu Y. Quantitative assessment of the influence of tumor necrosis factor alpha polymorphism with gastritis and gastric cancer risk. Tumour Biol. 2014;35(2):1495–502.
160. Loh M, Koh KX, Yeo BH, et al. Meta-analysis of genetic polymorphisms and gastric cancer risk: variability in associations according to race. Eur J Cancer. 2009;45(14):2562–8.
161. Silva-Fernandes IJ, da Silva TA, Agnez-Lima LF, et al. Helicobacter pylori genotype and polymorphisms in DNA repair enzymes: where do they correlate in gastric cancer? J Surg Oncol. 2012;106(4):448–55.
162. Goto Y, Ando T, Yamamoto K, et al. Association between serum pepsinogens and polymorphismof PTPN11 encoding SHP-2 among Helicobacter pylori seropositive Japanese. Int J Cancer. 2006;118(1):203–8.
163. Kawai S, Goto Y, Ito LS, et al. Significant association between PTPN11 polymorphism and gastric atrophy among Japanese Brazilians. Gastric Cancer. 2006;9(4):277–83.

164. Hishida A, Matsuo K, Goto Y, et al. Associations of a PTPN11 G/A polymorphism at intron 3 with Helicobactor pylori seropositivity, gastric atrophy and gastric cancer in Japanese. BMC Gastroenterol. 2009;9:51.
165. He C, Tu H, Sun L, et al. Helicobacter pylori-related host gene polymorphisms associated with susceptibility of gastric carcinogenesis: a two-stage case-control study in Chinese. Carcinogenesis. 2013;34(7):1450–7.
166. Wang GY, Lu CQ, Zhang RM, et al. The E-cadherin gene polymorphism 160C->A and cancer risk: a HuGE review and meta-analysis of 26 case-control studies. Am J Epidemiol. 2008;167(1):7–14.
167. Gao L, Nieters A, Brenner H. Meta-analysis: tumour invasion-related genetic polymorphisms and gastric cancer susceptibility. Aliment Pharmacol Ther. 2008;28(5):565–73.
168. Wang Q, Gu D, Wang M, et al. The E-cadherin (CDH1) -160C>A polymorphism associated with gastric cancer among Asians but not Europeans. DNA Cell Biol. 2011;30(6):395–400.
169. Chen B, Zhou Y, Yang P, et al. CDH1 -160C>A gene polymorphism is an ethnicity-dependent risk factor for gastric cancer. Cytokine. 2011;55(2):266–73.
170. Cui Y, Xue H, Lin B, et al. A meta-analysis of CDH1 C-160A genetic polymorphism and gastric cancer risk. DNA Cell Biol. 2011;30(11):937–45.
171. Li YL, Tian Z, Zhang JB, et al. CDH1 promoter polymorphism and stomach cancer susceptibility. Mol Biol Rep. 2012;39(2):1283–6.
172. Wang L, Wang G, Lu C, et al. Contribution of the -160C/A polymorphism in the E-cadherin promoter to cancer risk: a meta-analysis of 47 case-control studies. PLoS One. 2012;7(7):e40219.
173. Miao X, Zhang X, Zhang L, et al. Adenosine diphosphate ribosyl transferase and x-ray repair cross-complementing 1 polymorphisms in gastric cardia cancer. Gastroenterology. 2006;131(2):420–7.
174. Fan H, Liu D, Qiu X, et al. A functional polymorphism in the DNA methyltransferase-3A promoter modifies the susceptibility in gastric cancer but not in esophageal carcinoma. BMC Med. 2010;8:12.
175. Ravishankar Ram M, Goh KL, Leow AH, et al. Polymorphisms at locus 4p14 of toll-like receptors TLR-1 and TLR-10 confer susceptibility to gastric carcinoma in Helicobacter pylori infection. PLoS One. 2015;10(11):e0141865.
176. Rigoli L, Di Bella C, Fedele F, et al. TLR4 and NOD2/CARD15 genetic polymorphisms and their possible role in gastric carcinogenesis. Anticancer Res. 2010;30(2):513–7.
177. Hold GL, Rabkin CS, Chow WH, et al. A functional polymorphism of toll-like receptor 4 gene increases risk of gastric carcinoma and its precursors. Gastroenterology. 2007;132(3):905–12.
178. Santini D, Angeletti S, Ruzzo A, et al. Toll-like receptor 4 Asp299Gly and Thr399Ile polymorphisms in gastric cancer of intestinal and diffuse histotypes. Clin Exp Immunol. 2008;154(3):360–4.
179. Jing JJ, Li M, Yuan Y. Toll-like receptor 4 Asp299Gly and Thr399Ile polymorphisms in cancer: a meta-analysis. Gene. 2012;499(2):237–42.
180. Hishida A, Matsuo K, Goto Y, et al. Toll-like receptor 4 +3725 G/C polymorphism, Helicobacter pylori seropositivity, and the risk of gastric atrophy and gastric cancer in Japanese. Helicobacter. 2009;14(1):47–53.
181. De Oliveira JG, Silva AE. Polymorphisms of the TLR2 and TLR4 genes are associated with risk of gastric cancer in a Brazilian population. World J Gastroenterol. 2012;18(11):1235–42.
182. Tahara T, Arisawa T, Wang F, et al. Toll-like receptor 2–196 to 174del polymorphism influences the susceptibility of Japanese people to gastric cancer. Cancer Sci. 2007;98(11):1790–4.
183. Tahara T, Arisawa T, Wang F, et al. Toll-like receptor 2 (TLR) -196 to 174del polymorphism in gastro-duodenal diseases in Japanese population. Dig Dis Sci. 2008;53(4):919–24.
184. Zeng HM, Pan KF, Zhang Y, et al. Genetic variants of toll-like receptor 2 and 5, helicobacter pylori infection, and risk of gastric cancer and its precursors in a chinese population. Cancer Epidemiol Biomark Prev. 2011;20(12):2594–602.
185. Hofner P, Gyulai Z, Kiss ZF, et al. Genetic polymorphisms of NOD1 and IL-8, but not polymorphisms of TLR4 genes, are associated with Helicobacter pylori-induced duodenal ulcer and gastritis. Helicobacter. 2007;12(2):124–31.
186. Kara B, Akkiz H, Doran F, et al. The significance of E266K polymorphism in the NOD1 gene on Helicobacter pylori infection: an effective force on pathogenesis? Clin Exp Med. 2010;10(2):107–12.
187. Wang P, Zhang L, Jiang JM, et al. Association of NOD1 and NOD2 genes polymorphisms with Helicobacter pylori related gastric cancer in a Chinese population. World J Gastroenterol. 2012;18(17):2112–20.
188. Kim EJ, Lee JR, Chung WC, et al. Association between genetic polymorphisms of NOD 1 and Helicobacter pylori-induced gastric mucosal inflammation in healthy Korean population. Helicobacter. 2013;18(2):143–50.
189. Li ZX, Wang YM, Tang FB, et al. NOD1 and NOD2 genetic variants in association with risk of gastric Cancer and its precursors in a Chinese population. PLoS One. 2015;10(5):e0124949.
190. Castaño-Rodríguez N, Kaakoush NO, Goh KL, et al. The NOD-like receptor signalling pathway in Helicobacter pylori infection and related gastric cancer: a case-control study and gene expression analyses. PLoS One. 2014;9(6):e98899.
191. Companioni O, Bonet C, Muñoz X, et al. Polymorphisms of Helicobacter pylori signaling pathway genes and gastric cancer risk in the European Prospective Investigation into Cancer-Eurgast cohort. Int J Cancer. 2014;134(1):92–101.
192. Wex T, Ebert MP, Kropf S, et al. Gene polymorphisms of the NOD-2/CARD-15 gene and the risk

of gastric cancer in Germany. Anticancer Res. 2008;28(2A):757–62.
193. Hnatyszyn A, Szalata M, Stanczyk J, et al. Association of c.802C>T polymorphism of NOD2/CARD15 gene with the chronic gastritis and predisposition to cancer in H. pylori infected patients. Exp Mol Pathol. 2010;88(3):388–93.
194. Angeletti S, Galluzzo S, Santini D, et al. NOD2/CARD15 polymorphisms impair innate immunity and increase susceptibility to gastric cancer in an Italian population. Hum Immunol. 2009;70(9):729–32.
195. Cooney R, Baker J, Brain O, et al. NOD2 stimulation induces autophagy in dendritic cells influencing bacterial handling and antigen presentation. Nat Med. 2010;16(1):90–7.
196. Salucci V, Rimoldi M, Penati C, et al. Monocyte-derived dendritic cells from Crohn patients show differential NOD2/CARD15-dependent immune responses to bacteria. Inflamm Bowel Dis. 2008;14(6):812–8.
197. Ying HY, Yu BW, Yang Z, et al. Interleukin-1B 31 C>T polymorphism combined with Helicobacter pylori-modified gastric cancer susceptibility: evidence from 37 studies. J Cell Mol Med. 2016;20(3):526–36.
198. Park MJ, Hyun MH, Yang JP, et al. Effects of the interleukin-1β-511 C/T gene polymorphism on the risk of gastric cancer in the context of the relationship between race and H. pylori infection: a meta-analysis of 20,000 subjects. Mol Biol Rep. 2015;42(1):119–34.
199. Persson C, Canedo P, Machado JC, et al. Polymorphisms in inflammatory response genes and their association with gastric cancer: a HuGE systematic review and meta-analyses. Am J Epidemiol. 2011;173(3):259–70.
200. Lu W, Pan K, Zhang L, et al. Genetic polymorphisms of interleukin (IL)-1B, IL-1RN, IL-8, IL-10 and tumor necrosis factor {alpha} and risk of gastric cancer in a Chinese population. Carcinogenesis. 2005;26(3):631–6.
201. Cheng D, Hao Y, Zhou W, et al. Positive association between Interleukin-8 -251A > T polymorphism and susceptibility to gastric carcinogenesis: a meta-analysis. Cancer Cell Int. 2013;13(1):100.
202. Wu MS, Wu CY, Chen CJ, et al. Interleukin-10 genotypes associate with the risk of gastric carcinoma in Taiwanese Chinese. Int J Cancer. 2003;104(5):617–23.
203. Yang JP, Hyun MH, Yoon JM, et al. Association between TNF-α-308 G/A gene polymorphism and gastric cancer risk: a systematic review and meta-analysis. Cytokine. 2014;70(2):104–14.
204. Yu JY, Li L, Ma H, et al. Tumor necrosis factor-α 238 G/A polymorphism and gastric cancer risk: a meta-analysis. Tumour Biol. 2013;34(6):3859–63.
205. Qin Q, Lu J, Zhu H, et al. PARP-1 Val762Ala polymorphism and risk of cancer: a meta-analysis based on 39 case-control studies. PLoS One. 2014;9(5):e98022.
206. Zhang WH, Wang XL, Zhou J, et al. Association of interleukin-1B (IL-1B) gene polymorphisms with risk of gastric cancer in Chinese population. Cytokine. 2005;30(6):378–81.
207. Yang JJ, Cho LY, Ma SH, et al. Oncogenic CagA promotes gastric cancer risk via activating ERK signaling pathways: a nested case-control study. PLoS One. 2011;6(6):e21155.
208. Yang JJ, Cho LY, Ko KP, et al. Genetic susceptibility on CagA-interacting molecules and gene-environment interaction with phytoestrogens: a putative risk factor for gastric cancer. PLoS One. 2012;7(2):e31020.
209. Arbour NC, Lorenz E, Schutte BC, et al. TLR4 mutations are associated with endotoxin hyporesponsiveness in humans. Nat Genet. 2000;25(2):187–91.
210. Rallabhandi P, Bell J, Boukhvalova MS, et al. Analysis of TLR4 polymorphic variants: new insights into TLR4/MD-2/CD14 stoichiometry, structure, and signaling. J Immunol. 2006;177(1):322–32.
211. Mommersteeg MC, Yu J, Peppelenbosch MP, et al. Genetic host factors in Helicobacter pylori-induced carcinogenesis: emerging new paradigms. Biochim Biophys Acta. 2018;1869(1):42–52.
212. Camargo MC, Mera R, Correa P, et al. Interleukin-1B and interleukin-1 receptor antagonist gene polymorphisms and gastric cancer: a meta-analysis. Cancer Epidemiol Biomark Prev. 2006;15:1674–87.
213. Kamangar F, Cheng C, Abnet CC, et al. Interleukin-1B polymorphisms and gastric cancer risk—a meta-analysis. Cancer Epidemiol Biomark Prev. 2006;15:1920–8.
214. Camargo MC, Mera R, Correa P, et al. IL1B polymorphisms and gastric cancer risk. Cancer Epidemiol Biomark Prev. 2007;16(3):635; author reply 635–6.

Genetic and Epigenetic Mechanisms in Gastric Cancer

2

Valli De Re and Riccardo Dolcetti

Introduction

Gastric cancer (GC) is the fifth most common cancer and the third leading cause of cancer-related deaths [1] and is a complex heterogeneous disease. Besides tumor node metastasis (TNM) staging, GC has two clinically accepted classifications based on histologic features: the Lauren's criteria, in which intestinal-type and diffuse-type adenocarcinomas are the two major histologic subtypes [2], and the World Health Organization (WHO) classification that differentiates GC into categories such as tubular, papillary, mucinous, and poorly cohesive, including signet ring cell carcinomas, plus uncommon histologic variants [3]. Both classifications enable a better understanding of the biology of the GC, but so far they had limited success in promoting the development of subtype-specific treatment options, due to the complex heterogeneity of the disease. More recently, genomic studies and comprehensive characterization of GC have confirmed this complex heterogeneity by providing further insights into the pathogenesis of GC, proposing genetic/molecular subclassifications of the disease and identifying new potential therapeutic targets. This may pave the way for the development of personalized prognostication and treatment [4].

V. De Re (✉)
Immunopathology and Biomarker Unit/Bio-proteomics Facility, Department of Research and Advanced Tumor Diagnostics, IRCCS, CRO Aviano, National Cancer Institute, Aviano, PN, Italy
e-mail: vdere@cro.it

R. Dolcetti
Immunopathology and Biomarker Unit/Bio-proteomics Facility, Department of Research and Advanced Tumor Diagnostics, IRCCS, CRO Aviano, National Cancer Institute, Aviano, PN, Italy

Translational Research Institute, University of Queensland Diamantina Institute, Brisbane, QLD, Australia
e-mail: rdolcetti@cro.it

Etiological Classification

Diverging trends in the incidence of GC by tumor location and histology have suggested that GC heterogeneity may result from differences in the etiology. During the past two decades, while there has been a marked decline in distal and primarily intestinal type (mainly antrum and pyloric regions of the stomach) [5], the incidence of proximal diffuse GC type (the first three parts of the stomach, cardia, fundus, and body) has been increasing, particularly in the Western countries and Asia (particularly Japan, China, and Korea) (Fig. 2.1) [6–8].

Incidence by tumor sub-site also varies widely based on geographic location, race, and socio-economic status. Distal GC predominates in the Republic of Korea, followed by Mongolia, Japan,

© Springer Nature Switzerland AG 2019

V. Canzonieri, A. Giordano (eds.), *Gastric Cancer In The Precision Medicine Era*, Current Clinical Pathology, https://doi.org/10.1007/978-3-030-04861-7_2

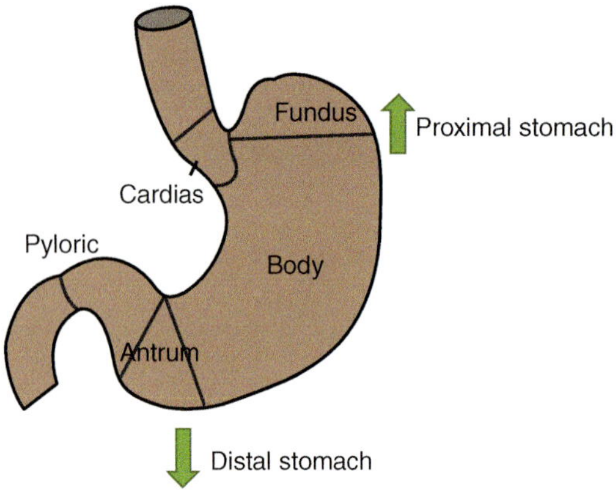

Fig. 2.1 The anatomical location of GC. During the last years, the numbers of proximal and diffuse types of tumors are increasing, while for the distal neoplasia, mainly of intestinal type, the number of cases is decreasing

and Colombia, and in lower socioeconomic groups, whereas proximal tumors are more common in developed countries, among whites, and in higher socioeconomic classes. The main risk factors for distal GC include *Helicobacter pylori* (*H. pylori*) infection and dietary factors, whereas gastroesophageal reflux disease and obesity play important roles in the development of proximal cardia/stomach cancer. Patients with immune deficiencies (i.e., immunodeficiency syndrome acquired and posttransplant immunodeficiency) have also an increased risk for GC [9]. Nonetheless, intrinsic genetic factors could play an additional key role in determining GC development since only a small part of *H. pylori*-infected individuals will progress to GC [10] and about 10% of cases occur in familial GC clusters with some cases showing specific germline mutations [11].

Inherited Genetic Predisposition

The first major inherited form of diffuse GC (HDGC) was found in linkage to the E-cadherin (CDH1) gene on chromosome 16q22.1 that encodes the epithelial cadherin protein (E-cad) (Fig. 2.2). CDH1 has been considered to be the prototypic gene of the cadherin family [14]. E-cad is a calcium-dependent cell-cell adhesion glycoprotein composed of five extracellular cadherin repeats, a single transmembrane domain, and a cytoplasmic domain with highly conserved binding sites for p120-catenin (also known as catenin-δ1) and β-catenin (Fig. 2.3). E-cad suppresses tumorigenicity and tumor dissemination by complex mechanisms that promote tissue organization and block of the apoptosis [16]. Moreover, the ectodomain of E-cad mediates bacterial adhesion to mammalian cells, and the cytoplasmic domain is required for bacterial internalization. Tumor pathogenesis are thought to involve biophysical adhesion processes and mechanotransduction-based intracellular signaling coupled to inhibition of molecules such as β-catenin and epidermal growth factor receptor (EGFR). EGFR belongs to a family of receptor tyrosine kinases that includes three other members (erbB2/HER-2, erbB3/HER-3, and erbB4/HER-4). These receptors are anchored in the cytoplasmic membrane and share a similar structure that is composed of an extracellular ligand-binding domain, a short hydrophobic transmembrane region, and an intracytoplasmic tyrosine kinase domain (Fig. 2.3). Malignant carcinoma cells abrogate CDH1 function in numerous ways [16]. In HDGC cases, the CDH1 gene showed a damaging mutation leading to the production of a truncated or incorrect E-cadherin protein (E-cad) [17]. Patients had an autosomal-dominant inheritance and an earlier age at onset of the disease (<40 years, range of 14–69 years). Tumors were primarily of diffuse-type histology, a poorly differentiated adenocarcinoma that infiltrates into the stomach wall causing solidity of the wall (*linitis plastica*) without forming a distinct mass. Diffuse GC is also referred to as signet ring carcinoma with increasing proliferation, invasion, and/or metastasis. The estimated cumulative risk of GC by age 80 years is 80% for both men and women. Women also have a 39–52% risk for lobular breast cancer. Somatic mutations in CDH1 had been also reported in GCs, and lobular breast cancers that were not necessarily familial and CDH1 gene mutations also correlated with the risk of colorectal, thyroid, and ovarian cancer.

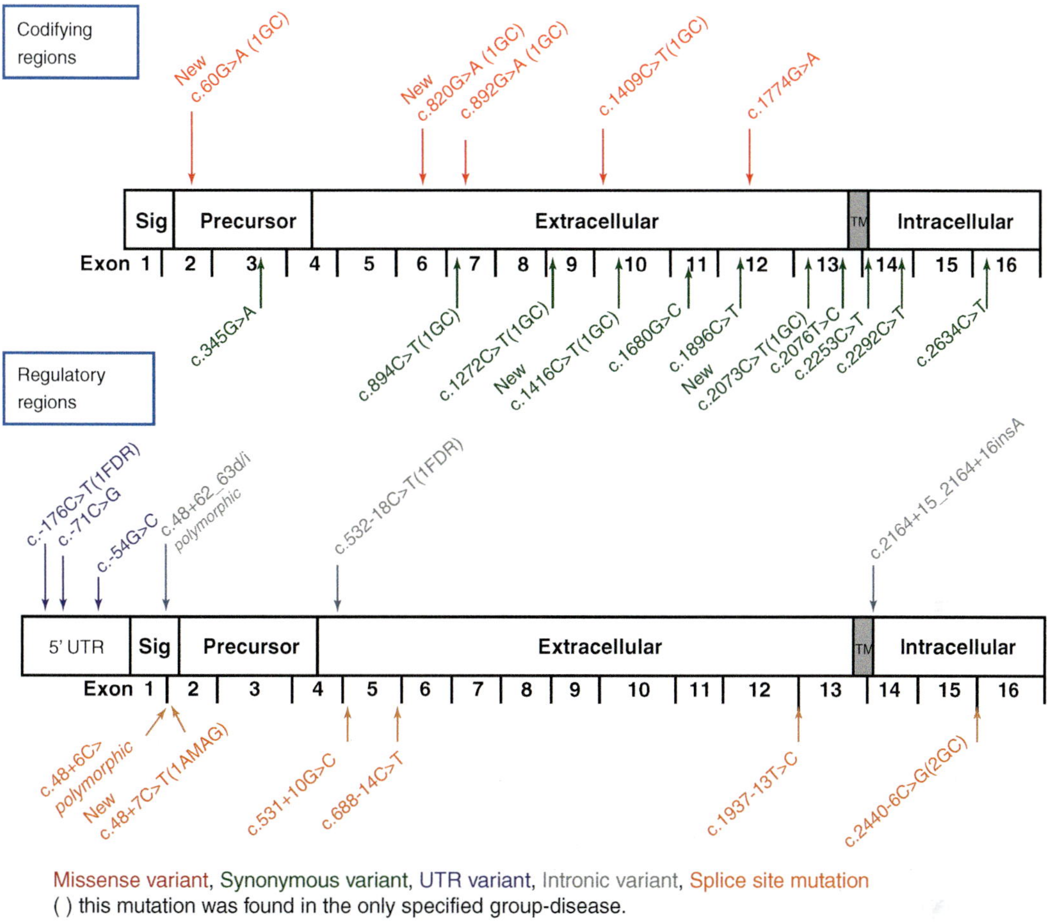

Fig. 2.2 CDH1 gene with some representative germline sense and missense mutations found in patients with gastric cancer [12]. The figure illustrates the high number of mutations, including new ones, their distribution along all the entire gene, and their potential impact on gene expression. Mutations had a different impact on the clinical status in patients, but only a few of them had a clear pathogenic role [13]

The HDGC syndrome was defined by the International Gastric Cancer Linkage Consortium (IGCLC) as the presence of two or more documented cases of diffuse GC in first- or second-degree relatives with at least one case diagnosed prior to age 50 years or three or more documented cases of diffuse GC in first- or second-degree relatives, regardless of age of onset [18]. Table 2.1 reports clinical criteria for the genetic screening of families with suspected hereditary gastric cancer according to the IGCLC guidelines updated in 2010.

Table 2.2 reports difference in the families with aggregation of GC and GC at early onset.

About 30–40% of HDGCs can be explained by defective germline alleles of CDH1, but for the remaining families, the factors driving susceptibility remain unknown even if in most cases, a reduced expression of the E-cad protein was present in the tumor tissue [20]. Of additional interest, in some cases of HDGC without CDH1 mutation, variants of genes encoding for CTNNA1, a truncated α-catenin [21], mitogen-activated protein kinase (MAP 3K6) [22], and insulin resistance receptor (INSR), FBXO24, and DOT1L [23], were discovered. Since α-catenin [24], MAP 3K6 [24], and INSR [25] function in complex with E-cad [25], genetic alterations of

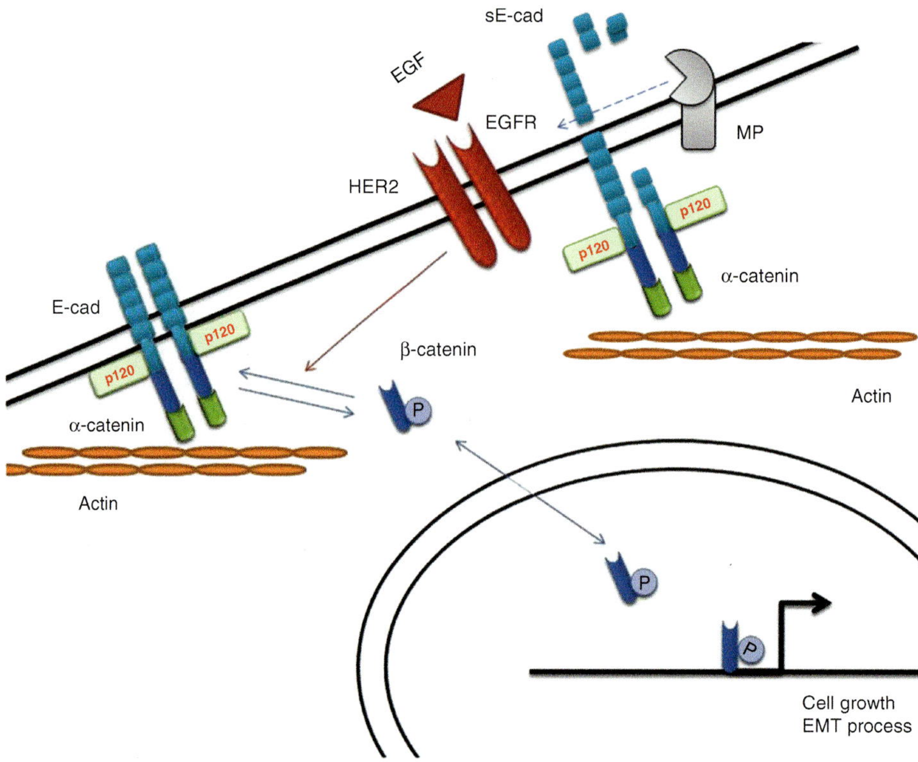

Fig. 2.3 Schematic diagram of E-cadherin-HER2 interaction. The mature E-cadherin contains three distinct domains: the highly conserved cytoplasmic domain, a single pass transmembrane domain, and an extracellular domain. The cytoplasmic tail of E-cadherin consists of two regions: the catenin-binding domain and the juxta-membrane domain. β-Catenin binds to the E-cadherin domain, and this complex via α-catenin connects and regulates E-cad interaction with the actin cytoskeleton. p120-catenin binds the CDH1 juxtamembrane domain and stabilizes E-cad expression at the cell surface. Activation of the HER2 receptor (e.g., by epidermal growth factor (EGF) ligation to the EGF receptor (EGFR) by inducing the phosphorylation of β-catenin directs the dissociation of β-catenin from the E-cad complex, thus leading to a decrease of E-cad-mediated cell adhesion, enhanced epithelial-mesenchymal transition (EMT), and increased translocation of β-catenin into the nucleus where it acts as a transcriptional regulator of genes involved in cell growth and EMT process. Metalloproteinases (MP) lead to production of soluble E-cadherin (sE-cad) through the cleavage of E-cad. HER2 phosphokinase activity favors the dissociation of β-catenin/E-cad complex leading to GC progression and metastasis. The production of sE-cad, as a paracrine/autocrine signaling molecule, not only undermines adherence junctions, causing a reduction in cell aggregation capacity, but its diffusion into the extracellular environment and the blood regulates multiple signaling pathways involved in GC progression [15]

Table 2.1 Criteria for the genetic screening of families with suspected HDGC; one of the following cases

Two GC cases in a family, in which one individual developed confirmed diffuse GC under age 50 years
Three confirmed individuals with diffuse GC in first- or second-degree relatives independent of age
One case of diffuse GC occurring before age 40 years
Personal or family history of diffuse GC and lobular breast cancer, one diagnosed before age 50 years

Table 2.2 Families with aggregation of GC and GC at early onset

Hereditary diffuse gastric cancer (HDGC): Families with aggregation of GC fulfilling the IGCLC criteria reported in Table 2.1
Familial diffuse gastric cancer (FDGC): Families with aggregation of GC and index cases with diffuse GC but not fulfilling the IGCLC criteria for HDGC
Familial intestinal gastric cancer (FIGC): Families with aggregations of GC and an index case with intestinal GC. No germline genetic defect has been found to date in this type of predisposing disease
GC at early onset: Patients who developed GC at an early age (<50 years old) without a familial history of GC [19]

these genes are particularly intriguing, but the exact contribution of these genes to GC predisposition remains unclear until a higher number of families with mutations in these genes will be reported and characterized.

Important observations in the last two decades allowed the identification of individuals who have inheredited a genetic mutation conferring susceptibility to syndromes including GC gene penetrance. While these individuals comprise a small portion of the overall burden of GC, the underlying inheredited genes identified are important to distinguish phonotypical features of GC and to better decipher the GC pathogenesis. Syndromes showing incomplete penetrance for GC include gastric adenocarcinoma and proximal polyposis of the stomach syndrome (GAPPS) [26], Lynch syndrome (or hereditary nonpolyposis colorectal cancer, HNPCC) [27], Li-Fraumeni syndrome (LFS) [28], hereditary breast and ovarian cancer [29], Peutz-Jeghers syndrome [30], and juvenile polyposis [24]. Of note, Asian ancestry of patients having one of these hereditary syndromes had showed a markedly increased risk of GC suggesting an interplay between genetic risk and environmental factors, e.g., *H. pylori* infection or food ingestion.

GAPPS is a phenotypic variant of the familial adenomatous polyposis (FAP) that is caused by a germline mutation in the 1B promoter region of the adenomatous polyposis coli (APC) gene. Interestingly, large deletions in the same APC gene region were observed both in families with more classic FAP phenotypes and in GAPPS, showing that APC promoter is a region of particular importance in gastric neoplasia [26].

The Lynch syndrome is a gastrointestinal disorder caused by germline mutation/deletion in one of the mismatch repair genes (MLH1, MSH2, MSH6, or PMS2) or in the EPCAM gene neighboring the MSH2 gene evidenced by gene microsatellite instability (MSI). EPCAM deletions cause additional methyl groups to be attached to the MSH2 promoter, thus reducing the expression of the MSH2 gene. GC is the third most common cancer in these individuals, with the intestinal subtype of antrum location being the predominant GC [31]. GC with MSI showed generally better survival rates, and it is particularly frequent in an area of Italy (Florence) with high GC risk [32].

The Li-Fraumeni syndrome is caused by germline mutations in the P53 tumor suppressor gene or the cell cycle checkpoint kinase (CHEK2) gene [31, 33]. Both diffuse and intestinal GC subtypes were observed.

Hereditary breast and ovarian cancer occurs in patients with germline mutations in the tumor suppressor genes BRCA1 and BRCA2. BRCA-related pathways safeguard genetic content such as DNA damage recognition, double-strand break repair, checkpoint control, transcription regulation, and chromatin remodeling; however despite the general nature of BRCA functions, tumors in mutation carriers predominantly target the breast and ovary. Some observational studies report elevations of the risk for certain cancers, including GC, besides breast or ovarian cancer in BRCA1 or BRCA2 mutation carriers [29].

Peutz-Jeghers and juvenile polyposis are two even more rare syndromes: the first caused by germline mutations in a serine/threonine kinase (STK11) [34] and the second one most frequently caused by mutations in the SMAD4 or BMPR1A genes [35].

Table 2.3 resumes the germline genetic alterations inheredited in syndromes predisposing to GC.

Table 2.3 Hereditary syndromes predisposing to gastric cancer

Syndromes	Gene inheredited
Hereditary diffuse gastric cancer [25]	CDH1
Gastric adenocarcinoma and proximal polyposis of the stomach (GAPPS) [26]	APC
Lynch or hereditary nonpolyposis colorectal cancer, (HNPCC) [27]	MLH1, MSH2, MSH6, PMS2 or EPCAM
Li-Fraumeni (LFS) [28]	P53 or CHEK2
Hereditary breast and ovarian cancer	BRCA1 or BRCA2
Peutz-Jeghers	STK11
Juvenile polyposis	SMAD4 or BMPR1A

Genetic Alterations and Epigenetic Changes in Precancerous Lesions and GC at Early Diagnosis

In most instances, GC represents the culmination of a precancerous lesion sequence, i.e., metaplasia-dysplasia-GC [36]. Several comparative molecular genetics profiles of precancerous lesions and GC were performed to identify the genes and the mechanisms responsible for GC onset. Due to heterogeneity of the tumor, however, a unique panel for genetic alterations had not been found yet. However, epigenetic silencing of tumor-related genes by methylation (in particular, CDH1, runx3, MGMT, DAPK, CDKN2A, MLH1) and histone modifications were found to be restricted to cancer lesions and demonstrated to play an important role in GC pathogenesis [37]. Among these genes, MLH1 and CDKN2A presented a lower methylation frequency in intestinal metaplasia than in carcinoma suggesting a potential pathogenic role of progressively increasing levels of methylation in these genes. Methylation influences gene expression by affecting the interactions with DNA, proteins, and transcription factors. Promoter hypermethylation of the mismatch repair gene MLH1 is considered the main mechanism responsible for microsatellite instability in GC. Precancerous lesions are also characterized by a high frequency of hypermethylation of the CDKN2A gene, encoding for the cyclin-dependent kinase inhibitor p16, which slows down the cell cycle by prohibiting progression from G1 to S phase (Fig. 2.4) [38].

Hypermethylation of promoter CpG islands, which correlated with silencing of the downstream genes, reflects microsatellite unstable GC subtypes in *H. pylori*-positive [39] and EBV-positive GC subtypes [40].

More recently, an association between EBV-positive GC with aberrant histone modifications and related DNA methylation alterations has also been reported [40]. Histones are highly alkaline proteins with a high content in amino acids with basic side chains (particularly lysine and arginine). Their tasks are packaging and ordering of DNA into structural units called nucleosomes (Fig. 2.5). Nucleosomes represent the main protein components of chromatin, which is used to pack the large eukaryotic genomes into the nucleus, ensuring the appropriate access to DNA and correct gene expression. Posttranslational modifications of histones include acetylation/deacetylation, and methylation may thus interfere with gene expression.

Precancerous lesions often carry cyclin-E and cyclin-dependent kinase dysregulations (i.e., p15, p16, p21, p27) (Fig. 2.4) and alteration of the RAS-MAPK pathway and HER2 gene amplification (Fig. 2.6).

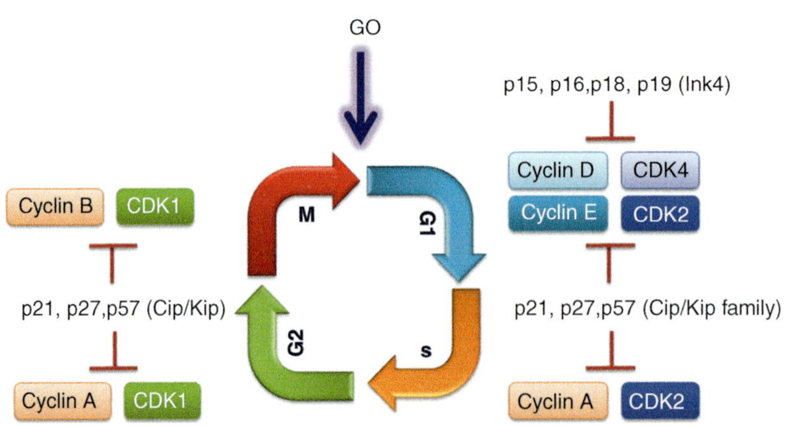

Fig. 2.4 Cell cycle progression. Orderly progression through the cell cycle involves passage through sequential checkpoints (i.e., G1, S, G2, M). Cyclin D1 binds to cdk4 and the assembly factor, p27, to create an active ternary complex. This complex can be inactivated by association with Ink4 or loss of cyclin D1 via proteasomal degradation. Through phosphorylation of intermediates, the complex induces genes involved in enhancing S-phase entry. The differential expression of cyclins and Cdks is highly coordinated and regulated through cell cycle progression

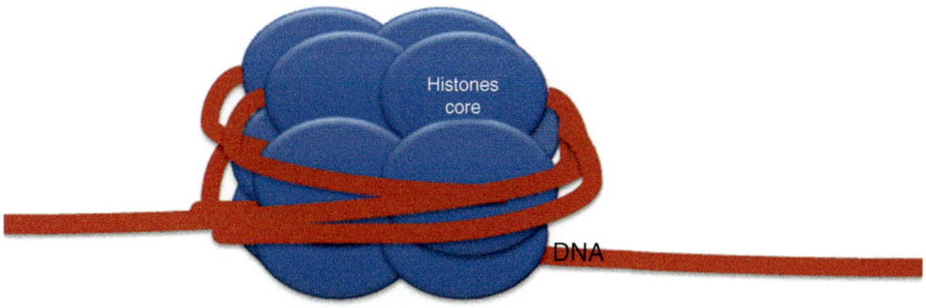

Fig. 2.5 Nucleosome is the basic unit of DNA packaging. It consists of a segment of DNA wound around a core of eight histone proteins. Histone modifications have a direct effect on nucleosome architecture. Posttranslational modifications of histones regulate DNA-templated processes, including replication, transcription, and repair. Acetylation, methylation, phosphorylation, and citrullination of the histone core may influence chromatin structure by affecting histone-histone and histone-DNA interactions

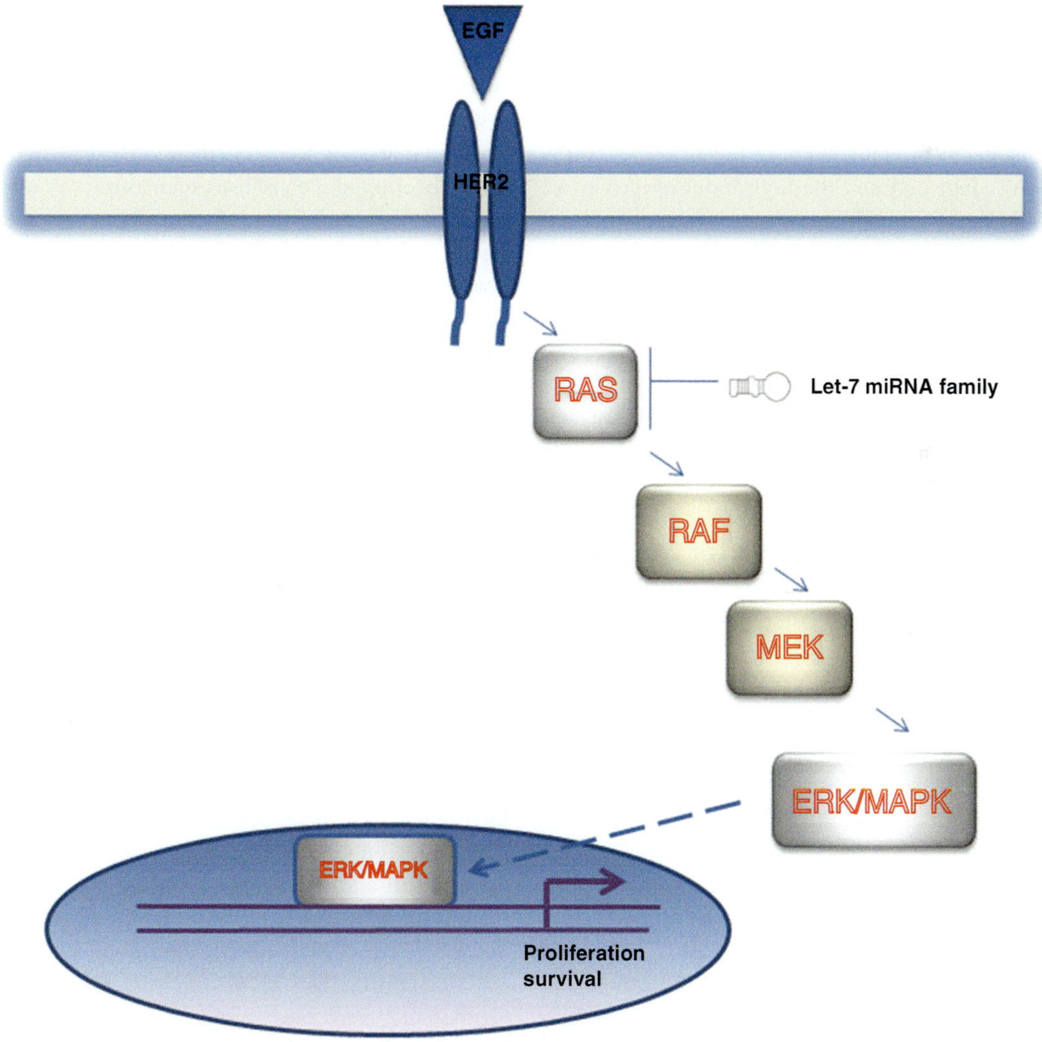

Fig. 2.6 RAS/RAF/MAPK pathway. Binding of a growth factor (e.g., EGF) to the tyrosine kinase HER2 activates the receptor activity. HER2 is activated either as a homo- or heterodimer and results in regulation of multiple pathways and in particular the RAS/RAF/MAPK pathway by downstream phosphorylation and activation of (H/N/K)-RAS, (A,B,C)-RAF, MEK1/2 (MAP 2K1), and ERK1/2 (MAPK1). Ultimately, ERK activation activates gene transcription that regulates cell proliferation and survival

Table 2.4 The most common molecular alterations found in precancerous lesions

Hypermethylation	MLH1 CDKN2A(p16)
Acetylation/deacetylation/methylation	Histone modifications
Gene dysregulations	Cyclin-E and cyclin-dependent kinases (i.e., P15, p16, p21, p27) RAS-MAPK pathway HER2 gene amplification
miRNA dysregulations	Let-7 family
Protein dysregulations	Tyrosine kinase (RAS)/HMGA2

An aberrant downregulation of microRNA expression, particular of the let-7 family members, has been observed in both gastritis and GC, especially during *H. pylori* infection [41, 42]. Importantly, their expression can be restored after *H. pylori* eradication [43]. Let-7 miRNA family is downregulated in various solid tumors and shows a key role in recognition of target oncogenic proteins such as the tyrosine kinase RAS (Fig. 2.4) and the high mobility group A2 (HMGA2), a non-histonic protein with structural DNA-binding domains acting as a transcriptional regulating factor.

Table 2.4 summarizes the most common molecular alterations often associated with premalignant lesions of the stomach and that become much more frequent in GC lesions, thus suggesting an association with malignant transformation.

Molecular Classification for GC

The first and most comprehensive molecular characterization for GC was proposed by the Cancer Genome Atlas (TCGA) project in 2014 [44]. Authors proposed a classification based on four subtypes: microsatellite instability-high (MSI-high), Epstein-Barr virus (EBV)-associated, chromosomal instability (CIN), and genomically stable (GS). The main distinctive characteristics of these subtypes are reported in Table 2.5.

The following year (2015), the Asian Cancer Research Group (ACRG work) provided a further molecular classification for GC, which also identified four subtypes with an increasing worse prognosis: microsatellite instability-high (MSI-high), microsatellite stable/TP53-positive (MSS/TP53-positive), MSS/TP53-negative, and MSS/epithelial-mesenchymal transition (MSS/EMT) [46]. ACRG introduced a role for P53, a key suppressor gene that responds to DNA damage and promotes apoptotic processes. Somatic P53 alterations have been reported in approximately 50% of overall human cancers [47]. The principal characteristics for ACRG subtypes are reported in Table 2.5.

ATCG and ACRG classifications showed a partial overlapping consensus such as microsatellite instability and EBV infection. However the ACRG is different for the demographic population and histologic subtype distribution, introduces the P53 mutations, and considers different baseline molecular mechanisms and prognostic factors [48]. Moreover, while microsatellite instability subtype showed a better prognosis in both these classifications, there were no prognostic differences in CIN and GS subtypes when TCGA classification was applied to the ACRG patient population. In addition, none of the two classifications takes into account the tumor microenvironment, the infiltrating immune cells, nor the role of tumor stage. Of note, both these molecular classifications failed to show significant survival differences in terms of OS or PFS when compared to simply staging tumor-nodes-metastases system (TNM – Union for International Cancer Control/American Joint Committee on Cancer) classification [49]. Thus, there is still an open debate about the reliability of current molecular classifications for GC prognosis. The use of more precise stratification criteria by combining TNM classification with histological and new molecular tools could achieve a more reliable classification impacting on therapeutic management of the patients in the near future.

Table 2.5 Molecular classification for GC

Classification	Subtypes			
ATCG	MSI (21.7%)	EBV (8.8%)	CIN (49.8%)	GS (19.7%)
	Prevalence female (56%) Older age at diagnosis (median age 72 years) Hypermutation (CpG island) MLH1 silencing Mitotic pathways	Prevalence in males (81%)[a] Fundus and body location (62%)[a] PIK3CA (80%), ARID1A (55%), BCOR (23%) mutations PD-L1/PD-L2 overexpression Hypermethylation CDKN2A (p16) silencing Immune cell signaling (Kak2, PD-1, PD-L) ARID1A and BCOR mutations	Intestinal GC Frequent gastroesophageal location (65%) TP53 mutation (71%) Receptor tyrosine kinase (RTK)/Ras amplification/activation (EGFR, HER2, HER3, VEGF-A, FGFR2, POCDILG2, PIK3CA, c-met) Amplification of cyclin genes (CCNE1, CCND1, CDK6). Constant activation of EGFR by phosphorylation/amplification	Invasiveness, diffuse histotype (73%) Younger age (median age 59 years) CDH1 (E-cad) (37%)/RHOA (15%) mutations CLDN18-ARHGAP fusion mutually exclusive with RHOA mutations Integrin and syndecan-1 pathway/angiogenesis
ACRG	MSI-high (22.7%)	MSS/TP53-positive (26.3%)	MSS/TP53-negative (35.7%)	MSS/EMT (15.3%)
	Intestinal histotype (60%) Antrum Location (75%) Hypermutation KRAS (23%), PI3K-PTEN-mTOR pathway (42%), ARID1A (44.2%), and ALK (16.3%) alterations	EBV Intact P53	Loss of functional P53 activity	Younger age Diffuse
	Best prognosis →		Worst prognosis	

Cin chromosomal instability, *EBV* Epstein-Barr virus, *EMT* epithelial-mesenchymal transition, *GS* genomically stable, *MSI* microsatellite instability
[a]*MSS* microsatellite stable, *PD-L* programmed death ligand; brown color indicates an overlapping between the ATCG and ACRG subtypes [45]

At present, the possible advantage deriving from the use of a molecular classification is starting to become evident in both research and clinical settings. Encouraging positive results obtained with the use of immune therapies in MSI and EBV-positive GC subtypes and with two targeted agents, ramucirumab targeting VEGF [50, 51] and trastuzumab targeting HER2 receptor [52], are some important examples.

It is now well accepted that the presence of immune-active cellular components in the tumor microenvironment may contribute to a better prognosis in various tumors also including GC [53]. Tumors with high mutation burden or carrying mismatch repair deficiencies showed better and durable response rates after treatment with agents that control immune response [54, 55]. Inhibitors of cytotoxic T lymphocyte-associated antigen 4 (CTLA-4), programmed cell death protein 1 (PD-1) receptor (pembrolizumab), or PD-L1 (avelumab), which restore T-cell activation, are now being used in several clinical trials [50]. Other agents targeting immune pathways are in clinical development (e.g., [56]). Notably, the load of tumor mutational burden was proposed as potentially suitable marker to predict the response to the anti-PD-1 treatment than expression of PD-L1 by immunohistochemistry [57, 58].

Available evidence indicates that EBV-positive GC, mainly associated with a MSI genotype, also showed encouraging response rates when treated with immune-based therapies [59]. EBV is a ubiquitous γ-herpesvirus distributed in the world's population with a high capacity in establishing immunoevasive latent infection (95%). EBV is also associated with mononucleosis and the development of both lymphoid and epithelial malignancies, particularly in immunodeficiency [60, 61] each characterized by a distinct pattern of viral protein expression [62–65]. Indeed during primary infection, EBV infects cells in a lytic form, and then the EBV genome is circularized, condensed, and methylated by host proteins to enter into a latent state in which only a small percentage of viral genes are expressed [66–70]. Several studies demonstrated that tumor cells of EBV-associated malignancies carry EBV as a latent infection [71–73]. It was then discovered that the switch of latent virus to lytic phase, leading to the expression of immediate-early, early, and then late protein through specific signaling cascade [74, 75], rendered the tumor cells more susceptible to the cytotoxic antiviral drugs and oncotherapies against EBV-associated malignancies such as GC [76–81]. In alternative, the discovery of lytic antigen (e.g., BARF1 antigen) abnormally expressed in EBV latent phase in some pathological situations including EBV-related nasopharyngeal carcinoma and GC could be also potentially appropriate targets for immune therapeutic treatment [82]. To identify GC subtypes that more likely respond to immunotherapy, a subclassification of GC has been recently proposed on the basis of PD-L1 expression, EBV status, MSI, and tumor-infiltrating lymphocytes (TILs) [83] or immune-related gene expression signatures, including interferon-gamma (6 genes) and expanded-immune (18 genes) signatures [84]. These findings are yet to be confirmed in prospective clinical trials.

The VEGF family consists of five ligands (VEGF-A, VEGF-B, VEGF-C, VEGF-D, and placental growth factor, PIGF) and three receptor tyrosine kinases (VEGF-R1,VEGF-R2, and VEGF-R3). VEGF is a signal protein that stimulates the formation of blood vessels (neoangiogenesis from pre-existing vasculature; vasculogenesis, for de novo formation), vasodilatation, and increased vascular permeability, overall mostly induced in hypoxic condition (release of HIF factor). All members of the VEGF family stimulate cellular responses by binding to tyrosine kinase receptors, such as the HER2 receptor (Fig. 2.7), and promoting their dimerization and the subsequent activation. Bevacizumab is the first anti-VEGF drug approved in 2004, while ramucirumab (AIFA 2014) is directed against the VEGF-R first FDA-approved therapy for advanced or metastatic GC after chemotherapy. Not all patients benefit from anti-VEGF treatment. Plasma VEGF-A and neuropilin-1 are emerging as potential predictive biomarkers for bevacizumab in GC, while biomarkers in patients treated with ramucirumab have yet to be identified.

HER2 is an oncogene encoded by the ERBB2 gene on chromosome 17. It belongs to the EGF receptor family and is overexpressed in 7–34% of GC. HER2 has no ligand-binding domain of its own, but it does bind closely to other ligand-bound EGF receptor family members to form a heterodimer, stabilizing ligand binding and enhancing kinase-mediated activation of downstream signaling pathways, such as those involving mitogen-activated protein kinase and phosphatidylinositol-3 kinase (PIK3CA) [85] (Fig. 2.6). Alterations of HER2 structure, dysregulation of HER2 downstream signal effectors, and interaction of HER2 with other membrane receptors may interfere with the response to treatment [86]. E-cad/β-catenin (Fig. 2.3), RAS/MAPK (Fig. 2.6), and PI3K-Akt (Fig. 2.7) pathways are the main downstream signaling pathways of HER2. PIK3CA mutations and phosphate and tensin homolog (PTEN) inactivation were found to induce a hyper-activation of the PI3K-Akt pathway without the necessity of an upstream signal deriving from HER2 activation. It has now become clear that HER2 is expressed in many normal tissues, including the breast, gastrointestinal tract, kidney, and heart. Its major role in these tissues is to promote cell proliferation and suppress apoptosis, which may facilitate excessive/uncontrolled cell growth and tumorigenesis if aberrantly activated. Overexpression/amplification of HER2/*ERBB2* in breast cancer is associated with poor prognosis, increased risk of local recurrence, and distant metastasis. Conversely, the potential prognostic relevance of HER2 in the setting of GC is still inconsistent. Treatment leading to the selective inhibition of the HER2 protein has led to a modest survival benefit in GC; indeed, likewise HER2-positive breast cancer, patients are primary refractory or acquire resistance to trastuzumab therapy. Novel HER2-directed therapies including pan-HER TKIs, MET and mTOR inhibitors, and dual HER2-blockade are under investigations [87]. Specific targeted agents toward other genes/pathways with a key role in GC emerging from the ATCG and ACRG classifications (Table 2.5) are currently under investigation [48]. A list of the most promising targetable genetic lesions and signaling pathways is reported in Table 2.6.

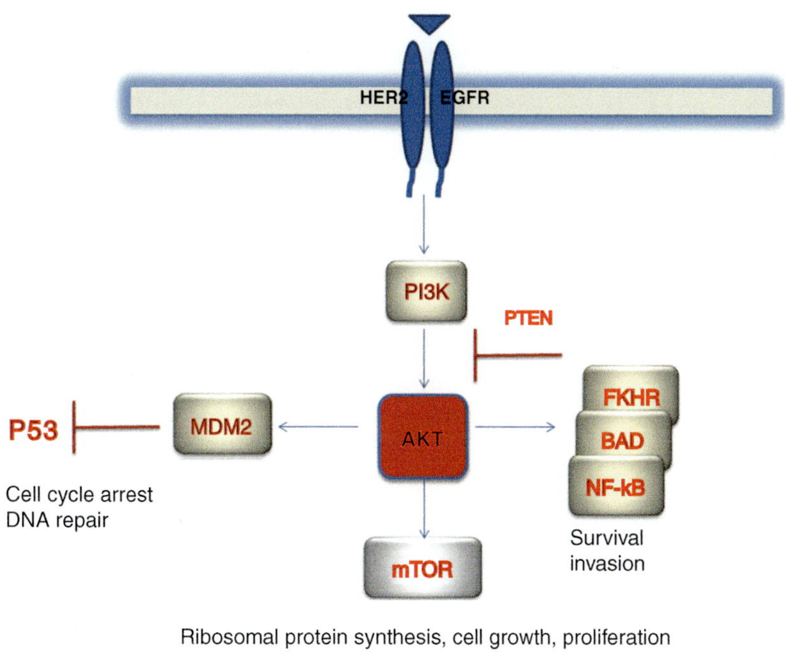

Fig. 2.7 Schematic representation of the PI3K/Akt pathway. HER2 activation leads to the activation of phosphatidylinositol-3 kinase (PI3K), which initiates activation of Akt by phosphorylation. Akt acts as a major source of activation to further downstream signaling genes involved in various cellular processes such as ribosomal protein synthesis and cell proliferation (through activation of mTOR), survival and invasion (through inhibition of BAD, FKHR and activation of NF-kB), metabolism (activation of GSK3β), cell cycle arrest, and DNA repair mediated by p53 (through MDM2)

Table 2.6 Emerging molecular markers and its targeted drug development

Gene	Activity	Positivity	Molecular alteration	Therapeutic agent
HER2	Member of the EGFR family, TYR kinase receptor	GC (7–34%) Intestinal (34%) Diffuse (6%) GJ (30%)	Amplification overexpression	Trastuzumab; other inhibitors had been tested: lapatinib, pertuzumab, trastuzumab emtansine; however benefit is modest. Resistance is under investigation
EGFR	TYR kinase receptor, most frequently form heterodimers with HER2	GC (24–27%) Intestinal (32.7%) Co-amplification (EGFR/HER2: 3.6%)	Amplification overexpression	Cetuximab; panitumumab. Disappointing results, but a possible lack of a proper selection of patients
P53	Cell cycle control, DNA repair, and apoptosis	GC (75%) Intestinal (50%) found also in adenoma and metaplasia	Mutation LOH	APR-246 and COTI-2 have progressed to clinical trials in some tumors
KRAS	RAS GTPase, recruits the cytosolic protein RAF	GC (5%) Intestinal (>50%) Associated with MSI	Mutation codon 12–13	No target therapies are currently approved. Other drugs, such as MEK (selumetinib), PI3K, or BCL-XL inhibitors, were tested in KRAS-mutated cancer cell lines with promising results
BRAF	Serine/threonine kinase	GC (2%)	Mutation, mostly V599M	Vemurafenib and dabrafenib have been approved for treatment of melanoma
FGFR2	Member of the fibroblast growth factor receptor family	GC (9%) Diffuse type (>50%)	Amplification	Several drugs and studies targeting this mutation are ongoing: AZD4547, dovitinib
MET	TYR kinase receptor, interacts with HGF (hepatocyte growth factor)	GC (8%) Diffuse (39%) Intestinal (19%)	Amplification Overexpression related to tumor stage and clinical outcome	Onartuzumab and an anti-HGF (rilotumumab) are studies discontinued (preliminary results were negative). By converse a positive tumor response to AMG337 was reported, but the study was interrupted for excess of agent toxicity. Study on LY2875358 is ongoing in other tumors
VEGF	Factor of angiogenesis	GC (50%)	Expression, prognostic for survival	Bevacizumab showed an improvement in progression-free survival and tumor response, but no overall survival benefit Ramucirumab and apatinib showed a significant improvement in the overall survival in subsequent line of treatments; their role in first-line therapy is still unclear
ATM	Serine/threonine kinase recruited and activated by DNA double-strand breaks	GC (13–22%)	Down expression Microsatellite mutation	Poli ADP-ribose polymerase inhibitor (olaparib)
Neo-antigens	MSI and MMR deficiency amplify the number of tumor neo-antigens	GC (30%)	Mismatch repair deficiency	Immunotherapies: pembrolizumab (PD-1); nivolumab plus/without ipilimumab preventive vaccine (against recurrent neo-antigens) is under study

Table 2.6 (continued)

CDH1	Tumor suppressor gene	GC (37% of GS subtype)	Mutations, hypermethylation downregulated expression	Treatments targeting epithelial-mesenchymal transition (EMT) are under study: emodin; an antimalarial agent ARS4, a steroidal alkaloid cyclopamine/IPI-269609; a well-tolerated treatment for type 2 diabetes mellitus, metformin A clinical trial in hormone metastatic prostate cancer targeting E-cadherin is ongoing (NCT02913859)
ARID1A	Tumor suppressor gene involved in chromatin remodeling	GC (8%) GC (20% GS subtype) may synergize with PIK3CA activation and mutually exclusive to TP53 mutation	Inactivating mutations	Under study: EZH2, residual SWI/SNF activity, PI3K/AKT pathway, tumor immunological microenvironment, and stabilizing wild-type p53
RHOA	Ras-related family. It regulates cytoskeletal organization, cell adhesion, intracellular membrane trafficking, gene transcription, apoptosis, and cell cycle progression. Activates Stat3	GC (30% GS) Diffuse type	CLDN18-ARHGAP26 fusion gene or mutations	IMAB362 antibody against CLDN18-positive cancer. Fasudil, in other tumors
AURKA	Aurora family gene controlling mitotic events Serine/threonine kinase, located on centrosome	GC (5%)	Amplification, mutations	Alisertib
PLK1	Polo like kinase involved in the regulation of mitosis	GC (95%)	Overexpression	Volasertib
CLDN18	Member of claudins, components of the tight junction	GC (48%) Intestinal (>50%)	Downregulated Fusion gene with ARHGAP26, a gene encoding a RHOA inhibitor Mutually exclusive with RHOA mutations	Claudiximab (IMAB362)
MEK	Fibroblast growth factor receptor	GC (4%)	Amplification	Trametinib for treatment of melanoma BRAF+ GSK1120212 and PD0325901 in vitro
EBV	Epstein-Barr virus	GC (8.7%) Diffuse (50%)	Presence of the virus in the tumor cells	Immunotherapies PD1/PD-L1, JAK2 (pembrolizumab, nivolumab, MPDL3280A, MEDI 4736, AZD1480)

Abbreviation: *GJ* gastroesophageal junction, *MSI* microsatellite instability, *GS* genome stable ATCG subtype
Other drugs targeting PI3K/Akt pathway (4–24% of all GC, AZD5363, MK-226, BYL719) target of mTOR pathway (everolimus), ERB3 (15%, pertuzumab, trastuzumab)

References

1. Torre LA, Bray F, Siegel RL. Global cancer statistics. CA Cancer J Clin. 2015;65:87–108.
2. Lauren P. The two histological main types of gastric carcinoma: diffuse and so-called intestinal-type carcinoma. An attempt at a histo-clinical classification. Acta Pathol Microbiol Scand. 1965;64:31–49.
3. Aaltonen LA, Hamilton SR. World Health Organization. Lyon: IARC Press/Oxford University Press; 2000; Hamilton SR, Aaltonen LA, editors. Pathology and genetics of tumours of the digestive system.
4. Corso S, Giordano S. How can gastric cancer molecular profiling guide future therapies? Trends Mol Med. 2016;22(7):534–44.
5. Jemal A, Siegel R, Xu J, et al. Cancer statistics. CA Cancer J Clin. 2010;60:277–300.
6. He YT, Hou J, Chen ZF. Trends in incidence of esophageal and gastric cardia cancer in high risk areas in China. Eur J Cancer Prev. 2008;17:71–6.
7. Devesa SS, Blot WJ, Fraumeni JF Jr. Changing patterns in the incidence of esophageal and gastric carcinoma in the United States. Cancer. 1998;83:2049–53.
8. Maeda H, Okabayashi T, Nishimori I. Clinicopathologic features of adenocarcinoma at the gastric cardia: is it different from distal cancer of the stomach. J Am Coll Surg. 2008;206:306–10.
9. Bosman FT, Carneiro F, Hruban RH, et al. World Health Organization classification of tumours of the digestive system. Lyon: IARC Press, International Agency for Research on Cancer. 2010;
10. Marshall BJ, Windsor HM. The relation of Helicobacter pylori to gastric adenocarcinoma and lymphoma: pathophysiology, epidemiology, screening, clinical presentation, treatment, and prevention. Med Clin North Am. 2005;89(2):313–44.
11. La Vecchia C, Negri E, Franceschi S, Gentile A. Family history and the risk of stomach and colorectal cancer. Cancer. 1992;70:50–5.
12. Garziera M, Canzonieri V, Cannizzaro R, et al. Identification and characterization of CDH1 germline variants in sporadic gastric cancer patients and in individuals at risk of gastric cancer. PLoS One. 2013;8:e77035.
13. Pinheiro H, Oliveira C, Seruca R, Carneiro F. Hereditary diffuse gastric cancer – pathophysiology and clinical management. Best Pract Res Clin Gastroenterol. 2014;28:1055–68.
14. van Roy F. Beyond E-cadherin: roles of other cadherin superfamily members in cancer. Nat Rev Cancer. 2014;14:121–34.
15. Repetto O, De Paoli P, De Re V, Canzonieri V, Cannizzaro R. Levels of soluble E-cadherin in breast, gastric, and colorectal cancers. Biomed Res Int. 2014;2014:408047.
16. Paredes J, Figueiredo J, Albergaria A, et al. Epithelial E- and P-cadherins: role and clinical significance in cancer. Biochim Biophys Acta. 1826;2012:297–311.
17. Guilford P, Hopkins J, Harraway J. E-cadherin germline mutations in familial gastric cancer. Nature. 1998;392:402–5.
18. Fitzgerald RC, Hardwick R, Huntsman D, et al. Hereditary diffuse gastric cancer: updated consensus guidelines for clinical management and directions for future research. J Med Genet. 2010;47:436–44.
19. Caggiari L, Miolo G, Canzonieri V, et al. A new mutation of the CDH1 gene in a patient with an aggressive signet-ring cell carcinoma of the stomach. Cancer Biol Ther. 2017;13:1–6.
20. Pinheiro H, Bordeira-Carrico R, Seixas S. Allele-specific CDH1 downregulation and hereditary diffuse gastric cancer. Hum Mol Genet. 2010;19:943–52.
21. Majewski IJ, Kluijt I, Cats A. An alpha-E-catenin (CTNNA1) mutation in hereditary diffuse gastric cancer. J Pathol. 2013;229:621–9.
22. Gaston D, Hansford S, Oliveira C, et al. Germline mutations in MAP 3K6 are associated with familial gastric cancer. PLoS Genet. 2014;10:e1004669.
23. Donner I, Kiviluoto T, Ristimaki A, Aaltonen LA, Vahteristo P. Exome sequencing reveals three novel candidate predisposition genes for diffuse gastric cancer. Fam Cancer. 2015;14:241–6.
24. Hinck L, Nathke IS, Papkoff J, Nelson WJ. Dynamics of cadherin/catenin complex formation: novel protein interactions and pathways of complex assembly. J Cell Biol. 1994;125:1327–40.
25. de-Freitas-Junior JC, Carvalho S, Dias AM, et al. Insulin/IGF-I signaling pathways enhances tumor cell invasion through bisecting GlcNAc N-glycans modulation. an interplay with E-cadherin. PLoS One. 2013;8:e81579.
26. Li J, Woods SL, Healey S, et al. Point mutations in Exon 1B of APC reveal gastric adenocarcinoma and proximal polyposis of the stomach as a familial adenomatous polyposis variant. Am J Hum Genet. 2016;98:830–42.
27. Aarnio M, Salovaara R, Aaltonen LA, Mecklin JP, Jarvinen HJ. Features of gastric cancer in hereditary non-polyposis colorectal cancer syndrome. Int J Cancer. 1997;74:551–5.
28. Varley JM, McGown G, Thorncroft M, et al. An extended Li-Fraumeni kindred with gastric carcinoma and a codon 175 mutation in TP53. J Med Genet. 1995;32:942–5.
29. Friedenson B. BRCA1 and BRCA2 pathways and the risk of cancers other than breast or ovarian. Med Gen Med. 2005;7:60.
30. Utsunomiya J, Gocho H, Miyanaga T, Hamaguchi E, Kashimure A. Peutz-Jeghers syndrome: its natural course and management. Johns Hopkins Med J. 1975;136:71–82.
31. Lynch HT, Grady W, Suriano G, Huntsman D. Gastric cancer: new genetic developments. J Surg Oncol. 2005;90:114–33.
32. D'Errico M, de Rinaldis E, Blasi MF, et al. Genome-wide expression profile of sporadic gastric cancers with microsatellite instability. Eur J Cancer. 2009;45:461–9.

33. Hong Y, Shi J, Ge Z, Wu H. Associations between mutations of the cell cycle checkpoint kinase 2 gene and gastric carcinogenesis. Mol Med Rep. 2017;16:4287–92.
34. Hemminki A, Markie D, Tomlinson I, et al. A serine/threonine kinase gene defective in Peutz-Jeghers syndrome. Nature. 1998;391:184–7.
35. Howe JR, Roth S, Ringold JC, et al. Mutations in the SMAD4/DPC4 gene in juvenile polyposis. Science. 1998;280:1086–8.
36. Rugge M, Genta RM, Di MF, et al. Gastric cancer as preventable disease. Clin Gastroenterol Hepatol. 2017;15:1833–43.
37. Padmanabhan N, Ushijima T, Tan P. How to stomach an epigenetic insult: the gastric cancer epigenome. Nat Rev Gastroenterol Hepatol. 2017;14:467–78.
38. He D, Zhang YW, Zhang NN, et al. Aberrant gene promoter methylation of p16, FHIT, CRBP1, WWOX, and DLC-1 in Epstein-Barr virus-associated gastric carcinomas. Med Oncol. 2015;32:92.
39. Maekita T, Nakazawa K, Mihara M, et al. High levels of aberrant DNA methylation in Helicobacter pylori-infected gastric mucosae and its possible association with gastric cancer risk. Clin Cancer Res. 2006;12:989–95.
40. Funata S, Matsusaka K, Yamanaka R, et al. Histone modification alteration coordinated with acquisition of promoter DNA methylation during Epstein-Barr virus infection. Oncotarget. 2017;8:55265–79.
41. Zabaleta J. MicroRNA: a bridge from H. pylori infection to gastritis and gastric cancer development. Front Genet. 2012;3:294.
42. Hayashi Y, Tsujii M, Wang J, et al. CagA mediates epigenetic regulation to attenuate let-7 expression in Helicobacter pylori-related carcinogenesis. Gut. 2013;62:1536–46.
43. Fassan M, Saraggi D, Balsamo L, et al. Let-7c downregulation in Helicobacter pylori-related gastric carcinogenesis. Oncotarget. 2016;7:4915–24.
44. Comprehensive molecular characterization of gastric adenocarcinoma. Nature. 2014;513:202–9.
45. Murphy G, Pfeiffer R, Camargo MC, Rabkin CS. Meta-analysis shows that prevalence of Epstein-Barr virus-positive gastric cancer differs based on sex and anatomic location. Gastroenterology. 2009;137:824–33.
46. Wong SS, Kim KM, Ting JC, et al. Genomic landscape and genetic heterogeneity in gastric adenocarcinoma revealed by whole-genome sequencing. Nat Commun. 2014;5:5477.
47. Silva TC, Leal MF, Calcagno DQ, et al. hTERT, MYC and TP53 deregulation in gastric preneoplastic lesions. BMC Gastroenterol. 2012;12:85.
48. Garattini SK, Basile D, Cattaneo M, et al. Molecular classifications of gastric cancers: novel insights and possible future applications. World J Gastrointest Oncol. 2017;9:194–208.
49. Edge SB, Compton CC. The American Joint Committee on Cancer: the 7th edition of the AJCC cancer staging manual and the future of TNM. Ann Surg Oncol. 2010;17:1471–4.
50. Fuchs CS, Tomasek J, Yong CJ, et al. Ramucirumab monotherapy for previously treated advanced gastric or gastro-oesophageal junction adenocarcinoma (REGARD): an international, randomised, multicentre, placebo-controlled, phase 3 trial. Lancet. 2014;383:31–9.
51. Shitara K, Muro K, Shimada Y, et al. Subgroup analyses of the safety and efficacy of ramucirumab in Japanese and Western patients in RAINBOW: a randomized clinical trial in second-line treatment of gastric cancer. Gastric Cancer. 2016;19:927–38.
52. Bang YJ, Van CE, Feyereislova A, et al. Trastuzumab in combination with chemotherapy versus chemotherapy alone for treatment of HER2-positive advanced gastric or gastro-oesophageal junction cancer (ToGA): a phase 3, open-label, randomised controlled trial. Lancet. 2010;376:687–97.
53. Yousefi H, Yuan J, Keshavarz-Fathi M, Murphy JF, Rezaei N. Immunotherapy of cancers comes of age. Expert Rev Clin Immunol. 2017;13:1001–15.
54. Le DT, Durham JN, Smith KN, et al. Mismatch repair deficiency predicts response of solid tumors to PD-1 blockade. Science. 2017;357:409–13.
55. Le DT, Uram JN, Wang H, et al. PD-1 blockade in tumors with mismatch-repair deficiency. N Engl J Med. 2015;372:2509–20.
56. Uyttenhove C, Pilotte L, Theate I, et al. Evidence for a tumoral immune resistance mechanism based on tryptophan degradation by indoleamine 2,3-dioxygenase. Nat Med. 2003;9:1269–74.
57. Rosenberg JE, Hoffman-Censits J, Powles T, et al. Atezolizumab in patients with locally advanced and metastatic urothelial carcinoma who have progressed following treatment with platinum-based chemotherapy: a single-arm, multicentre, phase 2 trial. Lancet. 2016;387:1909–20.
58. Chalmers ZR, Connelly CF, Fabrizio D, et al. Analysis of 100,000 human cancer genomes reveals the landscape of tumor mutational burden. Genome Med. 2017;9(1):34.
59. Panda A, Mehnert JM, Hirshfield KM, et al. Immune activation and benefit from avelumab in EBV-positive gastric cancer. J Natl Cancer Inst. 2018;110(3):316–20.
60. Dolcetti R, Gloghini A, De VS, et al. Characteristics of EBV-infected cells in HIV-related lymphadenopathy: implications for the pathogenesis of EBV-associated and EBV-unrelated lymphomas of HIV-seropositive individuals. Int J Cancer. 1995;63:652–9.
61. De Re V, Boiocchi M, De VS, et al. Subtypes of Epstein-Barr virus in HIV-1-associated and HIV-1-unrelated Hodgkin's disease cases. Int J Cancer. 1993;54:895–8.
62. Young LS, Rickinson AB. Epstein-Barr virus: 40 years on. Nat Rev Cancer. 2004;4:757–68.
63. Ali AS, Al-Shraim M, Al-Hakami AM, Jones IM. Epstein-Barr virus: clinical and epidemiological

revisits and genetic basis of oncogenesis. Open Virol J. 2015;9:7–28.
64. Dolcetti R, Zancai P, De Re V, et al. Epstein-Barr virus strains with latent membrane protein-1 deletions: prevalence in the Italian population and high association with human immunodeficiency virus-related Hodgkin's disease. Blood. 1997;89:1723–31.
65. Dolcetti R, Quaia M, Gloghini A, et al. Biologically relevant phenotypic changes and enhanced growth properties induced in B lymphocytes by an EBV strain derived from a histologically aggressive Hodgkin's disease. Int J Cancer. 1999;80:240–9.
66. Cohen JI, Bollard CM, Khanna R, Pittaluga S. Current understanding of the role of Epstein-Barr virus in lymphomagenesis and therapeutic approaches to EBV-associated lymphomas. Leuk Lymphoma. 2008;49:27–34.
67. Boiocchi M, De Re V, Gloghini A, et al. High incidence of monoclonal EBV episomes in Hodgkin's disease and anaplastic large-cell KI-1-positive lymphomas in HIV-1-positive patients. Int J Cancer. 1993;54:53–9.
68. Hammerschmidt W. The epigenetic life cycle of Epstein-Barr virus. Curr Top Microbiol Immunol. 2015;390:103–17.
69. Tempera I, Lieberman PM. Epigenetic regulation of EBV persistence and oncogenesis. Semin Cancer Biol. 2014;26:22–9.
70. Lieberman PM. Chromatin structure of Epstein-Barr virus latent episomes. Curr Top Microbiol Immunol. 2015;390:71–102.
71. Boiocchi M, Carbone A, De Re V, Dolcetti R. Is the Epstein-Barr virus involved in Hodgkin's disease? Tumori. 1989;75:345–50.
72. Grywalska E, Rolinski J. Epstein-Barr virus-associated lymphomas. Semin Oncol. 2015;42:291–303.
73. He C, Huang X, Su X, et al. The association between circulating tumor cells and Epstein-Barr virus activation in patients with nasopharyngeal carcinoma. Cancer Biol Ther. 2017;18:888–94.
74. Ersing I, Nobre L, Wang LW, et al. A temporal proteomic map of Epstein-Barr virus lytic replication in B cells. Cell Rep. 2017;19:1479–93.
75. Chiu YF, Sugden B. Epstein-Barr virus: the path from latent to productive infection. Annu Rev Virol. 2016;3:359–72.
76. Ghosh SK, Perrine SP, Faller DV. Advances in virus-directed therapeutics against Epstein-Barr virus-associated malignancies. Adv Virol. 2012;2012:509296.
77. Hui KF, Cheung AK, Choi CK, et al. Inhibition of class I histone deacetylases by romidepsin potently induces Epstein-Barr virus lytic cycle and mediates enhanced cell death with ganciclovir. Int J Cancer. 2016;138:125–36.
78. Wildeman MA, Novalic Z, Verkuijlen SA, et al. Cytolytic virus activation therapy for Epstein-Barr virus-driven tumors. Clin Cancer Res. 2012;18:5061–70.
79. Wang M, Wu W, Zhang Y, Yao G, Gu B. Rapamycin enhances lytic replication of Epstein-Barr virus in gastric carcinoma cells by increasing the transcriptional activities of immediate-early lytic promoters. Virus Res. 2017;244:173–80. https://doi.org/10.1016/j.virusres.2017.11.021.
80. Murata T. Regulation of Epstein-Barr virus reactivation from latency. Microbiol Immunol. 2014;58:307–17.
81. Wu CC, Fang CY, Hsu HY, et al. EBV reactivation as a target of luteolin to repress NPC tumorigenesis. Oncotarget. 2016;7:18999–9017.
82. Turrini R, Merlo A, Martorelli D, et al. A BARF1-specific mAb as a new immunotherapeutic tool for the management of EBV-related tumors. Oncoimmunology. 2017;6:e1304338.
83. Park C, Cho J, Lee J, et al. Host immune response index in gastric cancer identified by comprehensive analyses of tumor immunity. Oncoimmunology. 2017;6:e1356150.
84. Ayers M, Lunceford J, Nebozhyn M, et al. IFN-gamma-related mRNA profile predicts clinical response to PD-1 blockade. J Clin Invest. 2017;127:2930–40.
85. Boku N. HER2-positive gastric cancer. Gastric Cancer. 2014;17:1–12.
86. Sukawa Y, Yamamoto H, Nosho K, et al. HER2 expression and PI3K-Akt pathway alterations in gastric cancer. Digestion. 2014;89:12–7.
87. Kelly CM, Janjigian YY. The genomics and therapeutics of HER2-positive gastric cancer-from trastuzumab and beyond. J Gastrointest Oncol. 2016;7:750–62.

Part II

Clinical and Pathological Characteristics

3 Diagnosis and Surveillance: Endoscopic Hallmarks

Renato Cannizzaro, Raffaella Magris, Stefania Maiero, Paola Spessotto, Valli De Re, and Mara Fornasarig

Introduction

There are some difficulties in early detection and diagnosis of stomach cancer because, usually, patients have non-specific symptoms as abdominal pain and a sense of fullness of the upper abdomen and in advanced stomach cancer poor appetite, weight loss, nausea and vomiting, and anemia. Patients presenting with the above-mentioned symptoms and patients with risk to develop gastric cancer require further workup [16]. Instrumental diagnostic tests, in patients with clinical symptoms or in presence of risk factors, include gastroscopy with biopsy, endoscopic ultrasound, computed tomography (CT), magnetic resonance imaging (MRI), positron emission tomography (PET), X-ray, laparoscopy and other laboratory tests [20]. Esophagogastroduodenoscopy (EGD) is the diagnostic imaging procedure of choice in initial step of diagnosis of gastric carcinoma (Fig. 3.1). An endoscope is used to visually examine the lining of the esophagus, stomach, and the upper portion of small intestine [6, 20]. EGD is performed with the patient in the left lateral position, usually under conscious sedation, mostly with benzodiazepines, sometimes in conjunction with a central analgesic and recently with propofol, and it is associated with very low complication rates [23]. After the general process of observation, differential diagnosis of minute mucosal changes found during the observational process should be conducted with caution by image-enhanced endoscopy (IEE). When judged to be necessary, the minimum necessary number of biopsy specimens should be obtained from the most suitable site. The presence of *H. pylori* infection, mucosal atrophy and intestinal metaplasia is closely associated with the risk of gastric cancer. Therefore, to recognize relevant endoscopic findings to these conditions, it is important to assess risk of gastric cancer and to detect early gastric cancer (EGC) efficiently [11]. The little adhesion of mucus, regular arrangement of collecting venules (RAC), and fundic gland polyps strongly suggest "*H. pylori* uninfected gastric

R. Cannizzaro (✉) · R. Magris · S. Maiero
M. Fornasarig
Oncological Gastroenterology Department, IRCCS, CRO Aviano, National Cancer Institute, Aviano, PN, Italy
e-mail: rcannizzaro@cro.it

P. Spessotto
Molecular Oncology Unit, IRCCS, CRO Aviano, National Cancer Institute, Aviano, PN, Italy

V. De Re
Immunopathology and Cancer Biomarkers/Bio-proteomics Facility, Department of Research and Advanced Tumor Diagnostics, IRCCS, CRO Aviano, National Cancer Institute, Aviano, PN, Italy

© Springer Nature Switzerland AG 2019
V. Canzonieri, A. Giordano (eds.), *Gastric Cancer In The Precision Medicine Era*, Current Clinical Pathology, https://doi.org/10.1007/978-3-030-04861-7_3

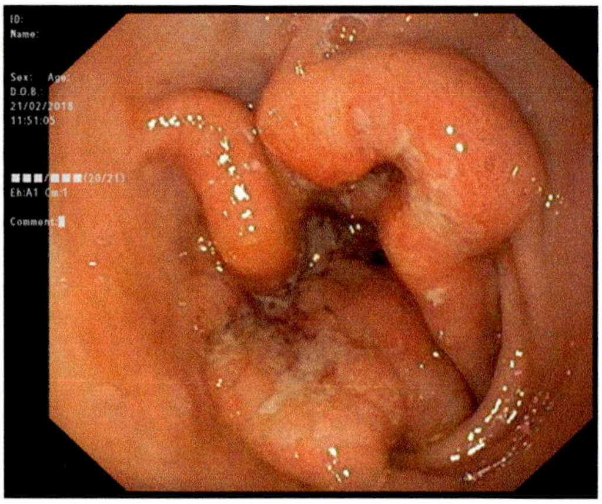

Fig. 3.1 Gastric cancer

mucosa." Atrophy of the gastric mucosa, meandering and thickening folds in the gastric corpus, xanthoma, or gooseflesh-like mucosa (nodular gastritis), indicates a "gastric mucosa with current or previous *H. pylori* infection" [11]. Undifferentiated carcinoma often originates from the region inside the endoscopic atrophic border or the intermediate zone (vicinity of the atrophic border). Well-differentiated carcinoma often arises from the external region of the endoscopic atrophic border.

The macroscopic aspect of gastric cancer is defined by Borrmann classification: polypoid lesions (type I); fungating, ulcerated with sharp raised margins (type II); ulcerated with poorly defined infiltrative margins (type III); and infiltrative, predominantly intramural lesion, and poorly demarcated (type IV).

EGD is a highly sensitive and specific diagnostic test, especially if combined with endoscopic macrobiopsies and histological examination of the tissue. The update Sydney system recommends at least five biopsies, two from the antrum, two from the corpus, and one from the incisura angularis, and multiple biopsies should be obtained from any suspicious areas. Gastroscopy must be performed with quality criteria, applying coloring methods (chromoendoscopy, NBI, etc.), magnification and endomicroscopy, which allow for high accuracy of diagnosis. There is no universal standard for the number of images to be recorded during EGD. The ESGE guideline recommends four images to be recorded for observation of the stomach [3]. This number is inconceivably low in comparison with the number of images usually taken in Japan. However, considering the low prevalence of gastric cancer in Europe, this number, reflecting moderate attention, may be appropriate and cause no clinical problems [11].

Recommendations for improving upper gastrointestinal (UGI) endoscopy in Western countries are:

- Focus training on early upper gastrointestinal cancer detection.
- Routine systematic mucosal washing with mucolytic and antifoam agents with or without use of antiperistaltic agents.
- Appropriate sedation to allow adequate examination.
- Systematic examination of upper gastrointestinal tract with routine high-definition white light photodocumentation using European Society of Gastrointestinal Endoscopy 2016 guidelines as a minimum standard.
- Minimum total procedure time 8 min: with 4 min gastric examination and 2 min oesophageal examination where detection of early upper gastrointestinal cancer is a diagnostic aim [31].
- When a gastric cancer is found, 6–8 biopsy specimens with macroforceps are recommended.
- This number of specimens provides a more correct evaluation of HER2 status.
- Further staging with endoscopic ultrasound in esophagogastric junctional tumors and selected gastric cancers is recommended (grade B) [2].

Chromoendoscopy and Magnification Endoscopy

Magnifying endoscopy in conjunction with chromoendoscopy is useful to improve visualization of mucosal details. Vital dyes in digestive endoscopy have been introduced 20 years ago for a better identification of mucosal surface abnormalities. In recent times, vital dyes can be associated to endoscopic high resolution and image magnification tools (zoom endoscopies).

The most commonly used dyes are methylene blue and contrasting dyes such as carmine indigo. Methylene blue is taken up by absorbent tissues such as the small intestinal epithelium; instead carmine indigo is not absorbed from cells but has the objective of delineating the edges and contour of a lesion accurately, to facilitate their detection.

Endoscopic magnification, with tools that enlarge the image up to 150 times with the use of electronic zoom, has allowed to improve the identification of preneoplastic lesions and early neoplasia (in particular non-protruding and small ones). The use of this technique permits to reduce the rate of lesions not detected during traditional endoscopy and to study, analyzing spatial arrangement of glandular crypt orifices (pit pattern), the histological type of the lesion (hyperplastic or adenomatic), and the depth of parietal invasion. Moreover, chromoendoscopy with methylene blue or acetic acid allowed the development of some superficial classifications that correlate with intestinal metaplasia and dysplasia. Regular or destructured patterns are related to the presence of high-grade dysplasia or carcinoma [14].

Narrow-band Imaging NBI

Narrow-band imaging (NBI) is based on the shrinking spectral bandwidth of RGB optical filters used in the sequential imaging method that creates video-endoscopic images. The NBI system is embedded in the endoscope and filters some wavelengths allowing only blue light to illuminate the tissue thus permitting an increased vascular-capillary network visibility and to process the endoscopic image in real time (Fig. 3.2). In this way, the endoscopist can evaluate the capillary pattern correlated with the degree of parietal infiltration of the neoplasm. This technology, with endoscopic magnification, can identify capillary or glandular mucosal alterations.

Other innovative technologies even if of more limited use are autofluorescence (AF), exogenous fluorescence or photodynamic diagnosis (PDD), reflection or light scattering spectroscopy (LSS), trimodal spectroscopy, Raman spectroscopy, and optical coherence tomography [14].

Finally, a very important point is the introduction of endoscopic macrobiopsy. The use of macrobiopsy, in addition to the electronic technology, allows taking tissue samples of about 0.5–0.7 cm against the "normal" pliers with 0.2–0.3 cm, reducing the number of inadequate samples for histological diagnosis.

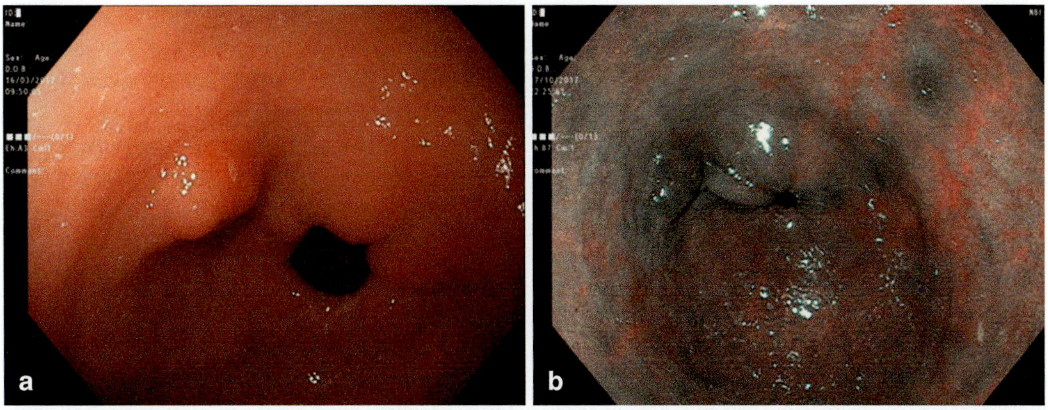

Fig. 3.2 (**a**) Endoscopic image of high-grade dysplasia; (**b**) NBI image of high-grade dysplasia

Confocal Laser Endomicroscopy

The confocal laser endomicroscopy (CLE) (CellVision, Mauna Kea Technologies, Paris, France) is a new endoscopic technique that is performed during a traditional endoscopic examination. It allows to examine mucous membranes and tissues during the diagnostic phase [14]. The confocal laser endomicroscope permits in vivo analysis of tissue microarchitecture, with cellular resolution, thus allowing a precise identification of areas to be biopsied. The analyzed region is enlarged 1000 times, so it permits to examine the mucosa and its glands, vessels, and microvessels at the same time and to interpret whether the alterations are inflammatory, preneoplastic, or neoplastic.

These features make pCLE potentially useful in early diagnosis of tumor or dysplastic lesions, as well as in biopsy optimization and targeted endoscopic treatment. The CLE probe is introduced into traditional endoscope during endoscopic examination. Endomicroscopic images are generated by the use of the contrast agent sodium fluorescein administered endovenously. After intravenous administration of 5–10 ml of 10% fluorescein sodium, cells, vascular system, and connective tissue can be well differentiated. During the acquisition of endomicroscopic images, the terminal of the probe should be gently rested on the mucosa/lesion to be investigated. 0.8 or 1.6 endomicroscopic images per second are displayed on the monitor and can be recorded in the database of the equipment.

The main indications to the endomicroscopic study are all those conditions in which it is possible to recognize alterations of cellular morphology or of vasculature in the superficial layers of the mucous membrane, especially the dysplastic lesions of the gastrointestinal tract, including the biliary duct.

Several clinical studies based on comparison with traditional histological examination have established the diagnostic confocal criteria for the diagnosis of normal gastric mucosa, chronic gastritis with intestinal metaplasia, and neoplasia. In the absence of pathology, the administration of fluorescein allows to identify in the gastric corpus a network of subepithelial honeycomb capillaries surrounding gastric foveole, while in the antrum, they have a spiral appearance. Early neoplastic well-differentiated lesions appear generally hypervascularized, with tortuous and dilated vessels with irregular form and dimensions. In contrast, undifferentiated tumor appears hypovascularized, and vessels have short and unconnected branches [8].

In a monocentric study conducted on 31 patients with 35 lesions, diagnostic accuracy of endomicroscopy was significantly higher than the histological diagnosis performed on standard biopsies (94% vs 86%), when the results were compared with the histological outcome of the entire post-ESD lesion. In the gastritis associated with the presence of *Helicobacter pylori*, CLE has demonstrated the presence of fluorescein outbreak through intercellular spaces. The eradication treatment reduced the fluorescein spill restoring the normal condition. Instead, the spill of contrast media persisted in the presence of morphological alterations, such as intestinal metaplasia, despite the success of eradication therapy. In this context CLE has highlighted the altered function of the in vivo mucous barrier, a factor that can contribute to carcinogenesis. Recently, due to the increasing interest in molecular imaging, specific biomarkers, also called molecular probes, have been developed. Typically, these are low molecular weight peptides, with variable affinity for specific structures, conjugated with fluorescein (e.g., fluorescent antibodies to the epidermal growth factor receptor – EGFR).

These antibodies allowed in vivo study of gastric cancer and possible response to targeted therapies in animal models and ex vivo on human tissues opening the way for new studies of markers that allow targeted use of drugs such as trastuzumab [13, 18].

Endomicroscopic observation is, however, time-consuming. Peristaltic visceral or transmitted (breath, heartbeat) movements and the remarkable enlargement of vision can generate artifacts. The depth of exploration, limited to a maximum of 250 microns, does not allow to evaluate the neoplastic infiltration of the submucosa.

A particular field of endomicroscopy concerns the study of tumor neoangiogenesis. The development of new blood vessels from pre-existing vessels (angiogenesis) is a phenomenon indispensable both in normal conditions and in pathological situations such as growth and tumor progression. Tumors cannot grow more than 2 mm unless they are in presence of an angiogenetic process. Be able to identify the onset in a relatively short time of new vessels in the intratumoral area can be crucial for a decisive and personalized anti-angiogenetic therapy.

The fluorescein as a contrasting medium is very useful in highlighting these neoformed vessels that often exhibit large structures and with defective flow and leakage areas (Fig. 3.3). Spessotto et al. demonstrate that in a total of 35 consecutive patients with gastric cancer that underwent endoscopy and pCLE during the same examination, the morphological neoangiogenesis was in agreement with histological and immunohistochemical analyses. They develop an arbitrary angiogenesis scale that can estimate the extent of intratumoral angiogenesis based on vessel shape and size, permeability, and blood flow and allowed the creation of an angiogenic score ranging from 0, for normal vasculature, to 4, for aberrant vasculature.

The study shows that the angiogenic score may be applied during endomicroscopy with a moderate grade of "consistency," at least for rectal cancer patients, thereby granting very rapid information on the vascularization pattern of a given patient. A lower concordance related to gastric cancer analyses could be due to the excess of fibrotic tissue in gastric tumors, which may render difficult the clear detection of the vascularized regions by pCLE in real time. They overcome this problem by off-line evaluation since the dedicated software allows the images to be corrected and stabilized after digital storage. In any case, they demonstrate that off-line evaluation can provide information more rapidly than histological procedures [28].

Endoscopic Ultrasound

Endoscopic ultrasound (EUS) is a modality that allows more accurate locoregional staging of early or locally advanced gastric cancer. The transducer is placed directly next to the gastric wall, so the depth of tumor invasion and local lymph node involvement, that usually influence survival, can be determined by high-frequency soundwaves [16].

EUS imaging is currently performed with radial or linear echoendoscope. These scope are video-endoscope coupled to electronic ultrasound processors for generation of electronic EUS images, endowed with special aspect including Doppler, contrast, and others: standard EUS usually utilizes high ultrasound frequencies that vary between 5 and 20 MHz [33] (Fig. 3.4). The transducer in most radial echoendoscopes generates radial images of 360°, oriented perpendicular to the shaft axis of the instrument. Indeed, linear echoendoscopes produce images directed parallel to the tube axis allowing for an effective

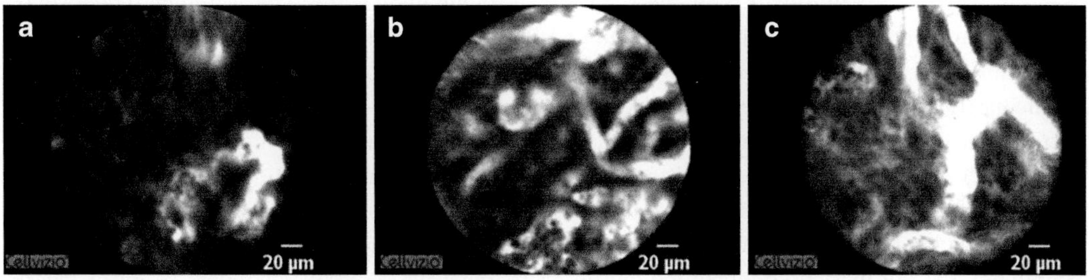

Fig. 3.3 Image of vasculature in gastric cancer obtained by probe confocal laser endomicroscopy

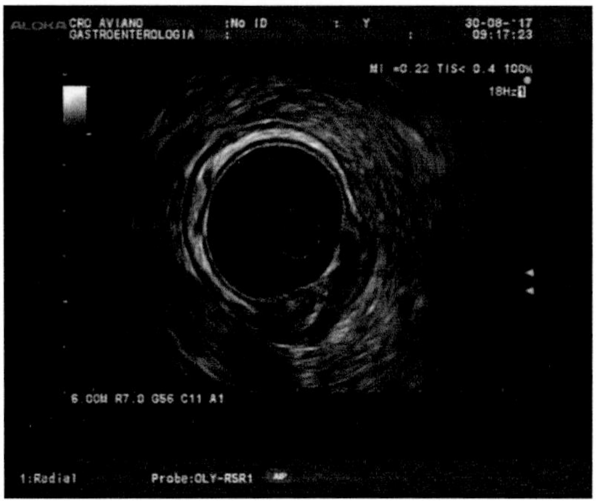

Fig. 3.4 Endoscopic ultrasound image of gastric cancer T3N0

and safe performance of EUS-guided fine needle aspiration puncture (EUS-FNA) when needed [33]. Acoustic coupling of the ultrasonic transducer to the GI wall requires application of fluid as interface between the wall and transducer. Usually water-filled balloon, placed around the tip of instrument, or instillation of water in the lumen is used to perform EUS [23, 33].

EUS can increase preoperative staging accuracy, but it cannot be used to assess distant lymph node involvement or to screen for lung or liver metastasis. EUS is useful in defining proximal and distal extent of the tumor and to evaluate T and N stage but is less useful for antral tumors [5, 27].

During echoendoscopy some scanning principles should be performed as scanning of target should be perpendicular to avoid erroneous diagnoses or overstaging due to broadening and blurring of structure; it should be kept an adequate focal distance; the use of higher frequencies may help to obtain a better visualization of structures and lesions [33].

The gastric wall normally consists of five distinct layers. The two inner layers (echo rich and echo poor) represent the interface/superficial mucosa and deep mucosa/muscularis mucosa. The third (echo rich) layer corresponds to the submucosa, the fourth (echo poor) to the muscularis propria, and the fifth (echo rich) to the serosa, which is difficult to distinguish from the surrounding tissue. For the orientation and other diagnostic purposes surrounding organs, vessels and other structures are very important [33].

EUS accuracy in determining infiltration degree of the wall ranges from 67% to 92%. A recent systematic review with meta-analysis has shown that the ability to accurately study gastric wall with EUS in cancer has a high accuracy compared to TAC or MRI in particular in the T1 and T4 stage, discriminating patients to be endoscopically resected and those in which surgery has little chance of treatment [17, 26].

Criterions to distinguish malignancy on EUS include hypoechogenicity, round shape, smooth, distinct margin, and size >1 cm [27].

EUS allows to perform a fine needle aspiration (FNA) or targeted needle biopsy on the suspicious lymph nodes.

Moreover, it has been demonstrated that EUS is useful in selecting patients who should undergo diagnostic laparoscopy; in fact, patients with EUS T1-T2, N0 staging have a 4% risk of peritoneal metastasis compared to the 25% risk in patients staged as T3-T4, N +, indicating how laparoscopy could be spared for subjects with EUS staging up to T2, N0 (negative predictive value of M1: 96%) [7, 22, 25]. Finally EUS is helpful in the diagnosis of linitis plastica.

Early Gastric Cancer

The Endoscopic Diagnosis of Early Gastric Cancer

The endoscopic diagnosis of early gastric cancer (EGC) requires good endoscopic techniques and thorough knowledge. The accuracy of endoscopy in the detection and diagnosis of EGC is reported to range between 90% and 96% [12]. Chromoendoscopy and magnifying endoscopy are promising image-enhanced endoscopic techniques for characterization. Early gastric cancer is defined as confined to the mucosa or submucosa, regardless of lymph node metastasis. To have an accurate diagnosis of early gastric cancer, it's very important to have a good knowledge of the characteristic of early-stage disease.

EGC can be divided into three types: elevated, superficial and excavated. The superficial type is further subdivided into superficial elevated, superficial flat and superficial depressed [32].

It is difficult to find superficial flat lesions in the conventional white light endoscopy (WLE), which often cause misdiagnosis and missed diagnosis. The most common lesions of EGC were usually manifested by erythema and erosion [34]. During white light endoscopy, it's important to pay attention to changes in color of mucosa (pale redness or fading of color), loss of visibility of underlying submucosal vessels, thinning of and interruptions in mucosal folds and spontaneous bleeding [32].

Most elevated EGCs are of the differentiated type, and some gastric superficial elevated type EGCs and adenomas appear whitish. Among the flat or depressed type EGCs, differentiated-type cancers look reddish, whereas undifferentiated types appear whitish because of a difference in hemoglobin content [11].

Chromoendoscopy

Several reports describe the magnification findings of early gastric cancer. The characteristic patterns of EGC are as follows: (i) a small regular pattern of sulci and ridges, (ii) an irregular pattern of sulci and ridges and (iii) a lack of visible structure. The presence of irregular minute vessels and the variation in the caliber of vessels are specific vascular patterns in EGC [4].

When mucosal changes are observed, chromoendoscopy can effectively aid to diagnosis. After spraying dye in lesion and over the mucosa surrounding the lesion, early gastric cancer is diagnosed through the comparison between the two parts. The detection of an irregular shape and distribution of microvessels make the difference between early cancer and focal gastritis. Irregular microvessels are tumorous vessels. The demarcation line between cancer and normal mucosa allowed the evaluation of the margin of the carcinoma before endoscopic resection [4].

It's important to wash the lesion accurately prior to spraying because the dye can make the lesion boundaries unclear when mucous is adherent to stomach wall. However, it's difficult to diagnose correctly gastric cancer smaller than 5 mm or superficial flat (IIb) gastric cancer using white light imaging or chromoendoscopy.

Narrow-band Image-Enhanced Endoscopy (NBI)

It enhances the superficial surface structure and vascular architecture of the mucous layer by illuminating blue and green narrowband lights. NBI is a promising technique for characterizing small or flat early gastric cancers. Microvascular and microsurface patterns on the gastric mucosa can be observed with NBI. Moreover it further reveals intestinal metaplasia by its whitish color. Intestinal metaplasia exists as a flat mucosa with subtle discoloration. Magnifying NBI images, a fine blue-white line of light is observed on the crests of the epithelial surface/gyri (light blue crest) of intestinal metaplasia. The "light blue crest" is thought to be caused by the reflection of short wavelength light at the brush border on the surface of the intestinal metaplasia [11].

Ultrasound Endoscopy

EUS can be used to make a more objective diagnosis. Through this diagnostic method, endoscopist can determine whether the patient can undergo endoscopic therapy and small diameter lesion is often targeted.

Therapeutic Endoscopy

Therapeutic endoscopy plays a major role in the management of gastric neoplasia. It is a local treatment of primary lesions, and it is totally ineffective if any metastatic lesions are present. It's indicated in cases of early gastric cancer if there are no lymph node metastasis [29]. Its indications can be broadly divided into four categories: to remove or obliterate the neoplastic lesion, to palliative recanalization of luminal obstruction, to treat bleeding and others [9, 10]. Two techniques are used to treat endoscopically early gastric cancer: endoscopic mucosal resection (EMR) and endoscopic submucosal dissection (ESD).

Endoscopic Mucosal Resection

Mucosectomy or endoscopic mucosal resection (EMR) is a minimally invasive technique safe, convenient and efficacious for T1 mucosal cancers [10, 21]. EMR is used in alternative to surgery in well-differentiated elevated lesions, intestinal type adenocarcinomas with no ulcer, confined to the mucosa, smaller than 20 mm in size with no lymphatic or vessel involvement [9, 10, 21]. Endoscopic resection is comparable in many aspects to conventional surgery, with the advantages of being less invasive, more economical [10] and to permit a complete pathological staging of the cancer. The risk of lymph node metastasis can be predicted, after endoscopic resection, thanks to the pathological assessment of cancer invasion depth, of cancer differentiation degree and of lymphovascular invasion extent [10]. After the submucosal injection of the lesion, a specialized crescent-shaped snare is deployed in the groove at the tip of the cap. The snare is closed and resection is performed by electrocauterization and then the lesion is drawn into the cap connected to the tip of a standard endoscope. Caps are available in different sizes according to the diameter of the endoscope and the size of the lesion [9, 10, 30]. Another EMR technique is the ligation EMR that uses ligation devices to capture the lesion and transform it into a polypoid lesion deploying the band underneath it [9].

Endoscopic Submucosal Dissection (ESD)

A subsequent technique developed in therapeutic endoscopy, called endoscopic submucosal dissection (ESD), allows the direct dissection of the submucosa and the resection en bloc of large lesions [9]. ESD is performed with special endoscopic knives and permit the en bloc resection with a standard single-channel gastroscope [9]. The lesions that should be considered for endoscopic resection which are at very low risk of lymph node metastasis are the following: noninvasive neoplasia (dysplasia) independently of size; intramucosal differentiated-type adenocarcinoma, without ulceration (size ≤2 cm absolute indication, >2 cm expanded indication); intramucosal differentiated-type adenocarcinoma, with ulcer, size ≤3 cm (expanded indication); intramucosal undifferentiated-type adenocarcinoma, size ≤2 cm (expanded indication); and differentiated-type adenocarcinoma with superficial submucosal invasion (sm1 ≤ 500 μm) and size ≤3 cm (expanded indication) [24]. The three are the steps involved in ESD technique: fluid injection into the submucosal layer to separate it from the muscle layer, circumferential cutting of the mucosa surrounding the lesion and finally submucosal dissection of the connective tissue of the submucosa under the lesion [9].

Surveillance

Approximately 40–60% of patients treated surgically develop a relapse, and in 80% it will happen within the first 2 years. Regional site relapses occur in 20–30% of cases, while the liver and peritoneum are the long distant organs that frequently show recurrence.

The risk of relapse at 5 years is lowered to 47% in patients who survived a year from the disease and 10% in patients who survived 5 years.

A regular follow-up may allow investigation and treatment of symptoms, psychological support, and early detection of recurrence, though there is no evidence that it improves survival outcome. Follow-up should be tailored to the individual patient and the stage of disease [27]. To date, there are no randomized controlled trials in gastric carcinoma that may indicate appropriate follow-up of patients after surgical resection or after treatment (Level of Evidence 3) [1]. The main purposes of a follow-up strategy are the early detection of anastomotic recurrences that can be treated surgically, the assessment of abnormalities concerning nutritional status (anemia, dumping syndrome), or identification of clinical signs related to recurrence. Given the lack of a significant impact on patients' survival using a regular follow-up of imaging, the international guidelines propose a clinical follow-up consisting only of the hematochemical parameters, leaving the instrumental investigations in relation to the symptomatology reported by the patient. In case of clinical suspicion of recurrence, CT appears to have higher sensitivity than ultrasound examinations (Level of Evidence 3).

The following scheme may be suggested:

- Every 3–4 months for the first 2 years (0–2 years): clinical examination including weight, blood tests (hemoglobin levels, sideremia, renal, and hepatic function), and instrumental to be performed on clinical need at the doctor's discretion.
- Every 6 months in the following 3 years (3–5 years): clinical examination including weight, blood tests (hemoglobin levels, sideremia, renal and hepatic function), and instrumental test to be performed on clinical need at the doctor's discretion.
- EGDS appears useful in particular in the case of subtotal gastrectomy for the search for local recurrences or cancer on the stump; it could be repeated every 2–3 years in the first 5 years and then every 3–5 years.

Although there are no published data, it is considered acceptable that after 5 years of specialist follow-up, surveillance may be continued annually, possibly by the general practitioner [15, 19, 27] (AIOM guidelines, 2015).

Acknowledgments The authors thank Francesca Masutti for her assistance in manuscript editing.

This work was supported by the following grant of Ministry of Health (*RF-2016-02361525* to R.C.).

References

1. Baiocchi GL, Marrelli D, Verlato G, Morgagni P, Giacopuzzi S, Coniglio A, Marchet A, Rosa F, Capponi MG, Di Leo A, Saragoni L, Ansaloni L, Pacelli F, Nitti D, D'Ugo D, Roviello F, Tiberio GA, Giulini SM, De Manzoni G. Follow-up after gastrectomy for cancer: an appraisal of the Italian research group for gastric cancer. Ann Surg Oncol. 2014;21(6):2005–11.
2. Bang YJ, Van Cutsem E, Feyereislova A, Chung HC, Shen L, Sawaki A, Lordick F, Ohtsu A, Omuro Y, Satoh T, Aprile G, Kulikov E, Hill J, Lehle M, Rüschoff J, Kang YK, Trial Investigators TGA. Trastuzumab in combination with chemotherapy versus chemotherapy alone for treatment of HER2-positive advanced gastric or gastro-oesophageal junction cancer (ToGA): a phase 3, open-label, randomised controlled trial. Lancet. 2010;376(9742):687–97.
3. Bisschops R, Areia M, Coron E, Dobru D, Kaskas B, Kuvaev R, Pech O, Ragunath K, Weusten B, Familiari P, Domagk D, Valori R, Kaminski MF, Spada C, Bretthauer M, Bennett C, Senore C, Dinis-Ribeiro M, Rutter MD. Performance measures for upper gastrointestinal endoscopy: a European Society of Gastrointestinal Endoscopy (ESGE) Quality Improvement Initiative. Endoscopy. 2016;48(9):843–64.
4. Boeriu A, Dobru D, Pascarenco O, Stoian M, Mocan S. Magnifying endoscopy and chromoendoscopy in upper gastrointestinal tract – clinical applications, new techniques in gastrointestinal endoscopy, prof. Oliviu Pascu (Ed.), InTech; 2011.
5. Cannizzaro R, Fornasarig M, Lacchin T. Endoscopic diagnosis and staging of gastric tumors. Suppl Tumori. 2003;2(5):S16–8. Review.
6. Cannizzaro R, Farinati F, Borzio M. Tumori dell'apparato digerente (esofago, stomaco, colonretto, pancreas, fegato). In: Bazzoli F, Buscarini E, Cannizzaro R, Conte D, De Boni M, Delle Fave G, Farinati F, Ravelli P, Spolaore P, Testoni PA, editors. Libro Bianco Della Gastroenterologia. Roma: Aigo Sied Sige; 2011.
7. Cannizzaro R, Marone P. Stomach and duodenum. In: De Angelis C, Bocus P, editors. IEC-atlas of endoscopic ultrasound. Turin: Edizioni Minerva Medica; 2012.
8. Cannizzaro R, Mongiat M, Canzonieri V, Fornasarig M, Maiero S, De Re V, Todaro F, De Paoli P, Spessotto P. Endomicroscopy and cancer: a new approach to the visualization of neoangiogenesis. Gastroenterol Res Pract. 2012;2012:537170.
9. Gotoda T, Yamamoto H, Soetikno RM. Endoscopic submucosal dissection of early gastric cancer. J Gastroenterol. 2006;41(10):929–42.
10. Gotoda T. Endoscopic resection of early gastric cancer. Gastric Cancer. 2007;10(1):1–11.
11. Gotoda T, Uedo N, Yoshinaga S, Tanuma T, Morita Y, Doyama H, Aso A, Hirasawa T, Yano T, Uchita K, Ho SH, Hsieh PH. Basic principles and practice of gastric cancer screening using high-definition white-light gastroscopy: eyes can only see what the brain knows. Dig Endosc. 2016;28 Suppl 1:2–15.
12. Hartgrink HH, Jansen EP, van Grieken NC, van de Velde CJ. Gastric cancer. Lancet. 2009;374(9688):477–90.
13. Hoetker MS, Kiesslich R, Diken M, Moehler M, Galle PR, Li Y, Goetz M. Molecular in vivo imaging of gas-

tric cancer in a human-murine xenograft model: targeting epidermal growth factor receptor. Gastrointest Endosc. 2012;76(3):612–20.
14. Kiesslich R, Goetz M, Hoffman A, Galle PR. New imaging techniques and opportunities in endoscopy. Nat Rev Gastroenterol Hepatol. 2011;8(10):547–53.
15. Kim JH, Jang YJ, Park SS, Park SH, Mok YJ. Benefit of post-operative surveillance for recurrence after curative resection for gastric cancer. J Gastrointest Surg. 2010;14(6):969–76.
16. Layke JC, Lopez PP. Gastric cancer: diagnosis and treatment options. Am Fam Physician. 2004;69(5):1133–40.
17. Lee YT, Ng EK, Hung LC, Chung SC, Ching JY, Chan WY, Chu WC, Sung JJ. Accuracy of endoscopic ultrasonography in diagnosing ascites and predicting peritoneal metastases in gastric cancer patients. Gut. 2005;54(11):1541–5.
18. Li Z, Zuo XL, Li CQ, Zhou CJ, Liu J, Goetz M, Kiesslich R, Wu KC, Fan DM, Li YQ. In vivo molecular imaging of gastric cancer by targeting MG7 antigen with confocal laser endomicroscopy. Endoscopy. 2013;45(2):79–85.
19. Linee guida AIOM, 2015, downloadable to: http://www.aiom.it/professionisti/documenti-scientifici/linee-guida/stomaco/1,712,1.
20. Page MR, Shriya P. Gastric cancer: understanding its burden, treatment strategies, and uncertainties in management. AJMC Supplements: The Current and Future Management of Gastric Cancer –Published on: June 29, 2017.
21. Miquel JM, Abad R, Souto J, Fabra R, Vila M, Bargalló D, Vázquez-Iglesia JL, Varas Lorenzo MJ. EUS-guided mucosectomy for gastrointestinal cancer. Rev Esp Enferm Dig. 2006;98(8):591–6.
22. Mocellin S, Marchet A, Nitti D. EUS for the staging of gastric cancer: a meta-analysis. Gastrointest Endosc. 2011;73(6):1122–34.
23. Papanikolaou IS, Triantafyllou M, Triantafyllou K, Rösch T. EUS in the management of gastric cancer. Ann Gastroenterol. 2011;24(1):9–15.
24. Pimentel-Nunes P, Dinis-Ribeiro M, Ponchon T, Repici A, Vieth M, De Ceglie A, Amato A, Berr F, Bhandari P, Bialek A, Conio M, Haringsma J, Langner C, Meisner S, Messmann H, Morino M, Neuhaus H, Piessevaux H, Rugge M, Saunders BP, Robaszkiewicz M, Seewald S, Kashin S, Dumonceau JM, Hassan C, Deprez PH. Endoscopic submucosal dissection: European Society of Gastrointestinal Endoscopy (ESGE) guideline. Endoscopy. 2015;47(9):829–54.
25. Power DG, Schattner MA, Gerdes H, Brenner B, Markowitz AJ, Capanu M, Coit DG, Brennan M, Kelsen DP, Shah MA. Endoscopic ultrasound can improve the selection for laparoscopy in patients with localized gastric cancer. J Am Coll Surg. 2009;208(2):173–8.
26. Puli SR, Batapati Krishna Reddy J, Bechtold ML, Antillon MR, Ibdah JA. How good is endoscopic ultrasound for TNM staging of gastric cancers? A meta-analysis and systematic review. World J Gastroenterol. 2008;14(25):4011–9.
27. Smyth EC, Verheij M, Allum W, Cunningham D, Cervantes A, Arnold D, ESMO Guidelines Committee. Gastric cancer: ESMO clinical practice guidelines for diagnosis, treatment and follow-up. Ann Oncol. 2016;27(Suppl 5):v38–49.
28. Spessotto P, Fornasarig M, Pivetta E, Maiero S, Magris R, Mongiat M, Canzonieri V, De Paoli P, De Paoli A, Buonadonna A, Serraino D, Panato C, Belluco C, Cannizzaro R. Probe-based confocal laser endomicroscopy for in vivo evaluation of the tumor vasculature in gastric and rectal carcinomas. Sci Rep. 2017;7(1):9819.
29. Tada M, Tanaka Y, Matsuo N, Shimamura T, Yamaguchi K. Mucosectomy for gastric cancer: current status in Japan. J Gastroenterol Hepatol. 2000;15(Suppl):D98–102. Review.
30. Torii A, Sakai M, Kajiyama T, Kishimoto H, Kin G, Inoue K, Koizumi T, Ueda S, Okuma M. Endoscopic aspiration mucosectomy as curative endoscopic surgery; analysis of 24 cases of early gastric cancer. Gastrointest Endosc. 1995;42(5):475–9.
31. Veitch AM, Uedo N, Yao K, East JE. Optimizing early upper gastrointestinal cancer detection at endoscopy. Nat Rev Gastroenterol Hepatol. 2015;12(11):660–7.
32. Yada T, Yokoi C, Uemura N. The current state of diagnosis and treatment for early gastric cancer. Diagn Ther Endosc. 2013;2013:241320.
33. Yasuda K. EUS in the detection of early gastric cancer. Gastrointest Endosc. 2002;56(4 Suppl):S68–75.
34. Zhu L, Qin J, Wang J, Guo T, Wang Z, Yang J. Early gastric Cancer: current advances of endoscopic diagnosis and treatment. Gastroenterol Res Pract. 2016;2016:9638041.

Pathological Diagnosis and Classification of Gastric Epithelial Tumours

4

Rossella Rotondo, Flavio Rizzolio, Tiziana Perin, Massimiliano Berretta, Fabrizio Zanconati, Antonio Giordano, and Vincenzo Canzonieri

Precancerous/Early Cancerous Lesions

Intra-epithelial Neoplasia/Dysplasia

The multistep process of gastric carcinogenesis has been postulated by Correa [1] as a sequence of events, referred to as Correa cascade, where dysplasia or intra-epithelial neoplasia represents the penultimate stage of sequence [2] (Fig. 4.1). In tumour pathology, dysplasia is a term that, literally, means abnormal growth. During the years, disagreements between American, European and Japanese pathologists lead to develop several classifications to standardize the definition of gastric dysplasia and neoplasia [3–5].

Nevertheless, despite the terminological differences between Western and Japanese pathologists, interpretative problems, including the distinction from inflammatory-related reactive or regenerative

R. Rotondo
Pathology Department, IRCCS, CRO Aviano, National Cancer Institute, Aviano, PN, Italy

F. Rizzolio
Pathology Department, IRCCS, CRO Aviano, National Cancer Institute, Aviano, PN, Italy

Department of Molecular Sciences and Nanosystems, Ca' Foscari University, Venice-Mestre, VE, Italy

Department of Biology, Temple University, Philadelphia, PA, USA

T. Perin
Pathology Department, IRCCS, CRO Aviano, National Cancer Institute, Aviano, PN, Italy

CRO Biobank, IRCCS, CRO Aviano, National Cancer Institute, Aviano, PN, Italy

M. Berretta
Medical Oncology Department, IRCCS, CRO Aviano, National Cancer Institute, Aviano, PN, Italy

F. Zanconati
Department of Medical, Surgical and Health Sciences, University of Trieste, Trieste, Italy

A. Giordano (✉)
Sbarro Institute for Cancer Research and Molecular Medicine, Department of Biology, Temple University, Philadelphia, PA, USA

Department of Medicine, Surgery and Neuroscience, Anatomic Pathology Section, University of Siena, Siena, Italy
e-mail: giordano@temple.edu

V. Canzonieri (✉)
Pathology Department, IRCCS, CRO Aviano, National Cancer Institute, Aviano, PN, Italy

Department of Medical, Surgical and Health Sciences, University of Trieste, Trieste, TS, Italy

CRO Biobank, IRCCS, CRO Aviano, National Cancer Institute, Aviano, PN, Italy

Department of Biology, Temple University, Philadelphia, PA, USA
e-mail: vcanzonieri@cro.it

© Springer Nature Switzerland AG 2019
V. Canzonieri, A. Giordano (eds.), *Gastric Cancer In The Precision Medicine Era*, Current Clinical Pathology, https://doi.org/10.1007/978-3-030-04861-7_4

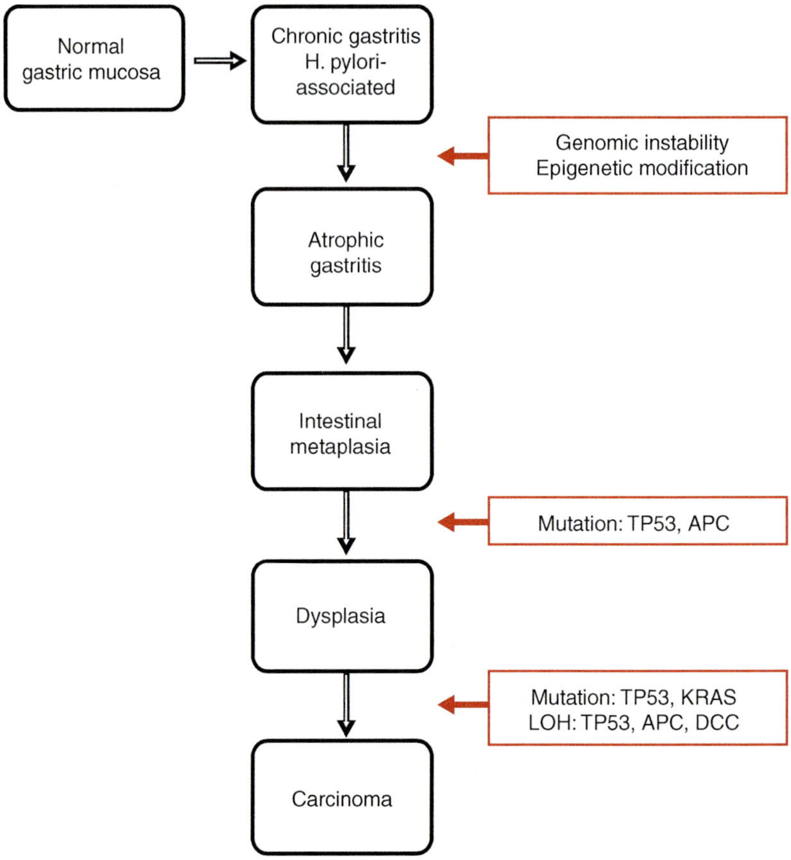

Fig. 4.1 The Correa cascade of gastric carcinogenesis

changes and the distinction between intra-epithelial and invasive carcinoma, limit the formulation of a correct diagnosis in grading gastric dysplasia/intra-epithelial neoplasia that is critical because it predicts the risk of both malignant transformation and metachronous gastric cancer [2].

On the basis of a consensus nomenclature, the so-called Vienna nomenclature, proposed in 1999 [5] and subsequently updated in 2003 [6] for the improvement in endoscopic techniques and their management implications, recently the World Health Organization (WHO) reiterated the classification of "dysplasia" and "intra-epithelial neoplasia" (IEN), using these terms as synonymous. The three following categories should, thus, be considered:

1. *Negative for intra-epithelial neoplasia/dysplasia*
   This category includes benign mucosal processes that are inflammatory, metaplastic or reactive in nature.
2. *Indefinite for intra-epithelial neoplasia/dysplasia*
   Although this term does not represent a final diagnosis, it is commonly used to indicate an ambiguous morphological pattern, especially in doubtful cases on the nature of a lesion, if neoplastic or not, particularly in small biopsies exhibiting inflammation. Taking into account the interpretative problems, it is not uncommon that regenerative changes could be misleading for intra-epithelial neoplasia/dysplasia, particularly in reactive gastritis and at the edge of a benign ulcer or in the postoperative stomach. Therefore, in those cases where inflammation raises the suspicion of an atypical regenerative process, the diagnosis may be clarified by cutting at deeper levels the tissue block, obtaining additional biopsies or after removing possible sources of cellular proliferative alterations.

   Epithelial proliferation may have the characteristics of indefinite dysplasia, when shows irregular and tubular structures with mucus depletion, high nuclear-cytoplasmic ratio and loss of cellular polarity. Mitotic activity may be brisk mainly near the proliferative zone in the mucous neck region. The glands are usually closely packed and lined by cells with large, hyperchromatic nuclei. An increasing gradient of alterations is appreciated from the base of the glands to their superficial portion.

3. *Intra-epithelial neoplasia/dysplasia*
   This category belongs to epithelial atypical/neoplastic proliferations characterized by variable cellular and architectural atypia but lacking clear evidence of invasive growth. They can have flat, polypoid or slightly depressed growth patterns.

Histologically, they can be distinguished into:

- *Low-grade intra-epithelial neoplasia/dysplasia*
  These lesions are characterized by a modified mucosal architecture, with distorted tubular structures, papillary formation, crypt lengthening with serration and cystic changes. Glands show various degree of mucin depletion.
  Nuclei are usually pseudostratified in the proliferation zone at the superficial portion of the dysplastic tubules.
- *High-grade intra-epithelial neoplasia/dysplasia*
  Important increasing of architectural distortion and prominent cellular atypia are seen in tubules with frequent irregular branching and folding; there is no stromal invasion. Mucin secretion is absent. Nuclei are often cigar-shaped with prominent nucleoli. Increased proliferative activity is present throughout the epithelium.
- *Intramucosal invasive neoplasia/intramucosal carcinoma*
  Carcinoma is diagnosed when the tumour invades into the lamina propria (intramucosal carcinoma).
  To distinguish intramucosal carcinoma from intra-epithelial neoplasia/dysplasia, absence or minimal desmoplasia accompanied by distinct structural anomalies, such as marked glandular crowding, excessive branching and budding, must be observed. Cells of intramucosal invasive neoplasia are usually cuboidal with a high nuclear-cytoplasmic ratio, round nuclei with prominent nucleoli and commonly show loss of cellular polarity.

Although variable, the diagnosis of gastric intra-epithelial neoplasia/dysplasia offers a relevant instrument to gastroenterologists into predicting an incremental risk of progression of these lesions to gastric cancer. If the progression from low-grade dysplasia to adenocarcinoma has been reported to 0–23% of cases within a mean interval from 10 months to 4 years, the rate of malignant transformation increases to 60–85% of cases within a median interval of 4–48 months for high-grade lesions [7–13]. Therefore, on the basis of the different malignant transformation rates of low-/high-grade dysplasia, patients will be treated with the appropriate therapy and included in a proper surveillance programme.

Benign Epithelial Tumours

Benign Gastric Epithelial Polyps

Gastric epithelial polyps are defined as lesions, which lay above the plain of the mucosal surface. The most common polyps are represented by fundic gland polyps that account for up to 77% of all gastric polyps, followed by hyperplastic polyps and adenomas [14, 15].

Fundic gland polyps (FGPs) occur in two different clinical settings: sporadic and syndromic. Development of dysplasia is extremely rare (<1%) in sporadic FGPs, and no association has been reported for progression in gastric cancer [16]. They also affect patients treated with long-term proton pump inhibitors [17, 18]. As sporadic manifestation of familial adenomatous polyposis (FAP) syndrome, numerous FGPs may be present in young patients. Contrary to sporadic FGPs, up to 48% of syndromic FGPs evolves into dysplasia, although progression to carcinoma remains rare [19, 20].

Recently, gastric adenocarcinoma and proximal polyposis syndrome has been identified as a new hereditary autosomal-dominant gastric cancer syndrome: it is characterized by the development of numerous FGPs and is associated with a significant risk of gastric carcinoma [21].

Hyperplastic polyps are often associated with chronic gastritis and *H. pylori* infection. Dysplasia may be found in 1–3% of hyperplastic polyps and is usually associated with lesions larger than 20 mm in diameter and prevalent in individuals over 50 years of age. Complete excision with entire histologic examination of large hyperplastic polyps is believed to be curative even if dysplasia or intramucosal carcinoma is well-documented [22].

Besides the conventional distinction between benign and malignant tumours, because most gastric tumours are epithelial in origin, they are also divided into two major categories [23]:

1. Exocrine, which comprises adenomas and adenocarcinomas
2. (N)endocrine, including carcinoid tumours and (N)endocrine cell carcinomas (NECC)

Gastric Adenomas

Gastric adenomas are characterized by lesions with raised polyps that by definition exhibit low- or high-grade epithelial dysplasia and comprise 0.5–3.75% of all gastric polyps in the Western Hemisphere, in contrast to 9–20% in areas of high-risk gastric cancer [14].

The risk of carcinoma progression of gastric adenomas is related to the size of the lesions and is increased in lesions larger than 2 cm in diameter.

Histologically, gastric adenomas may be classified as tubular, tubulovillous or villous based on the architecture. Gastric adenomas may be also subtyped, based on the epithelial phenotype, into intestinal and gastric types. The intestinal type of adenoma (adenomatous, type I) is more common and contains absorptive, goblet and Paneth cells [24, 25]. It is similar to colonic adenomas with crowded, tubular glands, lined by atypical columnar cells with overlapping, pencillate, hyperchromatic and/or pleomorphic nuclei with pseudostratification and inconspicuous nucleoli, mucin depletion and lack of surface maturation [26].

Gastric phenotype (foveolar, type II) contains cuboidal or low columnar cells, with clear or eosinophilic cytoplasm and showing round-to-oval nuclei [26].

Adenomatous and foveolar types can be immunohistochemically distinguished, since the first type expresses MUC2, CDX2 and CD10, whereas the second one expresses MUC5AC, lacks CD10 expression and exhibits low level of CDX2 [24, 27, 28].

Interestingly, other types of adenoma have been described:

- Pyloric adenomatous lesions in the body/fundus of the stomach of elderly patients, commonly associated with autoimmune gastritis. These lesions are characterized by eosinophilic cuboidal cells with finely granular cytoplasm with round nuclei and limited mitotic activity.
- Paneth cell adenoma, a rare variant composed exclusively of Paneth cells [29, 30].
- Oxyntic gland polyp or adenoma, which likely represents a morphological link to the previously described variant of gastric adenocarcinoma with chief cell differentiation [31].

The clinical and pathological characteristics of gastric adenomas are presented in Table 4.1.

Malignant Epithelial Tumours

Adenocarcinomas

Most gastric malignancies (95%) originate from glandular epithelium and are classified as adenocarcinoma. A multiplicity of environmental and genetic factors influences the aetiologies of this heterogeneous group of tumours, characterized by different morphologies, molecular backgrounds and histogenesis.

Epidemiology

Gastric carcinoma is the fifth most common malignancy worldwide and remains the third cause of death of all malignancies worldwide [32]. Since the disease remains asymptomatic until reaching the advanced stage, 5-year survival rate is relatively good only in Japan, where it

Table 4.1 Clinicopathologic characteristics of gastric adenomas according to histologic subtypes

Adenoma type	Location	Histological features	Association	Malignant transformation
Intestinal (Type I)	Antrum	Elongated hyperchromatic nuclei, focal globet cells and Paneth cells	Gastritis and IM	High
Foveolar (Type II)	Body	Round to oval nuclei, pale or clear cytoplasm, apical mucin	FAP	Controversial
Pyloric	Body	Round bland or atypical nuclei, ground glass cytoplasm	Autoimmune gastritis and IM	High
Paneth cell adenoma		Paneth cells	Gastritis and IM	Controversial
Oxyntic	Fundus/ cardia	Chief cells, mucous neck cells	Some with mild chronic gastritis	None

Modified from Ref. [39]
Abbreviations: *FAP* Familial Adenomatous Polyposis, *IM* intestinal metaplasia

reaches 90% [33], mainly due to early detection, while in European countries, survival rates vary from ~10% to 30% [34]. The incidence shows wide geographical variation: the distribution shifts from areas at high incidence (>60 per 100 000 males), such as in Eastern Asia, Eastern Europe and Latin America, to zones at low incidence (<15 per 100,000 population) as in North America, Northern Europe and most countries in Africa and in Southeast Asia [35]. A predominance of the cancers of antrum and pylorus occurs in high-risk areas, while proximal stomach and oesophagogastric junction adenocarcinomas are relatively more common in low-risk areas [36].

Nevertheless, a general declining incidence of gastric cancer has been observed worldwide in the last few decades, probably also due to the higher standards of hygiene, improvement in food conservation, a high intake of fresh fruits and vegetables and *Helicobacter pylori* (*H. pylori*) eradication [37].

Aetiology and Pathogenesis

The Correa cascade of gastric carcinogenesis [1] shows the progressive changes in the gastric mucosa with metamorphosis of normal gastric mucosa into carcinoma through the subsequent development of inflammation, atrophy, metaplasia and dysplasia [38], involving several genetic alterations (Fig. 4.1).

Several precancerous conditions have been reported, including atrophic gastritis and intestinal metaplasia due to *H. pylori* infection or autoimmunity, gastric ulcers, gastric polyps, previous gastric surgery and Ménétrier's disease. Moreover, associations with environmental agents such as dietary constituents and the generation of carcinogenic N-nitroso compounds within the stomach, in addition to inherited disposition, have also been recognized.

Chronic Gastritis and Intestinal Metaplasia

Chronic gastritis is the most important and well-studied risk factor for the intestinal type of gastric cancer [39]. Even though *H. pylori*-associated and autoimmune gastritis are two different etiologic agents of chronic inflammation, they result into atrophic gastritis that has been shown to precede the development of malignancy [40, 41].

For routine histopathological evaluation, the Sydney Classification System (later updated in Houston) was developed to provide information on the grade, topography (antrum, corpus, incisura) and origin of chronic gastritis [42].

To characterize the degree of chronicity, an international group of gastroenterologists and pathologists (Operative Link on Gastritis Assessment [OLGA]) developed a system for reporting the stage of gastritis, termed the OLGA Staging System [43]. The stage of gastritis is obtained by combining the extent of atrophy as scored histologically with the sites of atrophy identified by multiple biopsies from the antrum, incisura angularis (junctional area between the anatomic antrum and body along the lesser curvature) and corpus according to the Sydney System protocol [42, 43]. A long-term follow-up study reveals that the combination of OLGA Staging System with *H. pylori* status provides relevant information to stratify and confidently manage patients in accordance with their cancer risk [44].

Intestinal metaplasia (IM) is characterized by wide heterogeneity. In this regard, three types of IM have been recognized:

- Type I (complete or small intestinal type) consists of mature enterocytes with brush borders, Paneth cells and goblet cells, the latter secreting sialomucins [45]. The genetic characterization of complete-type IM evidences the expression of intestinal mucin MUC2 and markedly decreased levels of gastric mucins MUC1, MUC5AC and MUC6 [46]. Among IM subtypes, type I has been reported to be the predominant (73%) in biopsies, and it has been seen as the most common in benign conditions, 70% in gastric ulcers and 76% in chronic gastritis [47].
- Type II IM (incomplete, immature or colonic type) is characterized by few or absent absorptive cells and the presence of columnar "intermediate" cells in various stages of differentiation, secreting neutral and acid sialomucins, and goblet cells secreting sialomucin or occasionally sulphomucins [45, 47]. Differently to type I, in incomplete-type IM, gastric mucins are co-expressed with intestinal mucin MUC2. These expression patterns indicate that incomplete-type IM is a phenotypic mixture of gastric and intestinal cells, reflecting differentiation anomalies [46].
- Type III IM, in which the predominant mucin secreted by the "intermediate" cells is acid sulphomucin rather than sialomucin as in type II IM [47, 48]. Both type II and III incomplete IMs maintain the expression of gastric mucins MUC1, MUC5AC and MUC6 [46]. At molecular level, all types of IM express the intestinal transcription factor CDX2, generally expressed in the normal bowel [49]. Type III IM, which has been identified in only 9.8% of all biopsies with IM, has a higher incidence in carcinoma (35%) than in benign conditions (7%) [47].

Albeit some studies have demonstrated that cancer risk is increased from type I to type III of IM [47, 48, 50, 51], currently, subtyping of IM is not recommended in routine practice, because there is no conclusive evidences of the association between these subtypes and the risk of gastric cancer [39].

Recently, OLGA system has been modified for the assessment of IM (OLGIM) for the staging of chronic gastritis [52]. With respect to OLGA system, essentially based on atrophy, OLGIM system provided a significantly higher agreement between pathologists. However, the practical value of this system in predicting the development of dysplasia or cancer needs to be addressed. At present, the reversibility of metaplasia involving the gastric mucosa is considered controversial. Although eradication of *H. pylori* has been associated with the reversibility of IM in some studies [53–55], in other studies cancer risk decreased only after eradication in patients with nonatrophic mucosa [56–58].

Another pattern of metaplasia, spasmolytic polypeptide-expressing metaplasia (SPEM), is a metaplastic mucous cell lineage with morphological features and the phenotype of deep antral glands, including strong expression of trefoil factor (TFF)2, a member of small secretory peptides, which plays a role in the protection and repair of the gastrointestinal mucosa [59], and MUC6.

It has been reported that SPEM is strongly associated with *H. pylori* infection, since it was detected in 68% of infected patients, and it has been also seen in the setting of autoimmune atrophic gastritis targeting parietal cells in the corpus [60]. Moreover, recent studies have shown that SPEM is associated with 90% of gastric adenocarcinomas and have suggested that SPEM may play a role in the preneoplastic process [60–62].

Helicobacter pylori **Infection and Gastric Cancer**

H. pylori is the most common chronic pathogen in humans, since more than 50% of the world population is infected. Nowadays, it is the only bacteria classified as a class I carcinogen by the WHO [63], as confirmed by numerous epidemiologic studies on the association of *H. pylori* infection and risk of gastric cancer. However, considering that only 1–3% of infected people actually develop gastric cancer, it has been suggested that other factors, including the host, may also play a role in carcinoma development [64, 65].

On the basis of the undoubted strong correlation between *H. pylori* infection and gastric cancer, the Maastricht III Guidelines recommend to treat the infection in peptic ulcer diseases, mucosa-associated lymphoid tissue lymphomas, atrophic gastritis, patients after resection of gastric cancer, first-degree relatives of gastric cancer patients, patients with unexplained iron deficiency anaemia, patients with idiopathic thrombocytopenia purpura, patients who require long-term non-steroidal anti-inflammatory drugs (NSAIDs) and patients who just wish to be treated [66].

Diet

Diet exerts an important role in gastric carcinogenesis, especially in intestinal-type adenocarcinoma and in combination with *H. pylori* infection [67–69]. In this regard, high intake of fresh fruits and vegetables, Mediterranean diet, a low-sodium diet, salt-preserved food, red and high cured meat, adequate alcohol intake and maintaining a proper body weight might be associated with a decreased risk of gastric cancer [70–72]. Functional foods such as fresh fruits and dark green, light green and yellow vegetables rich in β-carotene, vitamins C and E and folate may exhibit a protective action in gastric cancer, probably due to their antioxidant effect. Among these compounds, β-carotene seems to be the leading risk reducer [73]. Nevertheless, the outcomes of a recent meta-analysis of randomized trials comparing the effect of antioxidant supplements with placebo or no intervention did not show a significant effect on the incidence of gastric cancer [74], even though the nutritional basic conditions of the populations seem to influence the results [75]. On the contrary, high plasma concentration of carotenoids, α-tocopherol and retinol was found to be associated with reduced risk of gastric cancer [76]. Therefore, further investigations are required.

Smoking

Several studies have confirmed that tobacco smoking increases the risk of gastric cancer, both cardia and non-cardia subtypes [77, 78]. The risk of gastric carcinoma is increased by 60% in male and 20% in female smokers compared to non-smokers. Moreover, this risk decreases in former smokers compared with occasional smokers, while smokers with higher consumption of cigarettes (>20 cigarettes per day) have a higher risk to develop gastric cancer [77].

The Operated Stomach and Cancer

Gastric stump cancer is a carcinoma that occurs in the gastric remnant at least 5 years after the surgery for peptic ulcer [79]. This gastric cancer subtype represents from 1.1% to 7% of all gastric carcinomas, with a prevalent disposition in male [80–82]. Gastrectomy is a well-documented risk factor for gastric stump cancer, even long time after the initial surgery [83, 84]: in fact, after 15 years from the gastrectomy, the risk to develop this cancer is increased from four- to sevenfold if compared with the general population [83, 85].

The infection with Epstein-Barr virus (EBV), a human herpesvirus for which a causal role in gastric carcinogenesis has been suggested [86], is more often present in gastric remnants than in intact stomachs [87] and may interact with the p53 protein [88]. In contrast, *H. pylori* infection in gastric stump cancer is less frequent [89]. Well-defined precursor lesions, mostly by dysplasia, commonly precede gastric stump cancer and therefore, endoscopic surveillance with multiple biopsies of the gastroenterostoma is recommended [90].

Pathology

Several systems have been proposed to classify gastric adenocarcinoma on the basis of macroscopic features (Borrmann) [91] or exclusively on the histological tumour growth pattern (Ming, Carneiro, Goseki) [92–94]. The two most commonly used histological classifications are the

Lauren and World Health Organization (WHO) systems (Table 4.2) [3, 95]. More recently, molecular classifications based on gene expression profiles and proteomics have been proposed; however, these have not yet used in routine [96–98].

Topography and Macroscopic Features of Gastric Adenocarcinoma

Adenocarcinoma may occur everywhere in the gastric mucosa. From the classification point of view, it is important to distinguish the oesophagogastric junction (OGJ) cancer from any other site in the gastric wall. The term oesophagogastric junction (OGJ) corresponds to the anatomical region where the oesophagus ends and the stomach begins. Several classification systems of OGJ tumours have been proposed on the basis of localization of tumour epicentre with respect of OGJ.

According to WHO classification:

1. Adenocarcinomas crossing the OGJ are considered as adenocarcinoma of OGJ, without taking into account the localization of remaining bulk of tumour.
2. Adenocarcinomas located entirely above the OGJ are considered to be oesophageal carcinomas.
3. Adenocarcinomas located entirely below the OGJ are considered as gastric carcinomas, also referred to as "adenocarcinoma of proximal stomach".

Table 4.2 Laurén and World Health Organization classification systems of gastric cancer

Laurén	World Health Organization 2010
Intestinal type	Papillary adenocarcinoma Tubular adenocarcinoma Mucinous adenocarcinoma
Diffuse type	Poorly cohesive carcinoma (including signet-ring cell carcinoma and other variants)
Mixed type	Adenocarcinoma and undifferentiated carcinoma
Indeterminate	Adenosquamous carcinoma Carcinoma with lymphoid stroma (medullary carcinoma) Hepatoid adenocarcinoma Squamouscell carcinoma

Modified from Ref. [39]

For the latter one, in 2017, the 8th Edition of Union for International Cancer Control (UICC) TNM classification [99] has proposed some modifications in the staging assessment, based on the tumour epicentre and tumour extension. Similarly, the TNM classification of the American Joint Committee on Cancer (AJCC) [100] refers to gastric or oesophageal staging systems, with a slight difference in the definition of anatomical limit of location of tumour epicentre (see also section "Staging of Gastric Carcinoma" in this chapter).

Advanced gastric carcinoma can display various macroscopic features. As previously mentioned, Borrmann's classification is the most commonly used. This classification divides gastric carcinoma into four distinct types [91] as reported in the Fig. 4.2.

Polypoid and fungating tumours typically consist of friable, ulcerated masses that bleed easily and project from a broad base in the gastric lumen. Characterized by sharp raised margins, they tend to develop in the body of stomach, in the region of greater curvature, posterior wall or fundus (see Fig. 4.2a, b).

Ulcerated carcinomas occur frequently in the OGJ, antrum or lesser curvature. They can be distinguished by benign ulcers for an irregular margin with raised borders and thickened, uneven and indurated surrounding mucosa. Furthermore, malignant ulcers tend to be larger than the benign ones. Nevertheless, in many malignant ulcers, these typical features are absent; thus endoscopic appearance should be supported by complemented biopsies (Fig. 4.2c).

Invasive adenocarcinoma may spread superficially in the mucosa and submucosa or infiltrates the wall (see Fig. 4.2d) which may become diffusely indurated as a consequence of an intense desmoplastic reaction (linitis plastica, Fig. 4.3). In such cases, there is usually non-visible localized growth.

Outer of classified types, other gastric carcinomas can secrete a considerable amount of mucins, which confers to tumours a gelatinous appearance at naked eye, such to be defined as mucinous or colloid carcinomas.

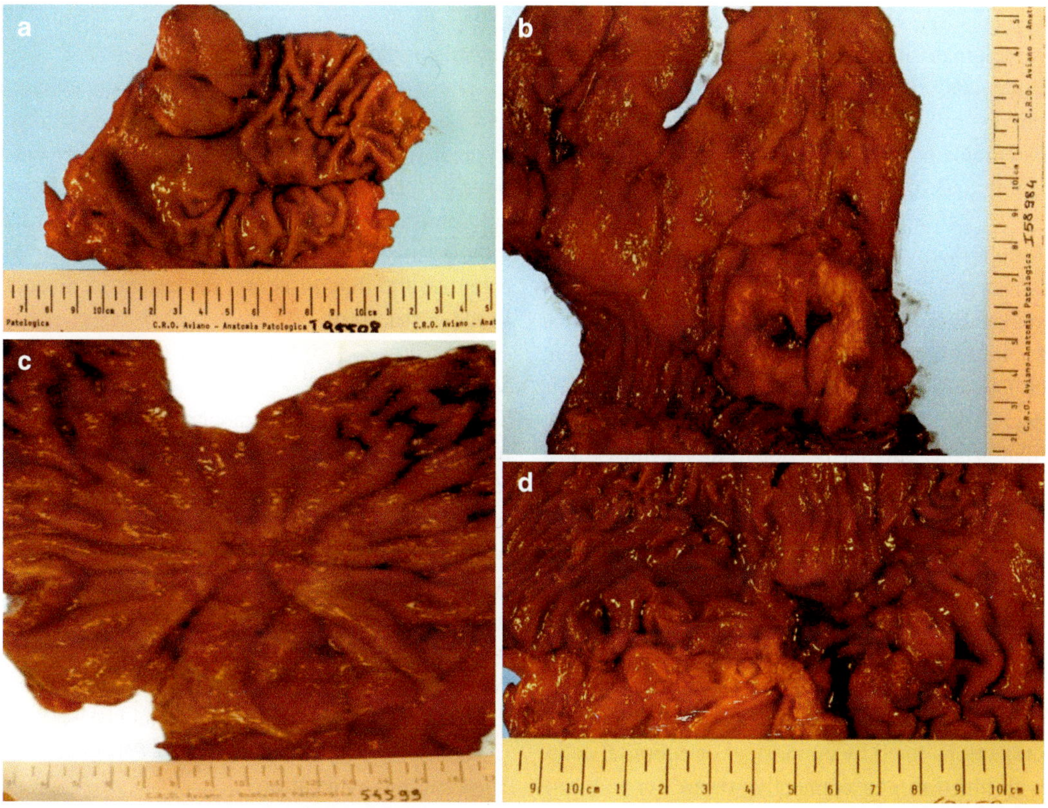

Fig. 4.2 Borrmann classification of gastric carcinomas. (**a**) type I, polypoid; (**b**) type II fungating, (**c**) type III ulcerated; (**d**) type IV, scirrhous, diffusely infiltrating

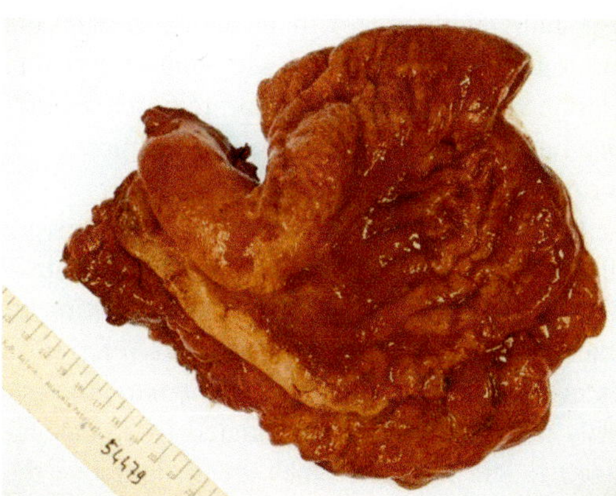

Fig. 4.3 Linitis plastic

Microscopic Features

At microscopic level, proximal and distal gastric adenocarcinomas show similar characteristics, despite their epidemiological differences. On the basis of contributions emerging from intratumoural variations in architecture and/or differentiation, several histological classifications have been proposed over the years.

The WHO Classification

In 2010, the WHO revised the classification of gastric adenocarcinoma, without taking into account the histogenesis and differentiation, but according to the morphological patterns commonly exhibited by tumours in other gastrointestinal sites, such as the small bowel, ampulla of Vater and colon [3]. The 2010 WHO classification recognizes five major types of gastric adenocarcinoma based on the predominant histological growth pattern: (1) papillary, (2) tubular, (3) mucinous (tumours with mucinous pools exceeding 50% of the tumour), (4) poorly cohesive (including signet-ring cell carcinoma and other variants) and (5) mixed adenocarcinomas

(Table 4.2) [3]. Uncommon variants of gastric carcinomas include the squamous cell, adenosquamous, hepatoid, parietal cell, Paneth cell, micropapillary, undifferentiated subtypes and carcinoma with lymphoid stroma (medullary carcinoma) [3, 101].

Tubular Adenocarcinomas

Branching tubules, varying in their diameter and acinar structures, are the main morphological features. Individual tumour cells are columnar, cuboidal or flattened by intraluminal mucin. The degree of cytological atypia varies from low- to high-grade. Tubular adenocarcinoma may show morphological variants, from a poorly differentiated, sometimes called solid carcinoma, to a lymphoid stroma-rich tumour (medullary carcinoma) or a desmoplastic tumour.

Papillary Adenocarcinomas

Papillary adenocarcinomas are well-differentiated exophytic carcinomas with elongated frond-like projections lined by cylindrical or cuboidal cells, with fibrovascular connective tissue cores. Some tumours show tubular differentiation (tubulo-papillary). The degree of cellular atypia and mitotic index may be variable.

Mucinous Adenocarcinomas

Extracellular mucinous pools must represent 50% or more of the tumour. Glands are lined by a columnar mucous-secreting epithelium, together with interstitial mucin, or the tumour is composed by chains or irregular cell clusters floating in mucinous lakes. A discrete component of signet-ring cells may be present but usually is not prominent.

Poorly Cohesive Carcinoma, Including Signet-Ring Cell Carcinomas

More than 50% of the tumour consists of isolated or small groups of malignant cells containing intracytoplasmic mucin that frequently displaces the nuclei at the periphery of the cytoplasm, creating a classical signet-ring cell appearance due to a globoid, optically clear cytoplasm. Other diffuse carcinomas contain cells with central nuclei resembling histiocytes, showing little or no mitotic activity; or small, deeply eosinophilic cells with or without mucins or finally anaplastic cells devoid of mucin.

These cell types intermingle with one another and constitute varying tumour proportions. Typically, signet-ring cell carcinomas may harbour diffuse desmoplasia with dispersed tumour cells in the stroma. Cytokeratin immunostaining may be useful in some difficult case in order to establish the diagnosis and the extent of disease in the gastric wall.

Mixed Carcinomas

These gastric carcinomas are composed of a mixture of morphologically identifiable glandular (tubular/papillary) and poorly cohesive cellular histological components. Mixed carcinomas have been shown to be clonal [102, 103] with phenotypic divergence attributed to somatic mutation in E-cadherin gene (CDH1) and restricted to the poorly cohesive component [104]. Epigenetic changes have also been seen to be implicated in the histogenesis of mixed carcinoma [105].

The Laurén Classification

The Laurén classification is applied in routine practice by pathologists, and it is commonly used by epidemiologists and clinicians for evaluating the natural history of gastric adenocarcinoma, especially with regard to incidence trends and etiologic precursors [106], although all existing classifications of gastric adenocarcinoma, including Laurén's one, are of limited significance in terms of therapeutic decisions [97].

In this classification system, the tumours are distinct in two types: intestinal or diffuse. Tumours which present an equal proportion of intestinal and diffuse components are referred to as mixed carcinomas. At the same way, tumour cells that are too undifferentiated to be categorized in the reported types are assigned in the indeterminate category.

Intestinal Carcinomas

As the most common subtype, the intestinal carcinoma occurs in about 54% of the cases, with a prevalence twofold higher in males compared to females and localized mostly in the antrum. Histopathologically, it is characterized by recognizable glands that range from well differentiated

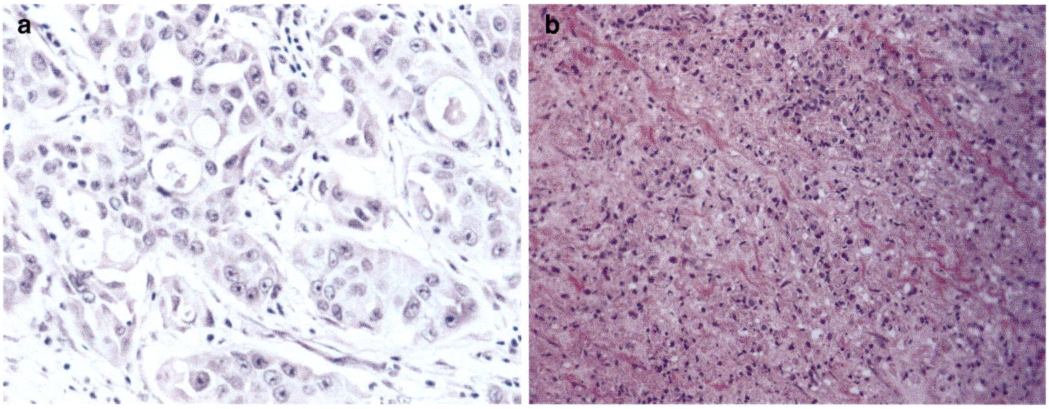

Fig. 4.4 Laurén classification of gastric adenocarcinomas. (**a**) Intestinal type; (**b**) diffuse type

to moderately differentiated, sometimes with poorly differentiated tumour areas (Fig. 4.4a). Intestinal carcinomas typically arise on a background of intestinal metaplasia. However, at cellular level, despite their classification into intestinal carcinomas, these cells may show morphological and immunological differentiation typical of gastric and gastrointestinal cells, or null differentiation, over the intestinal type. For this reason, the prognostic relevance of Laurén classification remains controversial [107].

Diffuse Carcinomas

By contrast, the diffuse subtype (32%) is characterized by tumour cells that are poorly cohesive and diffusely infiltrating the gastric wall with little or no gland formation (Fig. 4.4b). Small amounts of interstitial mucin may be present. Desmoplasia is more pronounced and associated inflammation is less evident in diffuse cancers than in the intestinal carcinomas.

This subtype occurs equally often in males and females, and these patients are on average younger than those with intestinal carcinomas. The intestinal type of gastric cancer is felt to be caused mainly by environmental (exogenous) factors, whereas the diffuse type is thought to be due to hereditary and genetic (endogenous) factors [108].

Albeit the intestinal and diffuse gastric carcinoma subtypes are pathologically considered as separate entities, from the clinical point of view, they are treated similarly. Clinically, the main difference is related to the distinct recurrence patterns, with the diffuse-mixed types more prone to peritoneal dissemination, especially when the serosa is involved, whereas the risk of liver metastases is higher in the intestinal type [108].

Comparing the Laurén and the WHO classifications, tubular and papillary adenocarcinomas fall within the intestinal type of stomach cancer, whereas signet-ring cell carcinoma and other poorly cohesive carcinomas correspond to the Laurén diffuse type (Table 4.2) [109].

Goseki Classification

The Goseki classification divides gastric cancer, based on intracellular mucin production and the degree of tubular differentiation, into four groups:

1. Group I: tubules well differentiated, intracellular mucin poor
2. Group II: tubules well differentiated, intracellular mucin rich
3. Group III: tubules poorly differentiated, intracellular mucin poor
4. Group IV: tubules poorly differentiated, intracellular mucin rich

Notably, prognostic value has been attributed to this classification system [94, 110].

The Dawn of Phenotypic Classification

A classification based on four histotypes has been proposed by Carneiro and colleagues in 1997 [111]:

1. Glandular and isolated cell carcinomas (approximately equivalent to the intestinal and diffuse carcinomas of Laurén classification)
2. A solid variety (composed of sheets, trabeculae or islands of undifferentiated cells with no glandular formation)
3. A mixed type consisting of glandular and isolated cell types mixture

This classification has been shown to have a prognostic significance [112].

The introduction of markers of cell differentiation allowed to obtain more information on the tumours histogenesis and classification. The following markers have been used:

- Mucin MUC5AC and trefoil peptide TFF1 as markers of surface gastric epithelium (foveolar cells) (Fig. 4.5a)
- MUC6 and TFF2 as markers of mucous neck cell, pyloric gland and Brunner's gland cells
- MUC2, CDX2 and CD10 as intestinal cell markers (Fig. 4.5b)

As a consequence, four phenotypes of gastric carcinomas have been identified:

1. Gastric
2. Mixed gastric and intestinal (further divisible in predominant gastric or intestinal type)
3. Intestinal
4. Unclassifiable or null phenotype (lack of these markers) [113–115]

Additionally, pepsinogen-1 staining helped to distinguish mucous neck/pseudo-pyloric type from true pyloric type [115].

This classification has evidenced the limit of Laurén classification into identifying tumours showing gastric phenotype (positive for selected markers) with the inappropriate term of "intestinal" carcinomas. Therefore, these findings had consequences also on the classical multistep process of gastric carcinogenesis [111, 116–118].

Although current histopathological systems influence endoscopic or surgical choices, they are still insufficient to guide precision treatments for individual patients. Not only new therapies, but a new classification for gastric carcinoma is needed as well [108].

The overwhelming majority of common gastric cancers are adenocarcinomas, for which the origin from a progenitor cell specializing towards an exocrine cell lineage has been hypothesized [119]. Nevertheless, several reports have shown that (neuro)endocrine markers chromogranin A (CgA) and/or synaptophysin (Syn) have been found immunohistochemically in about 15–70% of conventional gastric adenocarcinomas, on the basis of different criteria applied or variation in the sensitivity of antibodies used [120–124].

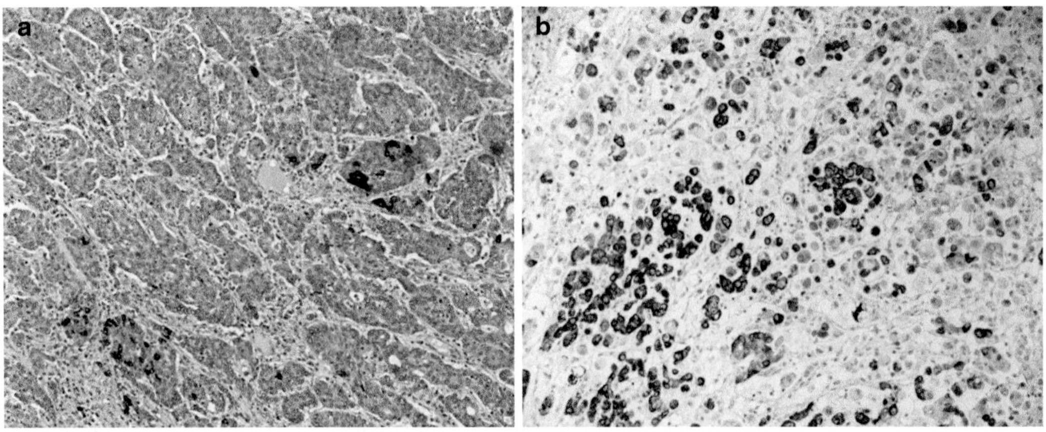

Fig. 4.5 Expression of (**a**) gastric mucin MUC5AC and (**b**) intestinal mucin MUC2 in two different cases of gastric adenocarcinoma

Jiang et al. [125] reported that adenocarcinomas of the stomach with more than 20% of the tumour cells expressing CgA and/or Syn, the so-called large cell neuroendocrine carcinomas (LCNEC), significantly correlated with a poorer overall survival rate than adenocarcinomas without endocrine differentiation or up to 20% of tumour cells expressing CgA and/or Syn (adenocarcinomas with neuroendocrine differentiation, ACNED).

Canzonieri et al. [23] evaluated the diagnostic and prognostic implications of endocrine differentiation in 103 common gastric adenocarcinomas (n = 71) and undifferentiated carcinomas (n = 32). Maturely differentiated exocrine and endocrine phenotypes were evaluated by using gastric exocrine markers (MUC5AC and MUC6) and endocrine markers (gastrin and somatostatin, in CgA- and/or Syn-positive tumours) along with intestinal exocrine (MUC2, villin and CD10) and endocrine markers (glucagon-like peptide-1, GLP-1, and gastric inhibitory polypeptide, GIP, in CgA- and/or Syn-positive tumours).

Immunohistochemical analysis revealed that 66 tumours (64%) were positive for generic endocrine markers such as CgA and/or Syn. The 14 patients with more than 20% tumour cells positive for at least 1 endocrine marker (LCNEC) experienced a poorer prognosis than patients with no (n = 37) or 1% to 20% (n = 52) positivity (ACNED). The 16 carcinomas expressing the maturely differentiated exocrine gastric phenotype significantly correlated with poorer outcome compared with carcinomas with mature exocrine intestinal (n = 22) or mixed/gastrointestinal phenotypes (at least 1 gastric and 1 intestinal exocrine phenotype marker simultaneously positive, n = 64).

Among tumours expressing CgA and/or Syn, the maturely differentiated endocrine gastric phenotype (n = 26) was a negative prognostic factor compared with mature endocrine intestinal (n = 21) and mixed/gastrointestinal (n = 5) phenotypes.

On the basis of these results, it has been demonstrated that endocrine differentiation and maturely exocrine/endocrine gastric phenotypes are associated with an unfavourable prognosis and may identify subsets of patients for tailored therapy [23].

Unusual Variants of Gastric Carcinoma

Several other uncommon histological variants of gastric carcinomas exist (5%) that are not an integral part of the above-mentioned classification system.

Adenosquamous and Squamous Cell Carcinoma

To be diagnosed, neoplastic squamous cells, characterized by keratin pearl formation and intercellular bridge, in addition to glandular element, must be detected in primary adenosquamous carcinoma [126]. At ultrastructural level, these neoplastic cells showed differentiation features typical of both squamous and adenosquamous cells, supporting the hypothesis of their origin from multipotent stem cells [127]. These tumours are often localized in the antrum and show lymphovascular permeation. This variant may pose some problems of interpretation of peculiar findings:

1. Metastases usually contain both glandular and squamous components, but, sometimes, only one component may be present.
2. A tumour with a distinct boundary between the two components may represent a collision tumour.
3. Tumours containing discrete foci of benign-appearing squamous metaplasia are termed adenocarcinomas with squamous differentiation (adenoacanthoma).

Pure squamous cell carcinomas develop rarely in the stomach [128, 129] and are usually diagnosed in advanced stages, thus having a poor prognosis [130]. Pure squamous cell carcinoma of the stomach possibly arises from squamous metaplasia of an adenocarcinoma, from heterotopic squamous epithelium or from multipotent stem cells showing bidirectional differentiation [130, 131].

Hepatoid Adenocarcinoma

Large polygonal eosinophilic hepatocyte-like neoplastic cells can be observed as interspersed elements in a small number of carcinomas of the stomach. These neoplastic cells may produce consistent amount of α-fetoprotein (AFP), as revealed by in situ detection and in the serum [132]. Hepatoid adenocarcinoma has generally been reported in patients older than 50 years, even though it has been occasionally diagnosed in younger patients [133, 134]. These carcinomas are characterized by advanced bulky polypoid tumours with ulceration, necrotic and haemorrhagic areas. Antrum is the most common site where the development of hepatoid adenocarcinoma has been described, followed by the fundus and, with a lower frequency, the cardia [133]. Tumour heterogeneity is demonstrated by hepatoid foci mixed with adenocarcinoma, often presenting papillary pattern, and less differentiated areas characterized by giant and spindle cells [132–136].

Since these cells express typical markers of intestinal cells, the histogenesis of hepatoid adenocarcinoma from an intestinal phenotype has been suggested [137]. Clinical evidences showed an extensive vascular infiltration of these adenocarcinomas, as demonstrated by the high incidence of liver and lymph node metastases and poorer prognosis compared with typical adenocarcinoma of the stomach [132, 134, 138, 139]. At molecular level, the presence of albumin, AFP, α_1-antichymotripsin and bile production have been demonstrated by immunohistochemical and in situ hybridization studies [140–142]. Recently, PLUNC (palate, lung and nasal epithelium carcinoma-associated protein) has been described as hepatoid adenocarcinoma marker [143].

Since it is difficult to distinguish a liver metastasis from gastric hepatoid adenocarcinoma and primary hepatocellular carcinoma (HCC) in a liver biopsy, it is useful adopting the immunostaining for Hep-Par-1 that extensively stains most HCCs, whereas only focal staining of Hep-Par-1 is observed in gastric hepatoid adenocarcinoma [144].

Gastric Choriocarcinoma

For a pathological diagnosis of choriocarcinoma of the stomach, the assessment of cytotrophoblast and syncytiotrophoblast is a prerequisite, and it can be confirmed by human chorionic gonadotropin (hCG)-positive cells in immunohistochemical tests [145–148] and by high levels of hCG in the blood [146, 147, 149]. Other histological features are intratumoural haemorrhage, necrosis and vascular invasion.

Gastric Carcinoma with Lymphoid Stroma

Infection with Epstein-Barr virus (EBV) has been detected in up to 18% of gastric carcinomas [150], and over 80% of gastric lymphomas are related to EBV infection [151]. These gastric carcinomas, with well-defined margins, prevalently occur at the proximal stomach, including at the stump of patients undergoing subtotal gastrectomy [152]. At histological level, the tumours are typically composed of irregular sheets, trabeculae, ill-defined tubules or syncytia of polygonal cells mixed with a prominent lymphocytic infiltrate.

As revealed by immunophenotypic analysis, the main component of the infiltrate is represented by CD8-positive T cells, followed in a minor extent by B lymphocytes, plasma cells, neutrophils and eosinophils and more rarely by giant cells [153]. The main differential diagnosis, in these cases, is with the gastric lymphomas. Compared to typical gastric carcinomas, gastric lymphomas occur in slightly younger age and prevalently in males [152, 154, 155] and has a better prognosis [87, 154, 156, 157].

Albeit it is not detected in normal gastric mucosa or intestinal metaplasia, EBV is revealed in dysplasia [158]. However, further investigations concerning the role of EBV are required to clarify if this virus intervenes directly in carcinogenesis process or occurs as secondary infection [159] in early stage.

Gastric Carcinosarcoma

Carcinosarcoma of the stomach is a rare biphasic tumour that consists of both carcinomatous and sarcomatous components. The sarcomatous components may be differentiated into leiomyosarcoma, rhabdomyosarcoma and osteosarcoma [160–163]. Occurrences of adenosquamous components combined with neuroendocrine cells have also been reported in these neoplasms [164–167]. Gastric carcinosarcoma is usually associated with poor prognosis [168].

Micropapillary Carcinoma

Micropapillary carcinoma is rare and histologically is characterized by irregular small clusters of neoplastic cells in clear lacunar spaces simulating lymphatic or vascular channels. Micropapillary carcinomas differ from tubular or papillary carcinomas because, histologically, they lack fibrovascular stalks and show an extensive lymphovascular tumour invasion and high metastatic potential. Moreover, the recognition of a micropapillary carcinoma component, which may range from 5% to 80%, is important, because it is associated with poorer prognosis in an otherwise common adenocarcinoma [101, 169].

Parietal Cell Carcinoma

Bulky lesions at both gastric body and antrum level have been reported as prevalent features of these exceedingly rare tumours [170]. With an expanding growth pattern, these neoplasms present sheets of cells containing small gland-like clefts. These tumour cells are similar to acid-secreting parietal cells, since they have eosinophilic granular cytoplasm and positively stain for PTAH (phosphotungstic acid haematoxylin) and Luxol fast blue. Moreover, they are immunopositive for parietal cell-specific antibodies, for H^+/K^+ ATPase and for human milk fat globule-2. Additionally, ultrastructural evaluation reveals numerous mitochondria and intracellular canaliculi [170–172]. Lymph node metastases are not particularly extensive, and the prognosis seems to be more favourable than other usual gastric adenocarcinomas [171].

Gastric Mucoepidermoid Carcinoma

These neoplasms are extremely rare and show mixed morphological features between mucus-producing and squamous epithelia [173].

Paneth Cell Carcinoma

As indicated by its designation, the predominant cells in these tumours are Paneth cells, which show eosinophilic cytoplasmic granules that are immunopositive for lysozyme [174, 175]. However, it must be noted that Paneth cells can be found dispersed among typical gastric adenocarcinomas [30, 176].

Gastric Malignant Rhabdoid Tumour

With poor prognosis, this carcinoma is characterized by poorly cohesive, round-to-polygonal cells with eosinophilic or clear cytoplasm and large nuclei with predominant nucleoli. In addition to a strong immunoreactivity to vimentin, these cancer cells are also immunopositive for cytokeratin, epithelial membrane antigen (EMA) and focal neuron-specific enolase (NSE) and immunonegative for carcinoembryonic antigen (CEA) [177–179].

Undifferentiated Carcinoma

With this terminology are indicated all gastric tumours that don't exhibit any differentiation, but only epithelial phenotype at least in part (e.g. cytokeratin expression) and that fall into indeterminate category of Laurén classification.

Staging of Gastric Carcinoma

Early Gastric Cancer

Early gastric cancer (EGC) is defined as intramucosal or submucosal tumour invasion independent of lymph node involvement [96]. Although the designation seems to be linked to the stage of cancer genesis, the term EGC indicates the possibility for these neoplasms to be cured [180]. Nevertheless, if not treated, 63% of EGC cases have been seen to evolve in advanced tumours within 5 years [181]. Albeit EGC represents 15–21% of all gastric cancers in the Western world, it accounts for more than 50% of the gastric carcinomas in Japan [3, 182, 183]. It could be speculated that these differences are probably related to endoscopic screening programmes implemented in Japan, although differences in diagnostic criteria may also play a role [39]. Specifically, most EGCs show dimensions ranging between 20 and 50 mm and occur in the lesser curvature and around the angulus [184, 185]. EGCs may exhibit different behaviours in terms of invasiveness: if some expanded only in the lateral sense, others, although the reduced size (3–5 mm), can invade into the submucosa [186, 187].

On the basis of endoscopic appearance, the Japanese Gastric Cancer Association classified EGCs as protruded (type I), elevated (type II), including the subtypes IIa (elevated type), IIb (flat type) and IIc (depressed type), and excavated (type III).

Histologically, especially for minute EGCs (<20 mm), a well-defined glandular differentiation can be observed, even though histological changes occur in the course of cancer development. Moreover, a weakly correlation of reported types with microscopic appearance could be observed: in fact, over 50% of EGCs corresponds to the tubular variant and 30% to the papillary one, which are, respectively, associated with types I and II of Japanese classification. Similarly, signet-ring cell carcinoma and poorly differentiated carcinoma represent 25% and 15% of EGCs and are usually associated with types IIc and III [182, 184, 188].

The risk of deep and multifocal penetration into the submucosa and the risk of lymphatic invasion are higher in type IIc, the depressed variant of type II.

Advanced Gastric Cancer

A substantial modification of TNM classification of gastric tumours has been operated in 2017 [99, 100].

As it has been reported in Table 4.3, the modification consists in the subdivision of T1 in two entities to distinguish the depth of tumour invasion in the mucosa and submucosa, the transition of stage T2a into T2 (muscularis propria) and T2b into T3 (subserosa), followed by the redefinition of tumour which penetrates the serosa or invades adjacent structures as, respectively, T4a and T4b, rather than as T3 and T4.

Concerning the staging of adenocarcinoma of the OGJ, it depends on the location of epicentre: if the centre of tumour, which extends into the oesophagus, is located within 2 cm of the OGJ, the adenocarcinoma is staged in accordance to the scheme of the oesophageal carcinoma. Alternatively, as it has been proposed by TNM classification of UICC, tumours of which epicentre in the stomach is more than 2 cm far from the OGJ are staged according to the scheme for gastric carcinoma, even if the OGJ is involved [99]. The TNM classification of AJCC is essentially in agreement with these definitions, but in the case of tumours centred within 2 cm of the OGJ, they can be staging by gastric carcinoma system, if they not cross the OGJ [100].

Pattern of Spread

Gastric carcinomas can spread by direct extension to adjacent organs, lymphatic and/or peritoneal dissemination.

Direct Extension of the Tumour

When the serosa was penetrated, gastric cancer cells can spread to the pancreas, liver, spleen, transverse colon and greater omentum. Often, an early transperitoneal dissemination can be observed. It has been reported that neoplasms at the OGJ infiltrate into the wall at the lower end of the oesophagus, whereas tumours at distal level tend to microscopically extend within the duodenum [189]. Carcinomas composed by poorly cohesive cells preferentially metastasize to serosal surface and show a widespread intramural permeation of small lymphovascular vessels. Therefore, these neoplasms commonly invade the duodenum via either submucosal or subserosal routes or the submucosal lymphatics [190]. Duodenal invasion occurs more frequently than expected based on gross examination. Therefore, resection margins should be monitored by intraoperative consultation.

Lymphatic Spread

A deeper invasiveness of tumour correlates with a major incidence of lymph node metastases [191], of which distribution differs according to the tumour location, but commonly involved nodes along the lesser and greater curves of the

Table 4.3 TNM classification of gastric tumours

Carcinoma of the stomach			
T – Primary tumour			
TX	Primary tumour cannot be assessed		
T0	No evidence of primary tumour		
Tis	Carcinoma in situ		
T1	Tumour invades lamina propria, muscularis mucosae or submucosa: T1a: Tumour invades lamina propria or muscularis mucosae T1b: Tumour invades submucosa		
T2	Tumour invades muscularis propria		
T3	Tumour penetrates subserosal tissue without invasion of visceral peritoneum or adjacent structures[a]		
T4	Tumour perforates serosa or adjacent structures T4a: Tumour penetrates serosa (visceral peritoneum)[b] T4b: Tumour directly invades adjacent organs or structures[c]		
N – Regional lymph nodes[d]			
NX	Regional lymph node(s) cannot be assessed		
N0	No regional lymph node metastases		
N1	Metastases in 1-2 regional lymph nodes		
N2	Metastases in 3-6 regional lymph nodes		
N3a	Metastases in 7-15 regional lymph nodes		
N3b	Metastases in 16 or more regional lymph nodes		
	Regional lymph nodes groups		
	Perigastric lymph nodes		
	Perigastric along greater curvature		
	Perigastric along lesser curvature		
	Right and left paracardial (cardio-oesophageal)		
	Suprapyloric		
	Infrapyloric		
	Second tier nodes		
	Left gastric artery		
	Celiac artery		
	Common hepatic artery		
	Hepatoduodenal (along proper hepatic artery, including portal)		
	Splenic artery		
	Splenic hilum		
M – Distant metastasis			
M0	No distant metastases		
M1[e,f]	Distant metastases Liver Peritoneum Non-regional lymph nodes Lung, CNS – less common		
Clinical Stage Groups (cTNM)			
Stage	**T**	**N**	**M**
Stage 0	Tis	N0	M0
Stage I	T1 T2	N0 N0	M0 M0
Stage IIA	T1 T2	N1, N2 or N3 N1, N2 or N3	M0 M0
Stage IIB	T3 T4a	N0 N0	M0 M0

(continued)

Table 4.3 (continued)

Stage III	T3 T4a	N1, N2 or N3 N1, N2 or N3	M0 M0
Stage IVA	T4b	Any N	M0
Stage IVB	Any T	Any N	M1
Pathological Stage Groups (pTNM)			
Stage	**T**	**N**	**M**
Stage 0	Tis	N0	M0
Stage IA	T1	N0	M0
Stage IB	T1 T2	N1 N0	M0 M0
Stage IIA	T1 T2 T3	N2 N1 N0	M0 M0 M0
Stage IIB	T1 T2 T3 T4a	N3a N2 N1 N0	M0 M0 M0 M0
Stage IIIA	T2 T3 T4a T4a T4b	N3a N2 N1 N2 N0	M0 M0 M0 M0 M0
Stage IIIB	T1 T2 T3 T4a T4b T4b	N3b N3b N3a N3a N1 N2	M0 M0 M0 M0 M0 M0
Stage IIIC	T3 T4a T4b T4b	N3b N3b N3a N3b	M0 M0 M0 M0
Stage IV	Any T	Any N	M1

Modified from Ref. [99]

[a]If the tumour invades greater or lesser omentum, gastrocolic or gastrohepatic ligaments without breach of peritoneum is classified as T3

[b]Beach of peritoneum corresponds to T4

[c]Intramural extension along alimentary canal into oesophagus or duodenum is not invasion of adjacent organ (ie. Not T4b)

[d]Metastatic carcinoma deposits in subserosal fat with no residual node and no vascular or neural structure are regarded as lymph node deposits

[e]Direct extension into liver, colon, pancreas, diaphragm is classified as T4b, not as M1

[f]Positive peritoneal cytology corresponds to M1

stomach. Mid-portion gastric carcinomas can metastasize into the pancreatic and splenic nodes, whereas lesions of the proximal stomach into mediastinal lymph nodes.

Haematogenous Spread

Even if lymph nodes are not involved, when gastric carcinomas invade the tributaries of the portal venous, spread through the bloodstream occurs and metastases can be commonly seen in liver, followed by the lung, peritoneum, adrenal glands, skin and ovaries.

Sometimes, the distribution of metastases depends on gastric histological type, since gland-forming carcinomas tend to form more likely metastases at liver by haematogenous spread than poorly cohesive carcinomas, whereas these latter are more likely to give rise to peritoneum and bone metastases than the gland-forming carcinomas [192].

Transperitoneal Spread

Secondary tumour deposits are frequently found in omentum, peritoneum and mesentery. Secondary ovarian deposits are well known as one form of Krukenberg's tumour more frequently associated with diffuse primary signet-ring carcinomas than gland-forming tumours. However, the presence of signet-ring cells within an ovarian mucinous tumour should not automatically exclude the extremely rare primary ovarian tumour.

In the Table 4.3 is reported the updated TNM classification of gastric carcinoma, with clinical and pathological stage groups. Clinical stage groups are different to pathological ones, since they are simplified for nodes, indicating only if they are involved or not, and as a consequence the stage cT4b NX M0, which has poor prognosis, is staged as IV. Furthermore, changes have also been introduced into pTNM groups with respect the previous edition, considering that pT4aN2 and pT4bN0 are now Stage IIIA rather than IIIB.

In addition to clinical and pathological stage, the AJCC also published post preoperative therapy prognostic groups for adenocarcinoma, classified as ypTNM.

Prognosis

Despite the ongoing decrease in morbidity and mortality, gastric cancer continues to be one of the leading types of fatal cancer worldwide. The majority of patients in the West are diagnosed with advanced disease, and only 6–10% of the cases is affected by early-stage cancer [108]. Therefore, in absence of a radical feasible surgery, the prognosis for these patients is poor. The late diagnosis can be due to absence of significant symptoms at an early stage and the lack of validated screening programmes. The expected 5-year survival rate for patients after surgery is approximately 26% in Western countries [193], whereas in Japan, it increases to 50% for T3 tumours and 60–80% for T2 adenocarcinoma [194, 195]. Furthermore, female sex and Japanase ethnicity are positively associated with survival rate as well as higher frequency of EGCs. Accurate staging and surgical expertise have been associated with improved survival in Japan compared to western countries [183, 196, 197]. A relevant feature in resectable cases is represented by complete tumour removal with negative edges [198]. However, despite the resection, it has been observed a local regional recurrence in 40% of the surgical cases and a systematic recurrence in 60% [199–201].

Hereditary Gastric Cancer Syndromes

Familial clustering represents about 10% of gastric cancers and approximately 1–3% arise from inhereted syndromes, which predispose to an incresed risk to develop this pathology [202]. These inherited syndromes include Familial Adenomatous Polyposis (FAP), Lynch syndrome [203–205], Li-Fraumeni syndrome and Peutz-Jeghers syndrome. In FAP patients, the risk to develop gastric cancer is sevenfold higher than the general population [206]. In Lynch syndrome, the high frequency to develop gastric carcinoma in earlier age than sporadic neoplasm is related to germline mutations of hMLH1 and hMSH2, genes of DNA mismatch repair (MMR) [203, 204, 207], as well as of TP53 in Li-Fraumeni syndrome [208]. Even though gastrointestinal cancer represents less than 10% of malignancies associated with syndrome, 50% of the cases are gastric cancer. Recently, it has also been reported that frameshift mutations in the STK11 gene in Peutz-Jeghers patients are responsible to the development of aggressive gastric cancers [209]. Moreover, a novel germline mutation of the LKB1 gene has been reported in a patient with sporadic Peutz-Jeghers syndrome with early onset of gastric cancer [210].

Criteria for Familial Gastric Cancer

Familial gastric cancers can be divided on the basis of knowledge of histopathology of the tumours: in absence of hystopathological characterization of carcinomas of individuals with familial aggregation, the carcinomas are simply referred to as familial gastric cancer (FGC), whereas when the histopathology of one or more neoplasms of individuals of familial aggregation are available, gastric cancers can be distinguished in hereditary diffuse gastric cancer (HDGC), familial diffuse gastric cancer (FDGC) and familial intestinal gastric cancer (FIGC).

Hereditary Diffuse Gastric Cancer (HDGC)

With this definition is indicated an autosomal-dominant syndrome associated with the development of signet-ring cell (diffuse) gastric cancer and lobular breast cancer. Germline mutations in the E-cadherin gene CDH1 are the genetic basis of the HDGC as discovered by Guilford in 1998 [211].

The International Gastric Cancer Linkage Consortium (IGCLC) defined families with HDGC syndrome on the basis of the meeting with one of the following clinical criteria:

1. Two or more documented cases of diffuse gastric cancer in first or second-degree relatives with at least one being diagnosed before the age of 50 years.
2. Three or more cases of documented diffuse gastric cancer in first- or second-degree relatives, independent of age of diagnosis [212].

Women of these mentioned families have an elevated risk of lobular breast cancer [213–217].

In 2010, the IGCLC criteria for genetic testing have been updated as reported in Table 4.4.

An alternative genetically-based nomenclature has been proposed, that restrains the term "HDGC" only to the families with germline mutations in the CDH1 gene [211, 218].

Table 4.4 Selected criteria for the genetic screening of suspected HDGC families

2 or more cases of diffuse gastric cancer in first or second-degree relatives, of which at least one diagnosed under the 50 years age
3 or more cases of confirmed diffuse type of gastric carcinoma in first- or second-degree relatives, independent of age of diagnosis
1 case of diffuse gastric cancer occurring before 40 years age, without a family history
Personal or family history of diffuse gastric carcinoma and lobular breast cancer, of which one diagnosed under the age of 50 years

In the clinically defined HDGC, mutations in the CDH1 gene have been reported in 30–40% of cases [216, 219, 220], most of which are truncating mutations and, in a minor extent, missense mutations [221, 222]. In absence of point mutations, large germline deletions have been described in 6.5% of HDGC families [220]. Furthermore, germline mutations can occur in the whole gene lenght of CDH1 and no hot spots have been identified.

A second CDH1 hit is required to initiate diffuse gastric carcinoma in mutant carriers. Most frequently, this occurs via promoter hypermethylation (epigenetic modification), and less frequently via CDH1 mutations and loss of heterozygosity (LOH) [223–225].

Because 60–70% of patients with HDGC are negative for CDH1 germline mutations, the attention is focused on the search for additional genes involved in HDGC.

Molecular Aspects of Gastric Carcinoma

The genomic changes involved in the multistep process of gastric carcinogenesis are the result of genetic and epigenetic abnormalities including (1) genomic instability through two distinct pathways: microsatellite instability (MSI) and chromosomal instability; (2) epigenetic alterations and (3) silencing of tumour-suppressor genes and activation of oncogenes.

Microsatellite Instability (MSI)

MSI is caused by defects in the DNA mismatch repair (MMR), a system able to recognize and correct nucleotide mismatches occurring during DNA replication. The MMR machinery consists of the MLH1, PMS2, MLH2, and MLH6 proteins.

Gastric cancers with MSI often show epigenetic silencing of the mutL homolog 1 (MLH1) gene. As member of MMR, when expressed, MLH1 protein plays an essential role in DNA mismatch repair and is responsible for fixing errors that occur during DNA replication. Furthermore, MSI-positive gastric cancers are often associated with activation of the epidermal growth factor receptor (EGFR) and PI3K pathways [226].

MSI has been detected in early stages of carcinogenesis including chronic gastritis, IM, dysplasia, and adenoma and in 15–49% of sporadic gastric cancers [227]. In gastric carcinomas, MSI is observed in 5–10% in diffuse type and in 15–40% of intestinal type.

Chromosomal Instability

About 80% of sporadic adenomas show chromosomal instability, which results in altered DNA copy numbers (aneuploidy) and various changes in chromosome regions, such as translocation, amplification, deletion or the loss of heterozygosity (LOH) [80]. Contrary to MSI, the mechanism underlying chromosomal instability is not well known. Aneuploidy results from alterations in mitotic segregation and centrosomal abnormalities [228]. Mechanisms and genes involved in aneuploidy have been reviewed by Aguilera and Gomez-Gonzalez [229].

Tumours characterized by chromosomal instability are frequently associated with activation of the RTK/RAS pathway and EGFR, HER2, HER3, JAK2, FGFR2, MET, PIK3CA and KRAS/NRAS amplifications [230].

Epigenetic Alterations

Several studies have proved that epigenetic alterations affected the cancer-related genes (i.e. APC, KRAS, TP53, hMLH1, CDKN2A/p16) even more commonly than genetic mutations [231–233]. Hypermethylation associated with gene silencing occurs at specific sites of the promoter sequences, defined as CpG islands [234]. The simultaneous hypermethylation of CpG island of multiple genes is referred to as CpG island methylator phenotype (CIMP). An increasing frequency of promoter methylation involving multiple genes has been shown to occur in the progression from chronic gastritis to carcinoma [235]. Tumours with multiple concurrently hypermethylated *loci* are described as high-CIMP. High-CIMP is frequently found in MSI-positive gastric cancers, and is associated with hypermethylation of MMR genes (hMLH1), as previously reported [232]. The CIMP phenotype is thought to be an early event in gastric cancer. Its presence in adjacent normal tissue may be associated with *H. pylori* infection, which points to the possible mechanism of its contribution to gastric carcinogenesis [232].

Moreover, recent studies revealed that CIMP is more prevalent in the diffuse as opposed to the intestinal type of gastric cancer [236, 237].

Tumour-Suppressor Genes

Several tumour-suppressor genes have been reported in the development of gastric cancers, such as CDH1 [238–242] and RB1 [243] in diffuse-type carcinomas and APC [244–247] and DCC [248, 249] in intestinal-type carcinomas. In this regard, somatic mutations in the APC gene are present in 6% of IM and in 20–40% of gastric adenomas and therefore are also considered as an early event in gastric carcinogenesis [3, 227].

Other genes such as PTEN and TP53 are deregulated in both types of gastric carcinoma, even though alteration of TP53 has been seen to be more common in intestinal-type carcinoma [246, 250–253]. As it has been reported for APC gene, alterations in TP53 were found in at least 30% of regions of IM, and in 33–58% of gastric dysplasia and adenomas, indicating that mutations in TP53 is an early event in gastric carcinogenesis [227].

Oncogenes

In intestinal type of gastric cancer, some oncogenes such as HER2 [254–256] and KRAS [257–260] are preferentially altered. Amplification and/or overexpression of HER2, a member of the human tyrosine kinase receptor family, is detected in 7–34% of gastric adenocarcinomas [39]. The overexpression of HER2 seems to occur in early event of gastric carcinogenesis, since its expression rises significantly from low-grade dysplasia to high-grade dysplasia to adenocarcinoma [261]. The increasing interest for HER2 expression in gastric carcinoma by immunohistochemical (IHC) and *in situ* hybridization assays is due to the positive responses of these neoplasms to treatment with Trastuzumab, a humanized monoclonal antibody targeting the HER2 receptor, as demonstrated by ToGA trial [262]. In this regard, in contrast to HER2 expression in breast cancer, HER2 immunohistochemical expression in gastric cancer is more heterogeneous and U shaped or lateral staining is more frequent in gastric cancer rather than a complete staining [263, 264].

Since the correlation between HER2 amplification and protein overexpression in gastric cancer is less stringent than in breast carcinoma [263], the European Medicines Agency (EMA) recommends to evaluate HER2 as first by immunohistochemistry, followed by fluorescence in situ hybridization (FISH) in IHC2-positive cases [265].

KRAS mutations have been detected in more than 50% of intestinal carcinoma, but not in diffuse carcinoma. Activating KRAS mutations result in RAS proteins that are constitutively active, leading to stimulation of downstream signalling pathway independent of EGFR signalling. EGFR is another member of the human tyrosine kinase receptor family that has been shown to be overexpressed by immunohistochemistry in 27% of gastric cancers, whereas gene amplification by FISH was evident in less than 3% of more than 500 cases of GC tissue analysed [266].

Differently to intestinal type, other oncogenes are preferentially altered in diffuse gastric carcinoma, among which BCL2 [267, 268] and FGFR2 [269, 270]. Oncogenes including CTNNB1 (encoding β-catenin) [271], MET [272] and MYC [273, 274] are deregulated both in intestinal and diffuse gastric cancers. Additionally, genes involved in the cell cycle regulation such as CDKN1B [275–277] and cyclin E [278], have been also reported to be altered in gastric cancer.

Conclusion

About 90–95% of gastric cancers (GC) are adenocarcinomas. These cancers develop within the cells of the mucosa, the inner most lining of the stomach. Other gastric cancer histotypes are lymphoma, gastrointestinal stromal tumours (GISTs), carcinoid tumours and other rare tumours.

The accurate and precise classification of gastric epithelial tumours is the prerequisite to better understanding the biology of this tumoural entity that deserves increasing attention due to early diagnosis reliability and more efficacious multimodal therapeutic approaches.

References

1. Correa P. A human model of gastric carcinogenesis. Cancer Res. 1988;48(13):3554–60.
2. Lauwers GY, Srivastava A. Gastric preneoplastic lesions and epithelial dysplasia. Gastroenterol Clin North Am. 2007;36(4):813–29, vi.
3. Lauwers GY, Carneiro F, Graham DY et al. Gastric carcinoma. In: Bosman FT, Carneiro F, Hruban RH. Theise ND, editors. WHO classification of tumours of the digestive system. 4th ed. Lyon: IARC; 2010. p. 48–58.
4. Rugge M, et al. Gastric dysplasia: the Padova international classification. Am J Surg Pathol. 2000;24(2): 167–76.
5. Schlemper RJ, et al. The Vienna classification of gastrointestinal epithelial neoplasia. Gut. 2000;47(2):251–5.
6. Stolte M. The new Vienna classification of epithelial neoplasia of the gastrointestinal tract: advantages and disadvantages. Virchows Arch. 2003;442(2):99–106.
7. Lansdown M, et al. High grade dysplasia of the gastric mucosa: a marker for gastric carcinoma. Gut. 1990;31(9):977–83.
8. Di Gregorio C, et al. Gastric dysplasia. A follow-up study. Am J Gastroenterol. 1993;88(10):1714–9.
9. Rugge M, et al. Gastric epithelial dysplasia: a prospective multicenter follow-up study from the Interdisciplinary Group on Gastric Epithelial Dysplasia. Hum Pathol. 1991;22(10):1002–8.
10. Saraga EP, Gardiol D, Costa J. Gastric dysplasia. A histological follow-up study. Am J Surg Pathol. 1987;11(10):788–96.
11. Fertitta AM, et al. Clinical significance of gastric dysplasia: a multicenter follow-up study. Gastrointestinal Endoscopic Pathology Study Group. Endoscopy. 1993;25(4):265–8.
12. Kokkola A, et al. Risk of gastric carcinoma in patients with mucosal dysplasia associated with atrophic gastritis: a follow up study. J Clin Pathol. 1996;49(12):979–84.
13. Yamada H, et al. Long-term follow-up study of gastric adenoma/dysplasia. Endoscopy. 2004;36(5):390–6.
14. Park DY, Lauwers GY. Gastric polyps: classification and management. Arch Pathol Lab Med. 2008;132(4):633–40.
15. Carmack SW, et al. The current spectrum of gastric polyps: a 1-year national study of over 120,000 patients. Am J Gastroenterol. 2009;104(6):1524–32.
16. Genta RM, et al. No association between gastric fundic gland polyps and gastrointestinal neoplasia in a

study of over 100,000 patients. Clin Gastroenterol Hepatol. 2009;7(8):849–54.
17. Fossmark R, et al. Serum gastrin and chromogranin A levels in patients with fundic gland polyps caused by long-term proton-pump inhibition. Scand J Gastroenterol. 2008;43(1):20–4.
18. Ally MR, et al. Chronic proton pump inhibitor therapy associated with increased development of fundic gland polyps. Dig Dis Sci. 2009;54(12):2617–22.
19. Attard TM, et al. Fundic gland polyposis with high-grade dysplasia in a child with attenuated familial adenomatous polyposis and familial gastric cancer. J Pediatr Gastroenterol Nutr. 2001;32(2):215–8.
20. Abraham SC, et al. Sporadic fundic gland polyps with epithelial dysplasia : evidence for preferential targeting for mutations in the adenomatous polyposis coli gene. Am J Pathol. 2002;161(5):1735–42.
21. Worthley DL, et al. Gastric adenocarcinoma and proximal polyposis of the stomach (GAPPS): a new autosomal dominant syndrome. Gut. 2012;61(5):774–9.
22. Carmack SW, et al. Management of gastric polyps: a pathology-based guide for gastroenterologists. Nat Rev Gastroenterol Hepatol. 2009;6(6):331–41.
23. Canzonieri V, et al. Exocrine and endocrine modulation in common gastric carcinoma. Am J Clin Pathol. 2012;137(5):712–21.
24. Park DY, et al. Adenomatous and foveolar gastric dysplasia: distinct patterns of mucin expression and background intestinal metaplasia. Am J Surg Pathol. 2008;32(4):524–33.
25. Abraham SC, et al. Gastric adenomas: intestinal-type and gastric-type adenomas differ in the risk of adenocarcinoma and presence of background mucosal pathology. Am J Surg Pathol. 2002;26(10):1276–85.
26. Jass JR. A classification of gastric dysplasia. Histopathology. 1983;7(2):181–93.
27. Nogueira AM, et al. Patterns of expression of trefoil peptides and mucins in gastric polyps with and without malignant transformation. J Pathol. 1999;187(5):541–8.
28. Park DY, et al. CDX2 expression in the intestinal-type gastric epithelial neoplasia: frequency and significance. Mod Pathol. 2010;23(1):54–61.
29. Rubio CA. Paneth cell adenoma of the stomach. Am J Surg Pathol. 1989;13(4):325–8.
30. Lev R, DeNucci TD. Neoplastic Paneth cells in the stomach. Report of two cases and review of the literature. Arch Pathol Lab Med. 1989;113(2):129–33.
31. Singhi AD, Lazenby AJ, Montgomery EA. Gastric adenocarcinoma with chief cell differentiation: a proposal for reclassification as oxyntic gland polyp/adenoma. Am J Surg Pathol. 2012;36(7):1030–5.
32. Torre LA, et al. Global cancer incidence and mortality rates and trends – an update. Cancer Epidemiol Biomarkers Prev. 2015;25(1):16–27.
33. Stock M, Otto F. Gene deregulation in gastric cancer. Gene. 2005;360(1):1–19.
34. Parkin DM, et al. Global cancer statistics, 2002. CA Cancer J Clin. 2005;55(2):74–108.
35. Curado MP, et al. Cancer incidence in five continents, vol. 9. Lyon: IARC Press International Agency for Research on Cancer; 2007.
36. Parkin DM. The global health burden of infection-associated cancers in the year 2002. Int J Cancer. 2006;118(12):3030–44.
37. Munoz N, Franceschi S. Epidemiology of gastric cancer and perspectives for prevention. Salud Publica Mex. 1997;39(4):318–30.
38. Correa P. Human gastric carcinogenesis: a multistep and multifactorial process – First American Cancer Society Award Lecture on Cancer Epidemiology and Prevention. Cancer Res. 1992;52(24):6735–40.
39. Yakirevich E, Resnick MB. Pathology of gastric cancer and its precursor lesions. Gastroenterol Clin North Am. 2013;42(2):261–84.
40. Siurala M, Varis K, Wiljasalo M. Studies of patients with atrophic gastritis: a 10-15-year follow-up. Scand J Gastroenterol. 1966;1(1):40–8.
41. Walker IR, et al. Simple atrophic gastritis and gastric carcinoma. Gut. 1971;12(11):906–11.
42. Dixon MF, et al. Classification and grading of gastritis. The updated Sydney System. International Workshop on the Histopathology of Gastritis, Houston 1994. Am J Surg Pathol. 1996;20(10):1161–81.
43. Rugge M, Genta RM. Staging and grading of chronic gastritis. Hum Pathol. 2005;36(3):228–33.
44. Rugge M, et al. Gastritis OLGA-staging and gastric cancer risk: a twelve-year clinico-pathological follow-up study. Aliment Pharmacol Ther. 2010;31(10):1104–11.
45. Jass JR, Filipe MI. The mucin profiles of normal gastric mucosa, intestinal metaplasia and its variants and gastric carcinoma. Histochem J. 1981;13(6):931–9.
46. Reis CA, et al. Intestinal metaplasia of human stomach displays distinct patterns of mucin (MUC1, MUC2, MUC5AC, and MUC6) expression. Cancer Res. 1999;59(5):1003–7.
47. Filipe MI, et al. Incomplete sulphomucin-secreting intestinal metaplasia for gastric cancer. Preliminary data from a prospective study from three centres. Gut. 1985;26(12):1319–26.
48. Jass JR, Filipe MI. Sulphomucins and precancerous lesions of the human stomach. Histopathology. 1980;4(3):271–9.
49. Barros R, et al. Gastric intestinal metaplasia revisited: function and regulation of CDX2. Trends Mol Med. 2012;18(9):555–63.
50. Pagnini CA, Bozzola L. Precancerous significance of colonic type intestinal metaplasia. Tumori. 1981;67(2):113–6.
51. Filipe MI, et al. Intestinal metaplasia types and the risk of gastric cancer: a cohort study in Slovenia. Int J Cancer. 1994;57(3):324–9.
52. Capelle LG, et al. The staging of gastritis with the OLGA system by using intestinal metaplasia as an accurate alternative for atrophic gastritis. Gastrointest Endosc. 2010;71(7):1150–8.

53. Correa P, et al. Chemoprevention of gastric dysplasia: randomized trial of antioxidant supplements and anti-helicobacter pylori therapy. J Natl Cancer Inst. 2000;92(23):1881–8.
54. Ley C, et al. Helicobacter pylori eradication and gastric preneoplastic conditions: a randomized, double-blind, placebo-controlled trial. Cancer Epidemiol Biomarkers Prev. 2004;13(1):4–10.
55. Zhou L, et al. A five-year follow-up study on the pathological changes of gastric mucosa after H. pylori eradication. Chin Med J (Engl). 2003;116(1):11–4.
56. Wong BC, et al. Helicobacter pylori eradication to prevent gastric cancer in a high-risk region of China: a randomized controlled trial. JAMA. 2004;291(2):187–94.
57. Asfeldt AM, et al. The natural course of Helicobacter pylori infection on endoscopic findings in a population during 17 years of follow-up: the Sorreisa gastrointestinal disorder study. Eur J Epidemiol. 2009;24(10):649–58.
58. Barros R, et al. Relevance of high virulence Helicobacter pylori strains and futility of CDX2 expression for predicting intestinal metaplasia after eradication of infection. Scand J Gastroenterol. 2010;45(7-8):828–34.
59. Wong WM, Poulsom R, Wright NA. Trefoil peptides. Gut. 1999;44(6):890–5.
60. Schmidt PH, et al. Identification of a metaplastic cell lineage associated with human gastric adenocarcinoma. Lab Invest. 1999;79(6):639–46.
61. Halldorsdottir AM, et al. Spasmolytic polypeptide-expressing metaplasia (SPEM) associated with gastric cancer in Iceland. Dig Dis Sci. 2003;48(3):431–41.
62. Yamaguchi H, et al. Identification of spasmolytic polypeptide expressing metaplasia (SPEM) in remnant gastric cancer and surveillance postgastrectomy biopsies. Dig Dis Sci. 2002;47(3):573–8.
63. Schistosomes, liver flukes and Helicobacter pylori. IARC Working Group on the Evaluation of Carcinogenic Risks to Humans. Lyon, 7-14 June 1994. IARC Monogr Eval Carcinog Risks Hum. 1994;61:1–241.
64. Fox JG, Wang TC. Inflammation, atrophy, and gastric cancer. J Clin Invest. 2007;117(1):60–9.
65. Uemura N, et al. Helicobacter pylori infection and the development of gastric cancer. N Engl J Med. 2001;345(11):784–9.
66. Malfertheiner P, et al. Current concepts in the management of Helicobacter pylori infection: the Maastricht III Consensus Report. Gut. 2007;56(6):772–81.
67. Ekstrom AM, et al. Dietary antioxidant intake and the risk of cardia cancer and noncardia cancer of the intestinal and diffuse types: a population-based case-control study in Sweden. Int J Cancer. 2000;87(1):133–40.
68. Epplein M, et al. Association of Helicobacter pylori infection and diet on the risk of gastric cancer: a case-control study in Hawaii. Cancer Causes Control. 2008;19(8):869–77.
69. Kono S, Hirohata T. Nutrition and stomach cancer. Cancer Causes Control. 1996;7(1):41–55.
70. Buckland G, et al. Healthy lifestyle index and risk of gastric adenocarcinoma in the EPIC cohort study. Int J Cancer. 2015;137(3):598–606.
71. Lin SH, et al. Salt processed food and gastric cancer in a Chinese population. Asian Pac J Cancer Prev. 2014;15(13):5293–8.
72. Massarrat S, Stolte M. Development of gastric cancer and its prevention. Arch Iran Med. 2014;17(7):514–20.
73. Nomura AM, et al. Case-control study of diet and other risk factors for gastric cancer in Hawaii (United States). Cancer Causes Control. 2003;14(6):547–58.
74. Bjelakovic G, et al. Systematic review: primary and secondary prevention of gastrointestinal cancers with antioxidant supplements. Aliment Pharmacol Ther. 2008;28(6):689–703.
75. Qiao YL, et al. Total and cancer mortality after supplementation with vitamins and minerals: follow-up of the Linxian General Population Nutrition Intervention Trial. J Natl Cancer Inst. 2009;101(7):507–18.
76. Jenab M, et al. Plasma and dietary carotenoid, retinol and tocopherol levels and the risk of gastric adenocarcinomas in the European prospective investigation into cancer and nutrition. Br J Cancer. 2006;95(3):406–15.
77. Ladeiras-Lopes R, et al. Smoking and gastric cancer: systematic review and meta-analysis of cohort studies. Cancer Causes Control. 2008;19(7):689–701.
78. Nishino Y, et al. Tobacco smoking and gastric cancer risk: an evaluation based on a systematic review of epidemiologic evidence among the Japanese population. Jpn J Clin Oncol. 2006;36(12):800–7.
79. Thorban S, et al. Prognostic factors in gastric stump carcinoma. Ann Surg. 2000;231(2):188–94.
80. Skierucha M, et al. Molecular alterations in gastric cancer with special reference to the early-onset subtype. World J Gastroenterol. 2016;22(8):2460–74.
81. Sons HU, Borchard F. Gastric carcinoma after surgical treatment for benign ulcer disease: some pathologic-anatomic aspects. Int Surg. 1987;72(4):222–6.
82. Sinning C, et al. Gastric stump carcinoma – epidemiology and current concepts in pathogenesis and treatment. Eur J Surg Oncol. 2007;33(2):133–9.
83. Offerhaus GJ, et al. Mortality caused by stomach cancer after remote partial gastrectomy for benign conditions: 40 years of follow up of an Amsterdam cohort of 2633 postgastrectomy patients. Gut. 1988;29(11):1588–90.
84. Toftgaard C. Gastric cancer after peptic ulcer surgery. A historic prospective cohort investigation. Ann Surg. 1989;210(2):159–64.
85. Tersmette AC, et al. Multivariate analysis of the risk of stomach cancer after ulcer surgery in an Amsterdam cohort of postgastrectomy patients. Am J Epidemiol. 1991;134(1):14–21.

86. Imai S, et al. Gastric carcinoma: monoclonal epithelial malignant cells expressing Epstein-Barr virus latent infection protein. Proc Natl Acad Sci U S A. 1994;91(19):9131–5.
87. Yamamoto N, et al. Epstein-Barr virus and gastric remnant cancer. Cancer. 1994;74(3):805–9.
88. van Rees BP, et al. Different pattern of allelic loss in Epstein-Barr virus-positive gastric cancer with emphasis on the p53 tumor suppressor pathway. Am J Pathol. 2002;161(4):1207–13.
89. Baas IO, et al. Helicobacter pylori and Epstein-Barr virus infection and the p53 tumour suppressor pathway in gastric stump cancer compared with carcinoma in the non-operated stomach. J Clin Pathol. 1998;51(9):662–6.
90. Offerhaus GJ, et al. The mucosa of the gastric remnant harboring malignancy. Histologic findings in the biopsy specimens of 504 asymptomatic patients 15 to 46 years after partial gastrectomy with emphasis on nonmalignant lesions. Cancer. 1989;64(3):698–703.
91. Borrmann R. Geshwulste des Magens und Duodenums. In: Henke F, Lubrasch O, editors. Handbuch der Speziellen Pathologischen Anatomie und Histologie. Berlin: Springer; 1926.
92. Ming SC. Gastric carcinoma. A pathobiological classification. Cancer. 1977;39(6):2475–85.
93. Carneiro F, Ribeiro MM, Sobrinho-Simoes M. Prognostic factors in gastric carcinoma. Br J Cancer. 1997;76(2):278.
94. Goseki N, Takizawa T, Koike M. Differences in the mode of the extension of gastric cancer classified by histological type: new histological classification of gastric carcinoma. Gut. 1992;33(5):606–12.
95. Lauren P. The two histological main types of gastric carcinoma: diffuse and so-called intestinal-type carcinoma. An attempt at a histo-clinical classification. Acta Pathol Microbiol Scand. 1965;64:31–49.
96. Tay ST, et al. A combined comparative genomic hybridization and expression microarray analysis of gastric cancer reveals novel molecular subtypes. Cancer Res. 2003;63(12):3309–16.
97. Tan IB, et al. Intrinsic subtypes of gastric cancer, based on gene expression pattern, predict survival and respond differently to chemotherapy. Gastroenterology. 2011;141(2):476–85.
98. Lee HS, et al. Protein expression profiling and molecular classification of gastric cancer by the tissue array method. Clin Cancer Res. 2007;13(14):4154–63.
99. Brierley JD, Gospodarowicz MK, Wittekind C, editors. TNM classification of malignant tumours. 8th ed. Chichester: Wiley-Blackwell; 2017.
100. Amin MB, et al., editors. AJCC cancer staging manual. 8th ed. New York: Springer International Publishing; 2017.
101. Eom DW, et al. Gastric micropapillary carcinoma: a distinct subtype with a significantly worse prognosis in TNM stages I and II. Am J Surg Pathol. 2010;35(1):84–91.
102. Carvalho B, et al. Mixed gastric carcinomas show similar chromosomal aberrations in both their diffuse and glandular components. Cell Oncol. 2006;28(5-6):283–94.
103. Zheng HC, et al. Mixed-type gastric carcinomas exhibit more aggressive features and indicate the histogenesis of carcinomas. Virchows Arch. 2008;452(5):525–34.
104. Machado JC, et al. E-cadherin gene mutations provide a genetic basis for the phenotypic divergence of mixed gastric carcinomas. Lab Invest. 1999;79(4):459–65.
105. Park SY, et al. Mixed-type gastric cancer and its association with high-frequency CpG island hypermethylation. Virchows Arch. 2010;456(6):625–33.
106. Fuchs CS, Mayer RJ. Gastric carcinoma. N Engl J Med. 1995;333(1):32–41.
107. Berlth F, et al. Pathohistological classification systems in gastric cancer: diagnostic relevance and prognostic value. World J Gastroenterol. 2014;20(19):5679–84.
108. Cislo M, et al. Distinct molecular subtypes of gastric cancer: from Lauren to molecular pathology. Oncotarget. 2018;9(27):19427–42.
109. Van Cutsem E, et al. Gastric cancer. Lancet. 2016;388(10060):2654–64.
110. Martin IG, et al. Goseki histological grading of gastric cancer is an important predictor of outcome. Gut. 1994;35(6):758–63.
111. Carneiro F. Classification of gastric carcinomas. Curr Diagn Pathol. 1997;4(1):51–59.
112. Carneiro F, Seixas M, Sobrinho-Simoes M. New elements for an updated classification of the carcinomas of the stomach. Pathol Res Pract. 1995;191(6):571–84.
113. Machado JC, et al. pS2 protein expression in gastric carcinoma. An immunohistochemical and immunoradiometric study. Eur J Cancer. 1996;32A(9): 1585–90.
114. Machado JC, et al. Gastric carcinoma exhibits distinct types of cell differentiation: an immunohistochemical study of trefoil peptides (TFF1 and TFF2) and mucins (MUC1, MUC2, MUC5AC, and MUC6). J Pathol. 2000;190(4):437–43.
115. Kushima R, et al. Gastric-type well-differentiated adenocarcinoma and pyloric gland adenoma of the stomach. Gastric Cancer. 2006;9(3):177–84.
116. Kushima R, Hattori T. Histogenesis and characteristics of gastric-type adenocarcinomas in the stomach. J Cancer Res Clin Oncol. 1993;120(1-2):103–11.
117. Tsukashita S, et al. MUC gene expression and histogenesis of adenocarcinoma of the stomach. Int J Cancer. 2001;94(2):166–70.
118. Shiroshita H, et al. Re-evaluation of mucin phenotypes of gastric minute well-differentiated-type adenocarcinomas using a series of HGM, MUC5AC, MUC6, M-GGMC, MUC2 and CD10 stains. Pathol Int. 2004;54(5):311–21.
119. Tatematsu M, Tsukamoto T, Mizoshita T. Role of Helicobacter pylori in gastric carcinogenesis: the

origin of gastric cancers and heterotopic proliferative glands in Mongolian gerbils. Helicobacter. 2005;10(2):97–106.
120. Blumenfeld W, et al. Neuroendocrine differentiation in gastric adenocarcinomas. An immunohistochemical study. Arch Pathol Lab Med. 1996;120(5):478–81.
121. Park JG, et al. Chromogranin-A expression in gastric and colon cancer tissues. Int J Cancer. 1992;51(2):189–94.
122. Sentani K, et al. Immunostaining of gastric cancer with neuroendocrine differentiation: Reg IV-positive neuroendocrine cells are associated with gastrin, serotonin, pancreatic polypeptide and somatostatin. Pathol Int. 2010;60(4):291–7.
123. Waldum HL, et al. Neuroendocrine differentiation in human gastric carcinoma. Cancer. 1998;83(3):435–44.
124. Yao GY, et al. Neuroendocrine markers in adenocarcinomas: an investigation of 356 cases. World J Gastroenterol. 2003;9(4):858–61.
125. Jiang SX, et al. Gastric large cell neuroendocrine carcinomas: a distinct clinicopathologic entity. Am J Surg Pathol. 2006;30(8):945–53.
126. Mori M, Iwashita A, Enjoji M. Adenosquamous carcinoma of the stomach. A clinicopathologic analysis of 28 cases. Cancer. 1986;57(2):333–9.
127. Mori M, Fukuda T, Enjoji M. Adenosquamous carcinoma of the stomach. Histogenetic and ultrastructural studies. Gastroenterology. 1987;92(4):1078–82.
128. Boswell JT, Helwig EB. Squamous Cell Carcinoma and Adenoacanthoma of the Stomach. A Clinicopathologic Study. Cancer. 1965;18:181–92.
129. Bonnheim DC, Sarac OK, Fett W. Primary squamous cell carcinoma of the stomach. Am J Gastroenterol. 1985;80(2):91–4.
130. Marubashi S, et al. Primary squamous cell carcinoma of the stomach. Gastric Cancer. 1999;2(2):136–41.
131. Yoshida K, et al. Early gastric cancer of adenosquamous carcinoma type: report of a case and review of literature. Jpn J Clin Oncol. 1996;26(4):252–7.
132. Ishikura H, et al. Hepatoid adenocarcinomas of the stomach. An analysis of seven cases. Cancer. 1986;58(1):119–26.
133. Nagai E, et al. Hepatoid adenocarcinoma of the stomach. A clinicopathologic and immunohistochemical analysis. Cancer. 1993;72(6):1827–35.
134. Chang YC, et al. Clinicopathologic features and long-term results of alpha-fetoprotein-producing gastric cancer. Am J Gastroenterol. 1990;85(11):1480–5.
135. Akiyama S, et al. Histogenesis of hepatoid adenocarcinoma of the stomach: molecular evidence of identical origin with coexistent tubular adenocarcinoma. Int J Cancer. 2003;106(4):510–5.
136. Petrella T, et al. Alphafetoprotein-producing gastric adenocarcinoma. Histopathology. 1995;26(2):171–5.
137. Kumashiro Y, et al. Hepatoid adenocarcinoma of the stomach: histogenesis and progression in association with intestinal phenotype. Hum Pathol. 2007;38(6):857–63.
138. Ishikura H, et al. Gastrointestinal hepatoid adenocarcinoma: venous permeation and mimicry of hepatocellular carcinoma, a report of four cases. Histopathology. 1997;31(1):47–54.
139. Liu X, et al. Analysis of clinicopathologic features and prognostic factors in hepatoid adenocarcinoma of the stomach. Am J Surg Pathol. 2010;34(10):1465–71.
140. Motoyama T, et al. alpha-Fetoprotein producing gastric carcinomas: a comparative study of three different subtypes. Acta Pathol Jpn. 1993;43(11):654–61.
141. Inagawa S, et al. Hepatoid adenocarcinoma of the stomach. Gastric Cancer. 2001;4(1):43–52.
142. Supriatna Y, et al. Evidence for hepatocellular differentiation in alpha-fetoprotein-negative gastric adenocarcinoma with hepatoid morphology: a study with in situ hybridisation for albumin mRNA. Pathology. 2005;37(3):211–5.
143. Sentani K, et al. Gene expression profiling with microarray and SAGE identifies PLUNC as a marker for hepatoid adenocarcinoma of the stomach. Mod Pathol. 2008;21(4):464–75.
144. Terracciano LM, et al. Hepatoid adenocarcinoma with liver metastasis mimicking hepatocellular carcinoma: an immunohistochemical and molecular study of eight cases. Am J Surg Pathol. 2003;27(10):1302–12.
145. Saigo PE, et al. Primary gastric choriocarcinoma. An immunohistological study. Am J Surg Pathol. 1981;5(4):333–42.
146. Liu AY, et al. Gastric choriocarcinoma shows characteristics of adenocarcinoma and gestational choriocarcinoma: a comparative genomic hybridization and fluorescence in situ hybridization study. Diagn Mol Pathol. 2001;10(3):161–5.
147. Smith FR, Barkin JS, Hensley G. Choriocarcinoma of the stomach. Am J Gastroenterol. 1980;73(1):45–8.
148. Yonezawa S, et al. Immunohistochemical localization of thrombomodulin in chorionic diseases of the uterus and choriocarcinoma of the stomach. A comparative study with the distribution of human chorionic gonadotropin. Cancer. 1988;62(3):569–76.
149. Krulewski T, Cohen LB. Choriocarcinoma of the stomach: pathogenesis and clinical characteristics. Am J Gastroenterol. 1988;83(10):1172–5.
150. Young LS, Rickinson AB. Epstein-Barr virus: 40 years on. Nat Rev Cancer. 2004;4(10):757–68.
151. Murphy G, et al. Meta-analysis shows that prevalence of Epstein-Barr virus-positive gastric cancer differs based on sex and anatomic location. Gastroenterology. 2009;137(3):824–33.
152. Lee JH, et al. Clinicopathological and molecular characteristics of Epstein-Barr virus-associated gastric carcinoma: a meta-analysis. J Gastroenterol Hepatol. 2009;24(3):354–65.
153. Willems S, Carneiro F, Geboes K. Gastric carcinoma with osteoclast-like giant cells and

lymphoepithelioma-like carcinoma of the stomach: two of a kind? Histopathology. 2005;47(3):331–3.
154. Minamoto T, et al. Medullary carcinoma with lymphocytic infiltration of the stomach. Clinicopathologic study of 27 cases and immunohistochemical analysis of the subpopulations of infiltrating lymphocytes in the tumor. Cancer. 1990;66(5):945–52.
155. Watanabe H, Enjoji M, Imai T. Gastric carcinoma with lymphoid stroma. Its morphologic characteristics and prognostic correlations. Cancer. 1976;38(1):232–43.
156. Wang HH, et al. Lymphoepithelioma-like carcinoma of the stomach: a subset of gastric carcinoma with distinct clinicopathological features and high prevalence of Epstein-Barr virus infection. Hepatogastroenterology. 1999;46(26):1214–9.
157. Matsunou H, et al. Characteristics of Epstein-Barr virus-associated gastric carcinoma with lymphoid stroma in Japan. Cancer. 1996;77(10):1998–2004.
158. Truong CD, et al. Characteristics of Epstein-Barr virus-associated gastric cancer: a study of 235 cases at a comprehensive cancer center in U.S.A. J Exp Clin Cancer Res. 2009;28:14.
159. Fukayama M, Chong JM, Kaizaki Y. Epstein-Barr virus and gastric carcinoma. Gastric Cancer. 1998;1(2):104–14.
160. Cho KJ, et al. Carcinosarcoma of the stomach. A case report with light microscopic, immunohistochemical, and electron microscopic study. APMIS. 1990;98(11):991–5.
161. Nakayama Y, et al. Gastric carcinosarcoma (sarcomatoid carcinoma) with rhabdomyoblastic and osteoblastic differentiation. Pathol Int. 1997;47(8):557–63.
162. Sato Y, et al. Gastric carcinosarcoma, coexistence of adenosquamous carcinoma and rhabdomyosarcoma: a case report. Histopathology. 2001;39(5):543–4.
163. Randjelovic T, et al. Carcinosarcoma of the stomach: a case report and review of the literature. World J Gastroenterol. 2007;13(41):5533–6.
164. Tsuneyama K, et al. A case report of gastric carcinosarcoma with rhabdomyosarcomatous and neuroendocrinal differentiation. Pathol Res Pract. 1999;195(2):93–7; discussion 98.
165. Yamazaki K. A gastric carcinosarcoma with neuroendocrine cell differentiation and undifferentiated spindle-shaped sarcoma component possibly progressing from the conventional tubular adenocarcinoma; an immunohistochemical and ultrastructural study. Virchows Arch. 2003;442(1):77–81.
166. Teramachi K, et al. Carcinosarcoma (pure endocrine cell carcinoma with sarcoma components) of the stomach. Pathol Int. 2003;53(8):552–6.
167. Kuroda N, et al. Gastric carcinosarcoma with neuroendocrine differentiation as the carcinoma component and leiomyosarcomatous and myofibroblastic differentiation as the sarcomatous component. APMIS. 2006;114(3):234–8.
168. Ikeda Y, et al. Gastric carcinosarcoma presenting as a huge epigastric mass. Gastric Cancer. 2007;10(1):63–8.
169. Roh JH, et al. Micropapillary carcinoma of stomach: a clinicopathologic and immunohistochemical study of 11 cases. Am J Surg Pathol. 2010;34(8):1139–46.
170. Capella C, et al. Gastric parietal cell carcinoma – a newly recognized entity: light microscopic and ultrastructural features. Histopathology. 1984;8(5):813–24.
171. Byrne D, Holley MP, Cuschieri A. Parietal cell carcinoma of the stomach: association with long-term survival after curative resection. Br J Cancer. 1988;58(1):85–7.
172. Yang GY, et al. Parietal cell carcinoma of gastric cardia: immunophenotype and ultrastructure. Ultrastruct Pathol. 2003;27(2):87–94.
173. Hayashi I, et al. Mucoepidermoid carcinoma of the stomach. J Surg Oncol. 1987;34(2):94–9.
174. Kazzaz BA, Eulderink F. Paneth cell-rich carcinoma of the stomach. Histopathology. 1989;15(3):303–5.
175. Ooi A, et al. Predominant Paneth cell differentiation in an intestinal type gastric cancer. Pathol Res Pract. 1991;187(2-3):220–5.
176. Caruso RA, Famulari C. Neoplastic Paneth cells in adenocarcinoma of the stomach: a case report. Hepatogastroenterology. 1992;39(3):264–6.
177. Ueyama T, et al. Vimentin-positive gastric carcinomas with rhabdoid features. A clinicopathologic and immunohistochemical study. Am J Surg Pathol. 1993;17(8):813–9.
178. Pinto JA, et al. Well differentiated gastric adenocarcinoma with rhabdoid areas: a case report with immunohistochemical analysis. Pathol Res Pract. 1997;193(11-12):801–5; discussion 806–8.
179. Rivera-Hueto F, et al. Early gastric stump carcinoma with rhabdoid features. Case report. Pathol Res Pract. 1999;195(12):841–6.
180. Murakami T. Pathomorphological diagnosis. In: Murakami T, editor. Early gastric cancer. Tokyo: University of Tokyo; 1971.
181. Tsukuma H, Mishima T, Oshima A. Prospective study of "early" gastric cancer. Int J Cancer. 1983;31(4):421–6.
182. Everett SM, Axon AT. Early gastric cancer in Europe. Gut. 1997;41(2):142–50.
183. Noguchi Y, et al. Is gastric carcinoma different between Japan and the United States? Cancer. 2000;89(11):2237–46.
184. Gotoda T. Endoscopic resection of early gastric cancer. Gastric Cancer. 2007;10(1):1–11.
185. Ming SC. Malignant epithelial tumours of the stomach. In: Ming SC, Goldman H, editors. Pathology of gastointestinal tract. Baltimore: Williams & Wilkins; 1998.
186. Oohara T, et al. Minute gastric cancers less than 5 mm in diameter. Cancer. 1982;50(4):801–10.
187. Kodama Y, et al. Growth patterns and prognosis in early gastric carcinoma. Superficially spreading and penetrating growth types. Cancer. 1983;51(2):320–6.

188. Xuan ZX, et al. Time trends of early gastric carcinoma. A clinicopathologic analysis of 2846 cases. Cancer. 1993;72(10):2889–94.
189. Zinninger MM, Collins WT. Extension of garcinoma of the stomach into the duodenum and esophagus. Ann Surg. 1949;130(3):557–66.
190. Fernet P, Azar HA, Stout AP. Intramural (tubal) spread of linitis plastica along the alimentary tract. Gastroenterology. 1965;48:419–24.
191. Maruyama K, et al. Lymph node metastases of gastric cancer. General pattern in 1931 patients. Ann Surg. 1989;210(5):596–602.
192. Duarte I, Llanos O. Patterns of metastases in intestinal and diffuse types of carcinoma of the stomach. Hum Pathol. 1981;12(3):237–42.
193. Marano L, et al. Surgical management of advanced gastric cancer: An evolving issue. Eur J Surg Oncol. 2016;42(1):18–27.
194. Ishigami S, et al. Clinical merit of subdividing gastric cancer according to invasion of the muscularis propria. Hepatogastroenterology. 2004;51(57):869–71.
195. Yoshikawa K, Maruyama K. Characteristics of gastric cancer invading to the proper muscle layer – with special reference to mortality and cause of death. Jpn J Clin Oncol. 1985;15(3):499–503.
196. Hundahl SA, Phillips JL, Menck HR. The National Cancer Data Base Report on poor survival of U.S. gastric carcinoma patients treated with gastrectomy: Fifth Edition American Joint Committee on Cancer staging, proximal disease, and the "different disease" hypothesis. Cancer. 2000;88(4):921–32.
197. Reid-Lombardo KM, et al. Treatment of gastric adenocarcinoma may differ among hospital types in the United States, a report from theNational Cancer Data Base. J Gastrointest Surg. 2007;11(4):410–9; discussion 419–20
198. Siewert JR, et al. Relevant prognostic factors in gastric cancer: ten-year results of the German Gastric Cancer Study. Ann Surg. 1998;228(4):449–61.
199. Wanebo HJ, et al. Cancer of the stomach. A patient care study by the American College of Surgeons. Ann Surg. 1993;218(5):583–92.
200. Karpeh MS, et al. Lymph node staging in gastric cancer: is location more important than Number? An analysis of 1,038 patients. Ann Surg. 2000;232(3):362–71.
201. Landry J, et al. Patterns of failure following curative resection of gastric carcinoma. Int J Radiat Oncol Biol Phys. 1990;19(6):1357–62.
202. Carneiro F. Hereditary gastric cancer. Pathologe. 2012;33 Suppl 2(2012):231–4.
203. Vasen HF, et al. MSH2 mutation carriers are at higher risk of cancer than MLH1 mutation carriers: a study of hereditary nonpolyposis colorectal cancer families. J Clin Oncol. 2001;19(20):4074–80.
204. Capelle LG, et al. Risk and epidemiological time trends of gastric cancer in Lynch syndrome carriers in the Netherlands. Gastroenterology. 2010;138(2): 487–92.
205. Lynch HT, et al. Review of the Lynch syndrome: history, molecular genetics, screening, differential diagnosis, and medicolegal ramifications. Clin Genet. 2009;76(1):1–18.
206. Jagelman DG, DeCosse JJ, Bussey HJ. Upper gastrointestinal cancer in familial adenomatous polyposis. Lancet. 1988;1(8595):1149–51.
207. Aarnio M, et al. Features of gastric cancer in hereditary non-polyposis colorectal cancer syndrome. Int J Cancer. 1997;74(5):551–5.
208. Varley JM, et al. An extended Li-Fraumeni kindred with gastric carcinoma and a codon 175 mutation in TP53. J Med Genet. 1995;32(12):942–5.
209. Shinmura K, et al. A novel STK11 germline mutation in two siblings with Peutz-Jeghers syndrome complicated by primary gastric cancer. Clin Genet. 2005;67(1):81–6.
210. Takahashi M, et al. A novel germline mutation of the LKB1 gene in a patient with Peutz-Jeghers syndrome with early-onset gastric cancer. J Gastroenterol. 2004;39(12):1210–4.
211. Guilford P, et al. E-cadherin germline mutations in familial gastric cancer. Nature. 1998;392(6674):402–5.
212. Caldas C, et al. Familial gastric cancer: overview and guidelines for management. J Med Genet. 1999;36(12):873–80.
213. Keller G, et al. Diffuse type gastric and lobular breast carcinoma in a familial gastric cancer patient with an E-cadherin germline mutation. Am J Pathol. 1999;155(2):337–42.
214. Brooks-Wilson AR, et al. Germline E-cadherin mutations in hereditary diffuse gastric cancer: assessment of 42 new families and review of genetic screening criteria. J Med Genet. 2004;41(7):508–17.
215. Suriano G, et al. Characterization of a recurrent germ line mutation of the E-cadherin gene: implications for genetic testing and clinical management. Clin Cancer Res. 2005;11(15):5401–9.
216. Kaurah P, et al. Founder and recurrent CDH1 mutations in families with hereditary diffuse gastric cancer. JAMA. 2007;297(21):2360–72.
217. Schrader KA, et al. Hereditary diffuse gastric cancer: association with lobular breast cancer. Fam Cancer. 2008;7(1):73–82.
218. Guilford PJ, et al. E-cadherin germline mutations define an inherited cancer syndrome dominated by diffuse gastric cancer. Hum Mutat. 1999;14(3):249–55.
219. Oliveira C, Seruca R, Carneiro F. Hereditary gastric cancer. Best Pract Res Clin Gastroenterol. 2009;23(2):147–57.
220. Oliveira C, et al. Germline CDH1 deletions in hereditary diffuse gastric cancer families. Hum Mol Genet. 2009;18(9):1545–55.
221. Blair V, et al. Hereditary diffuse gastric cancer: diagnosis and management. Clin Gastroenterol Hepatol. 2006;4(3):262–75.
222. Carneiro F, et al. Molecular pathology of familial gastric cancer, with an emphasis on hereditary diffuse gastric cancer. J Clin Pathol. 2008;61(1):25–30.

223. Grady WM, et al. Methylation of the CDH1 promoter as the second genetic hit in hereditary diffuse gastric cancer. Nat Genet. 2000;26(1):16–7.
224. Oliveira C, et al. Quantification of epigenetic and genetic 2nd hits in CDH1 during hereditary diffuse gastric cancer syndrome progression. Gastroenterology. 2009;136(7):2137–48.
225. Barber M, et al. Mechanisms and sequelae of E-cadherin silencing in hereditary diffuse gastric cancer. J Pathol. 2008;216(3):295–306.
226. Guo J, et al. Genomic landscape of gastric cancer: molecular classification and potential targets. Sci China Life Sci. 2017;60(2):126–37.
227. Tahara E. Genetic pathways of two types of gastric cancer. IARC Sci Publ. 2004;157:327–49.
228. Kawauchi S, et al. Genomic instability and DNA ploidy are linked to DNA copy number aberrations of 8p23 and 22q11.23 in gastric cancers. Int J Mol Med. 2010;26(3):333–9.
229. Aguilera A, Gomez-Gonzalez B. Genome instability: a mechanistic view of its causes and consequences. Nat Rev Genet. 2008;9(3):204–17.
230. Terada T. An immunohistochemical study of primary signet-ring cell carcinoma of the stomach and colorectum: II. Expression of MUC1, MUC2, MUC5AC, and MUC6 in normal mucosa and in 42 cases. Int J Clin Exp Pathol. 2013;6(4):613–21.
231. Yoda Y, et al. Integrated analysis of cancer-related pathways affected by genetic and epigenetic alterations in gastric cancer. Gastric Cancer. 2015;18(1):65–76.
232. Toyota M, et al. Aberrant methylation in gastric cancer associated with the CpG island methylator phenotype. Cancer Res. 1999;59(21):5438–42.
233. Enomoto S, et al. Lack of association between CpG island methylator phenotype in human gastric cancers and methylation in their background non-cancerous gastric mucosae. Cancer Sci. 2007;98(12):1853–61.
234. Fu DG. Epigenetic alterations in gastric cancer (Review). Mol Med Rep. 2015;12(3):3223–30.
235. Kang GH, et al. Profile of aberrant CpG island methylation along the multistep pathway of gastric carcinogenesis. Lab Invest. 2003;83(5):635–41.
236. Kang GH, et al. DNA methylation profiles of gastric carcinoma characterized by quantitative DNA methylation analysis. Lab Invest. 2008;88(2):161–70.
237. Park SY, et al. CpG island hypermethylator phenotype in gastric carcinoma and its clinicopathological features. Virchows Arch. 2010;457(4):415–22.
238. Becker KF, et al. E-cadherin gene mutations provide clues to diffuse type gastric carcinomas. Cancer Res. 1994;54(14):3845–52.
239. Jawhari A, et al. Abnormal immunoreactivity of the E-cadherin-catenin complex in gastric carcinoma: relationship with patient survival. Gastroenterology. 1997;112(1):46–54.
240. Ascano JJ, et al. Inactivation of the E-cadherin gene in sporadic diffuse-type gastric cancer. Mod Pathol. 2001;14(10):942–9.
241. Machado JC, et al. E-cadherin gene (CDH1) promoter methylation as the second hit in sporadic diffuse gastric carcinoma. Oncogene. 2001;20(12):1525–8.
242. Chan AO. E-cadherin in gastric cancer. World J Gastroenterol. 2006;12(2):199–203.
243. Feakins RM, et al. Abnormal expression of pRb, p16, and cyclin D1 in gastric adenocarcinoma and its lymph node metastases: relationship with pathological features and survival. Hum Pathol. 2003;34(12):1276–82.
244. Nakatsuru S, et al. Somatic mutation of the APC gene in gastric cancer: frequent mutations in very well differentiated adenocarcinoma and signet-ring cell carcinoma. Hum Mol Genet. 1992;1(8):559–63.
245. Tamura G, et al. Mutations of the APC gene occur during early stages of gastric adenoma development. Cancer Res. 1994;54(5):1149–51.
246. Seruca R, et al. p53 alterations in gastric carcinoma: a study of 56 primary tumors and 204 nodal metastases. Cancer Genet Cytogenet. 1994;75(1):45–50.
247. Lee JH, et al. Inverse relationship between APC gene mutation in gastric adenomas and development of adenocarcinoma. Am J Pathol. 2002;161(2):611–8.
248. Nishizuka S, et al. Loss of heterozygosity during the development and progression of differentiated adenocarcinoma of the stomach. J Pathol. 1998;185(1):38–43.
249. Uchino S, et al. Frequent loss of heterozygosity at the DCC locus in gastric cancer. Cancer Res. 1992;52(11):3099–102.
250. Li YL, et al. Loss of heterozygosity on 10q23.3 and mutation of tumor suppressor gene PTEN in gastric cancer and precancerous lesions. World J Gastroenterol. 2005;11(2):285–8.
251. Kakeji Y, et al. Gastric cancer with p53 overexpression has high potential for metastasising to lymph nodes. Br J Cancer. 1993;67(3):589–93.
252. Yonemura Y, et al. Correlation of p53 expression and proliferative activity in gastric cancer. Anal Cell Pathol. 1993;5(5):277–88.
253. Ikeguchi M, et al. Mutated p53 protein expression and proliferative activity in advanced gastric cancer. Hepatogastroenterology. 1999;46(28):2648–53.
254. Oda N, et al. DNA ploidy pattern and amplification of ERBB and ERBB2 genes in human gastric carcinomas. Virchows Arch B Cell Pathol Incl Mol Pathol. 1990;58(4):273–7.
255. Varis A, et al. Coamplified and overexpressed genes at ERBB2 locus in gastric cancer. Int J Cancer. 2004;109(4):548–53.
256. Barros-Silva JD, et al. Association of ERBB2 gene status with histopathological parameters and disease-specific survival in gastric carcinoma patients. Br J Cancer. 2009;100(3):487–93.
257. Brennetot C, et al. Frequent Ki-ras mutations in gastric tumors of the MSI phenotype. Gastroenterology. 2003;125(4):1282.
258. Kim IJ, et al. Mutational analysis of BRAF and K-ras in gastric cancers: absence of BRAF mutations in gastric cancers. Hum Genet. 2003;114(1):118–20.

259. Oliveira C, et al. BRAF mutations characterize colon but not gastric cancer with mismatch repair deficiency. Oncogene. 2003;22(57):9192–6.
260. Wu M, et al. BRAF/K-ras mutation, microsatellite instability, and promoter hypermethylation of hMLH1/MGMT in human gastric carcinomas. Gastric Cancer. 2004;7(4):246–53.
261. Fassan M, et al. Early HER2 dysregulation in gastric and oesophageal carcinogenesis. Histopathology. 2012;61(5):769–76.
262. Bang YJ, et al. Trastuzumab in combination with chemotherapy versus chemotherapy alone for treatment of HER2-positive advanced gastric or gastro-oesophageal junction cancer (ToGA): a phase 3, open-label, randomised controlled trial. Lancet. 2010;376(9742):687–97.
263. Ruschoff J, et al. HER2 diagnostics in gastric cancer-guideline validation and development of standardized immunohistochemical testing. Virchows Arch. 2010;457(3):299–307.
264. Albarello L, Pecciarini L, Doglioni C. HER2 testing in gastric cancer. Adv Anat Pathol. 2010;18(1):53–9.
265. Available at: www.ema.europa.eu/pdfs/human/opinion/Herceptin_82246709en.pdf. (Accessed 9 May 2012), in European Medicines Agency, Opinion 2009.
266. Kim MA, et al. EGFR in gastric carcinomas: prognostic significance of protein overexpression and high gene copy number. Histopathology. 2008;52(6):738–46.
267. Ayhan A, et al. Loss of heterozygosity at the bcl-2 gene locus and expression of bcl-2 in human gastric and colorectal carcinomas. Jpn J Cancer Res. 1994;85(6):584–91.
268. Lee HK, et al. Prognostic significance of Bcl-2 and p53 expression in gastric cancer. Int J Colorectal Dis. 2003;18(6):518–25.
269. Hattori Y, et al. K-sam, an amplified gene in stomach cancer, is a member of the heparin-binding growth factor receptor genes. Proc Natl Acad Sci U S A. 1990;87(15):5983–7.
270. Smith MG, et al. Cellular and molecular aspects of gastric cancer. World J Gastroenterol. 2006;12(19):2979–90.
271. Wang L, et al. Disordered beta-catenin expression and E-cadherin/CDH1 promoter methylation in gastric carcinoma. World J Gastroenterol. 2006;12(26):4228–31.
272. Kuniyasu H, et al. Frequent amplification of the c-met gene in scirrhous type stomach cancer. Biochem Biophys Res Commun. 1992;189(1):227–32.
273. Kozma L, et al. C-myc amplification and cluster analysis in human gastric carcinoma. Anticancer Res. 2001;21(1B):707–10.
274. Calcagno DQ, et al. Interrelationship between chromosome 8 aneuploidy, C-MYC amplification and increased expression in individuals from northern Brazil with gastric adenocarcinoma. World J Gastroenterol. 2006;12(38):6207–11.
275. Yasui W, et al. Reduced expression of cyclin-dependent kinase inhibitor p27Kip1 is associated with advanced stage and invasiveness of gastric carcinomas. Jpn J Cancer Res. 1997;88(7):625–9.
276. Xiangming C, et al. The cooperative role of p27 with cyclin E in the prognosis of advanced gastric carcinoma. Cancer. 2000;89(6):1214–9.
277. Kim DH, et al. Reduced expression of the cell-cycle inhibitor p27Kip1 is associated with progression and lymph node metastasis of gastric carcinoma. Histopathology. 2000;36(3):245–51.
278. Akama Y, et al. Frequent amplification of the cyclin E gene in human gastric carcinomas. Jpn J Cancer Res. 1995;86(7):617–21.

5 Diagnostic, Prognostic, Predictive and Therapeutic Tissue Biomarkers in Gastric Cancer

Vincenzo Canzonieri, Federica Rao, Tiziana Perin, Lara Alessandrini, Angela Buonadonna, Giulio Bertola, Claudio Belluco, Renato Cannizzaro, Antonino De Paoli, and Antonio Giordano

Introduction

Gastric cancer is one of the most common lethal cancers worldwide. Every year worldwide, there are 723,000 cancer-related deaths caused by gastric cancer according to the World Health Organization (WHO). It is the third leading cause of death by cancer and the fifth most common cancer in the world [1].

V. Canzonieri (✉)
Pathology Department, IRCCS, CRO Aviano, National Cancer Institute, Aviano, PN, Italy

Department of Medical, Surgical and Health Sciences, University of Trieste, Trieste, TS, Italy

CRO Biobank, IRCCS, CRO Aviano, National Cancer Institute, Aviano, PN, Italy

Department of Biology, Temple University, Philadelphia, PA, USA
e-mail: vcanzonieri@cro.it

F. Rao
Pathology Department, IRCCS, CRO Aviano, National Cancer Institute, Aviano, PN, Italy

T. Perin
Pathology Department, IRCCS, CRO Aviano, National Cancer Institute, Aviano, PN, Italy

CRO Biobank, IRCCS, CRO Aviano, National Cancer Institute, Aviano, PN, Italy

L. Alessandrini
Pathology Department, IRCCS, CRO Aviano, National Cancer Institute, Aviano, PN, Italy

Department of Medicine (DIMED), Surgical Pathology & Cytopathology Unit, University Hospital of Padova, Padova, Italy

A. Buonadonna
Medical Oncology Department, IRCCS, CRO Aviano, National Cancer Institute, Aviano, PN, Italy

G. Bertola · C. Belluco
Surgical Oncology Department, IRCCS, CRO Aviano, National Cancer Institute, Aviano, PN, Italy

R. Cannizzaro
Oncological Gastroenterology Department, IRCCS, CRO Aviano, National Cancer Institute, Aviano, PN, Italy

A. De Paoli
Radiation Oncology Department, IRCCS, CRO Aviano, National Cancer Institute, Aviano, PN, Italy

A. Giordano
Sbarro Institute for Cancer Research and Molecular Medicine, Department of Biology, Temple University, Philadelphia, PA, USA

Department of Medicine, Surgery and Neuroscience, Anatomic Pathology Section, University of Siena, Siena, Italy

© Springer Nature Switzerland AG 2019

V. Canzonieri, A. Giordano (eds.), *Gastric Cancer In The Precision Medicine Era*, Current Clinical Pathology, https://doi.org/10.1007/978-3-030-04861-7_5

The incidences and mortality rates are higher in men than in women.

Stomach cancer is common in different parts of the world, including Europe, the United States, Korea, China and Japan [2].

There are different factors that increase the risk of gastric cancer. They can be divided into genetics factors, such as mutations of the BRCA1 and BRCA2 genes, and non-genetic factors, such as age, sex, family history, smoking, alcohol consumption, obesity, physical inactivity, stress and infections. A relevant role has been recognized for *Helicobacter pylori* infection in the onset of gastric cancer [3, 4].

Despite progress in the diagnosis and treatment of advanced gastric cancer, the prognosis remains poor, mainly due to difficulty in diagnosing the disease in its early stages. Patients diagnosed with advanced GC have a dismal prognosis with a high mortality rate. Therefore, early detection of cancer can reduce the probability of disease progression, advanced cancer and death and increase the chances of treatment success.

In this chapter, the classification of gastric cancer into various histological subtypes and their biological characteristics, disease predictions by immunohistochemistry and in situ hybridization and gastric cancer assessments with standard and new tissue biomarkers are discussed.

Gastric Carcinoma

Precursor Lesions

Gastric Intestinal Metaplasia (GIM)

Gastric intestinal metaplasia (GIM) (Fig. 5.1) is an intermediate precancerous gastric lesion in the gastric cancer cascade of chronic gastritis, atrophic gastritis, intestinal metaplasia, dysplasia and adenocarcinoma. Although the risk of gastric cancer is increased in patients with intestinal metaplasia, the absolute risk is low. GIM can be divided into two subtypes: the complete type (type I) that morphologically resembles the normal small intestinal mucosa with absorbing cells, Paneth cells and goblet cells; the incomplete sulphomucin-negative type (type II), consisting of goblet cells scattered among gastric foveolar and neck cells; and the incomplete sulphomucin-positive type (type III), showing goblet cells scattered among sulphomucin-producing columnar cells. Another classification has been proposed by Tatematsu et al., in which IM can be divided into gastric-and-intestinal mixed (GI) and solely intestinal (I) types [5], expressing different tissue markers, so that IM might also be evidenced by the progressive intestinalization of stem cells from the GI-type to I-type. In this context, precocious identification of the early stages of GIM may be achieved with LI cadherin, (liver-intestine (LI) cadherin or CDH17, see below) which has higher sensibility and specificity than villin. However, specific subsets of patients with intestinal metaplasia might have a greater risk of progression. Hence, it is necessary to identify new biomarkers to better identify high-risk subgroups and to determine the optimal interval for surveillance in patients at increased risk for gastric cancer.

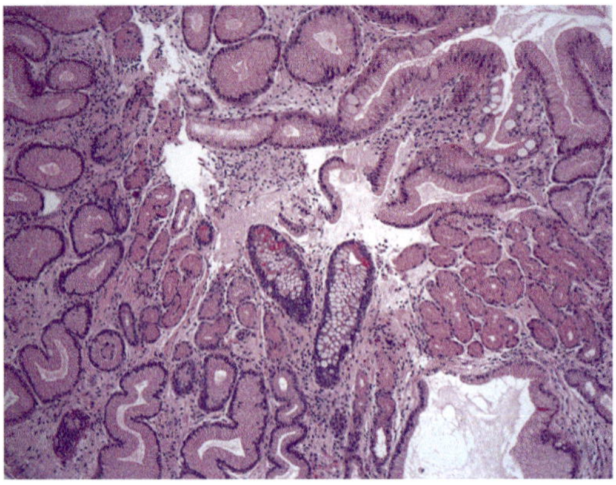

Fig. 5.1 Gastric intestinal metaplasia (GIM). Original Magnification 100×

Gastric Epithelial Dysplasia (GED)

Gastric epithelial dysplasia (GED) refers to neoplastic noninvasive proliferation widely accepted as a precursor to gastric adenocarcinoma. The frequency of GED increases with age, especially in men in their fifth decade of life or above. This tendency may be related to atrophic changes, especially intestinal metaplasia of the gastric mucosa, among the elderly. The prevalence of GED shows considerable geographic differences, and it seems to be associated with the regional prevalence of *Helicobacter pylori* infection [6].

Based on its morphological characteristics, GED is divided into three subtypes: low-grade, high-grade and indefinite dysplasia. It seems that 15% of low-grade dysplasia can evolve to carcinoma, while high-grade dysplasia has an 85% chance of progression (Fig. 5.2).

Gastric Adenocarcinoma (GA)

Gastric adenocarcinoma (GAC) is the most common histological type (~95%) of all malignancies originating in the stomach. It is a heterogeneous disease with different histological characteristics (phenotypes) and genotypes.

According to the most recent WHO classification (Bosman et al., 2010), GAC can be divided into five main types: papillary adenocarcinoma, tubular adenocarcinoma, mucinous adenocarcinoma, poorly cohesive carcinoma and mixed adenocarcinoma [7]. In addition, the Lauren classification divides GC into four histological types: intestinal gastric, diffuse gastric cancer, mixed and indeterminate types with distinct clinicopathological features. Intestinal gastric cancer is more associated with environmental factors such as infection of *H. pylori*, a high-salt diet, smoking and obesity [8], while diffuse gastric cancer comprises non-cohesive cells and is more commonly observed in younger patients, with an apparent hereditary feature. It has been reported that approximately 10% of gastric cancer cases show familial clustering [9]. The diffuse type of GA usually develops de novo and is usually not associated with *H. pylori*.

Rare hereditary forms of GAC are associated with germline mutations in various genes, such as CDH1, which encodes the tumour suppressor and cell adhesion protein cadherin 1 (also known as E-cadherin). Additionally, impaired function in mismatch repair genes (such as MLH1) or in CTNNA1 (which encodes catenin α1, a cell adhesion protein) or inactivating mutations in BRCA genes (which encode DNA damage repair proteins) can increase the risk. Furthermore, infection with *Helicobacter pylori* and Epstein-Barr virus (EBV), as well as exposure to other carcinogens, is known to contribute to the development of GAC [10] (Figs. 5.3 and 5.4).

Tissue Biomarkers of Gastric Cancer

The search for various antigens is critical in the diagnosis, prognosis and prediction of cancer. Different subtypes of gastric carcinoma show different antigenic patterns. Recently, several mole-

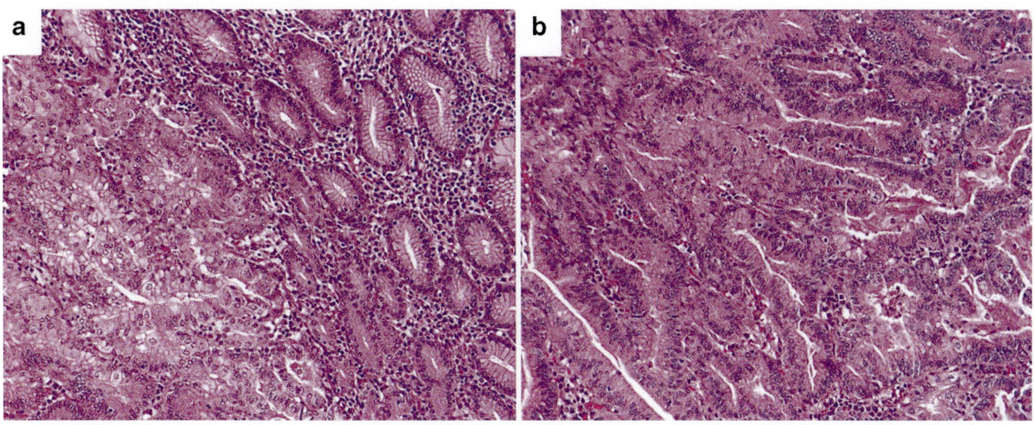

Fig. 5.2 Gastric epithelial dysplasia (GED): (**a**) Transition from normal tissue (right) to high-grade glandular dysplasia (left). Original magnification 200×; (**b**) High-grade dysplasia. Original magnification 200×

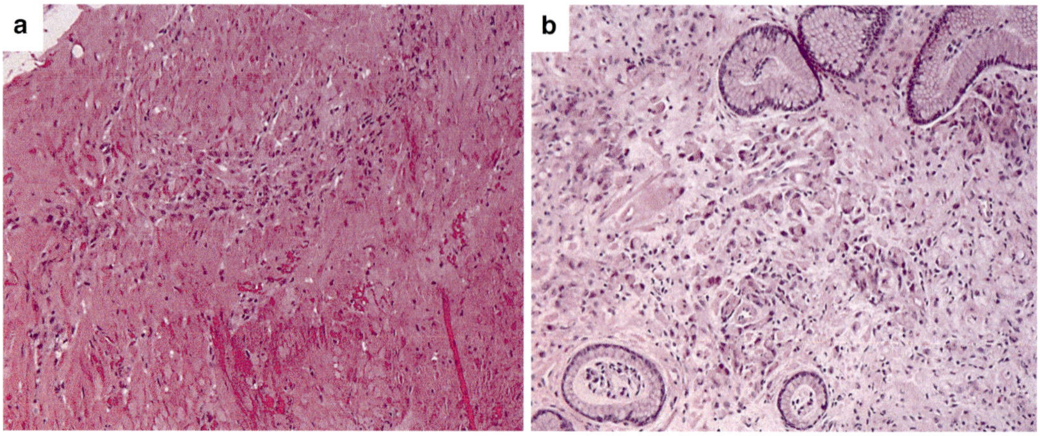

Fig. 5.3 Gastric adenocarcinoma (GA): (**a**) Diffuse-type gastric adenocarcinoma with infiltration of the muscular wall, original magnification 200×; and (**b**) neoplastic infiltration of lamina propria, original magnification 200×

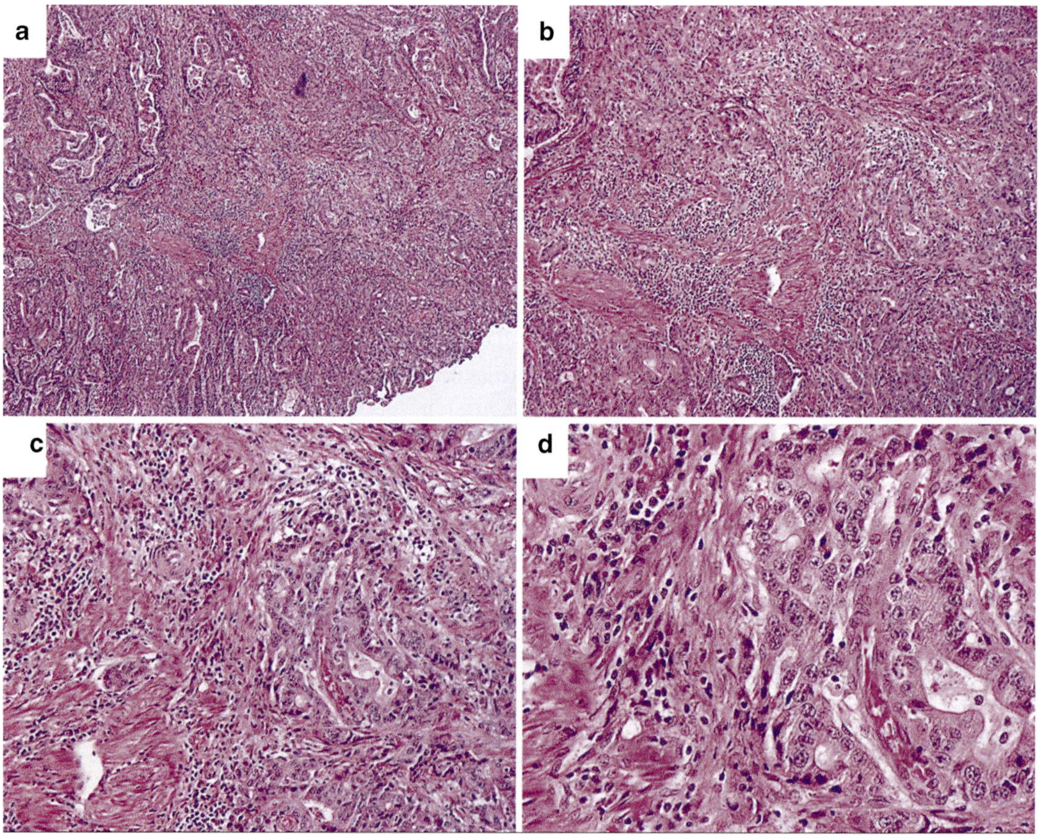

Fig. 5.4 Tubulo-papillary adenocarcinoma of the stomach at different original magnifications. (**a**) 50×; (**b**) 100×, (**c**) 200×; (**d**) 400×

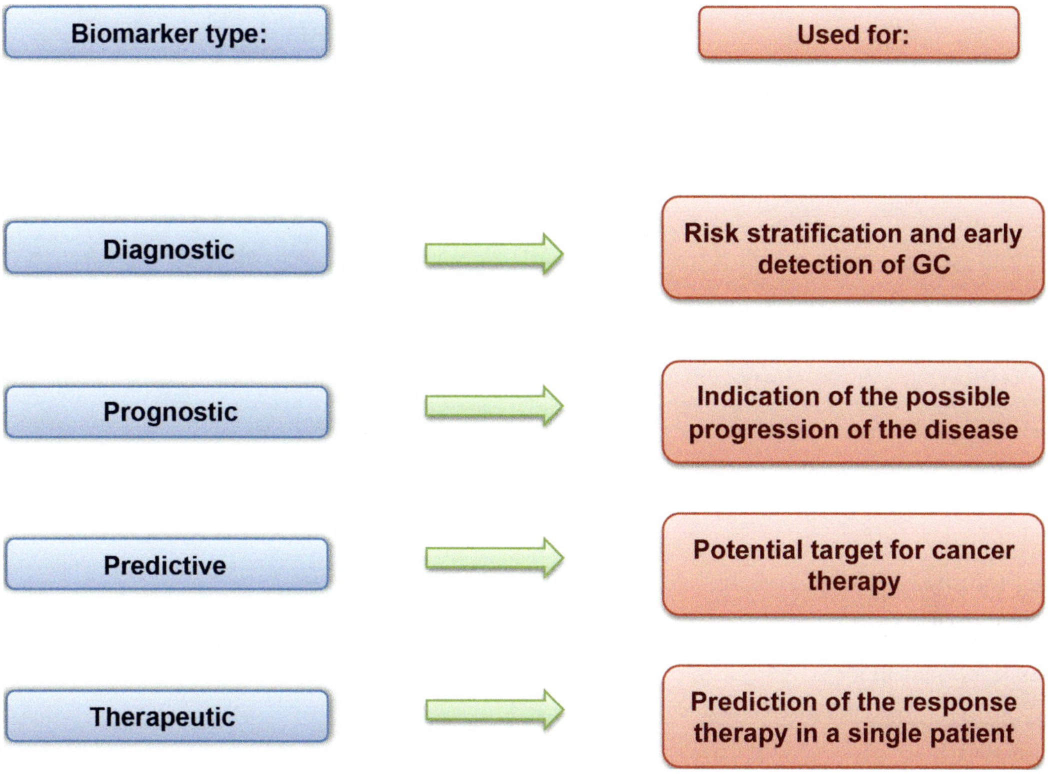

Fig. 5.5 Biomarker types and their utilization in clinical practice

cules have been proposed as novel biomarkers. They can be classified into four types: diagnostic, prognostic, predictive and therapeutic (Fig. 5.5). Notably, some markers might have an inclusive theranostic multirole in gastric cancer.

Diagnostic Tissue Biomarkers

Cytokeratins

Cytokeratins (CKs) are keratin proteins found in the intracytoplasmic cytoskeleton of epithelial tissue. They are important components of intermediate filaments, and they are involved in fixation of the nucleus and maintenance of cell morphology. There are at least 20 known cytokeratins, and they can be expressed differentially in healthy and neoplastic tissues. Thus, they are useful diagnostic tools.

Gastric adenocarcinomas stain with low- and high-molecular-weight cytokeratins (L-HMWCKs).

CK7 is expressed in approximately 80% of gastric adenocarcinomas, and it is observed in various ductal epithelial cell carcinomas, arising in the pancreatobiliary tract and renal collecting ducts. Otherwise, CK20 expression is reported in approximately 40% of gastric adenocarcinomas in a patchy or diffuse distribution. CK20 is specific to certain types of cancer and is typically used in combination with CK7 to distinguish different types of tumours (Fig. 5.6). However, the CK7/CK20 coordinate staining pattern has been considered of little utility for the differential diagnosis of primary gastric adenocarcinoma versus

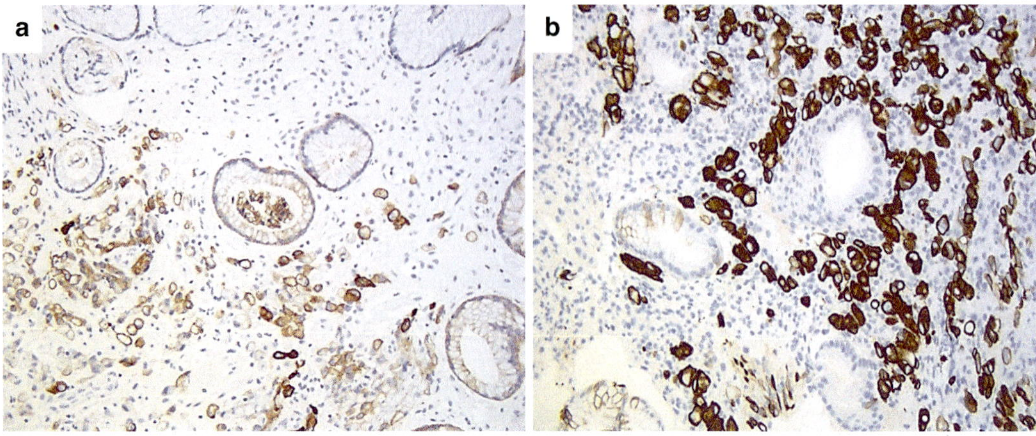

Fig. 5.6 (**a**) Immunohistochemical expression of CK7 in tubulo-papillary adenocarcinoma, original magnification 200×; (**b**) immunohistochemical expression of CK20 in tubulo-papillary adenocarcinoma, original magnification 200×

Fig. 5.7 Coordinate immunostaining pattern in gastric adenocarcinoma. Its use is not useful in the differential diagnosis with other adenocarcinomas

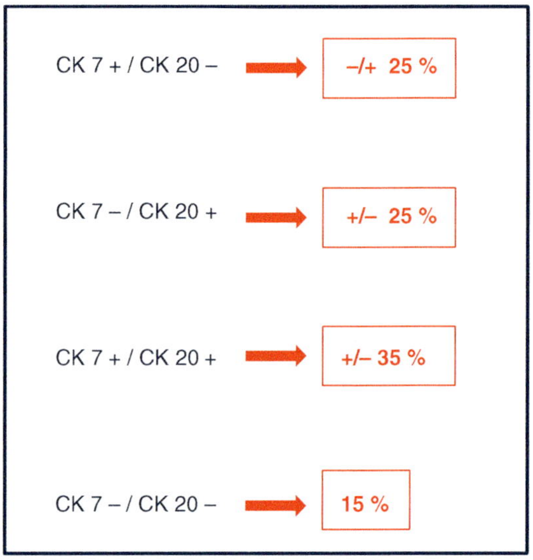

metastatic adenocarcinomas to the stomach (Fig. 5.7).

Other cytokeratins, strongly expressed in gastric adenocarcinomas, are CK18 and CK19. There is evidence that CK18 is involved in the invasion, growth and metastasis of tumours. Therefore, it can be used as a biomarker of gastric carcinoma aggressiveness [11]. Moreover, CK8 and cytokeratin Cam.5.2 are strongly expressed in gastric adenocarcinoma, whereas CK17 expression is constantly negative [12].

CDX2

CDX2 is a homeobox gene that encodes an intestine-specific transcription factor, and it is expressed in the nuclei of epithelial cells throughout the GI tract. It is considered a tumour suppressor gene in different tumour types, including gastric adenocarcinoma, where it is variably expressed (positivity ranges from 20% to 90%), and its expression is heterogeneous in diffuse-type cancers compared with strong and diffuse staining in tubular adenocarcinomas.

CK7 and the CK20 or CDX2 markers constitute an important panel for the diagnosis of GI tumours versus tumours of unknown origin. However, in some cases, the patterns of expression may vary, and the presence or absence of these markers may not lead to a definitive diagnosis [13] (Fig. 5.8).

Mucin Core Polypeptides (MUC)

Mucin core polypeptides (MUC) are high-molecular-weight glycoproteins expressed throughout the gastrointestinal tract, with a key role in mucosal protection and function. They are responsible for the mucus gel layer, which covers the mucosa. Immunohistochemistry specific to various mucins (MUC1, MUC2 MUC5AC and MUC6) has been used to evaluate the mucin phenotypes of gastric cancer. MUC1 is normally expressed by enterocytes and intestinal goblet cells, and it is present in rare cases; MUC2 is normally secreted by intestinal goblet cells, and it is expressed in approximately 50% of cases; MUC5AC is expressed by gastric foveolar mucus cells and neoplastic goblet cells, but it is positive in 38–70% of cases; MUC6 is secreted by gastric antral and fundic

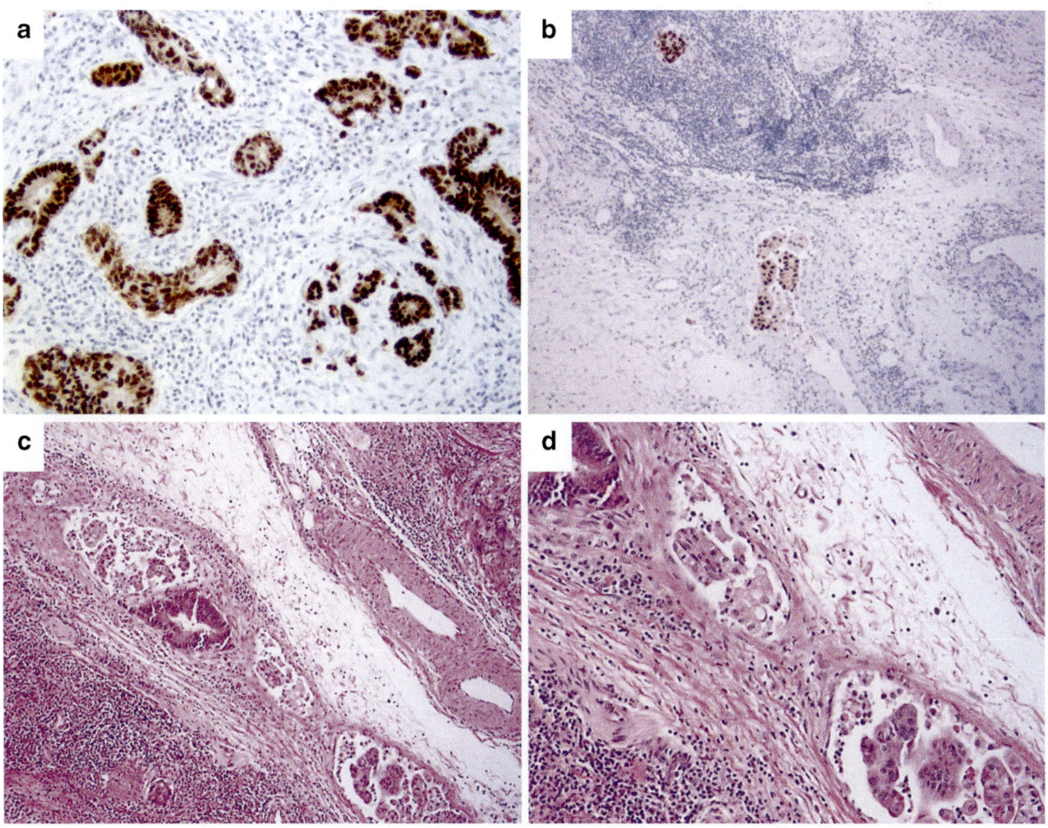

Fig. 5.8 (**a**) Immunohistochemical expression of CDX2 in a gastric tubulo-papillary adenocarcinoma, original magnification 200× (haematoxylin counterstain); (**b**) immunohistochemical expression of CDX2 with vascular invasion in a gastric tubulo-papillary adenocarcinoma, original magnification 100× (haematoxylin counterstain); (**c**) vascular invasion in a gastric tubulo-papillary adenocarcinoma (H&E), original magnification 100×; (**d**) same case at higher magnification (H&E), 200×

gland cells, and it is positive in 30–40% of cases [14] (Fig. 5.9).

β-catenin

β-catenin is an 88-kD member of the catenin family of proteins, which are important constituents of the cytoskeleton. It regulates gene expression and is an important component of the Wnt signalling cascade. Aberrant activation of the Wnt/β-catenin signalling pathway is involved in the development and progression of gastric cancer. The accumulation of β-catenin in the cytoplasm causes abnormal translocation to the nucleus and defects in gene expression. Thus, it seems that it is involved in tumour initiation, tumour growth, metastasis and resistance to therapy [15] (Fig. 5.10).

Chromogranin A and Synaptophysin

Chromogranin A and synaptophysin are two neuroendocrine markers. Chromogranin A is a member of the granin family of neuroendocrine secretory proteins. It is widely distributed in the secretory granules of most polypeptide-producing endocrine tissues and is considered very useful as a diagnostic aid for neuroendocrine normal and tumour cells. It is the most valuable marker of neuroendocrine tumours and is highly specific but less sensitive than synaptophysin. Synaptophysin is an integral membrane glycoprotein that was originally isolated from bovine neuronal presynaptic vesicles and is considered a significant neuroendocrine marker. Both chromogranin and synaptophysin play roles in characterizing some subsets of common gastric adenocarcinoma with expression of neuroendocrine markers (Fig. 5.11) [16].

Cyclooxygenase 2 (COX2)

Cyclooxygenase 2 (COX2) is an enzyme encoded by the PTGS2 gene; in humans, only one isoform is present. It is involved in the conversion of arachidonic acid to prostaglandin H2, an important precursor of prostacyclin. The expression of COX-2 in gastric cancer is upregulated, and its molecular mechanisms have been investigated. COX-2 likely plays a role in the promotion of proliferation in GC cells while inhibiting apoptosis, assisting angiogenesis and lymphatic metastasis and participating in cancer invasion and immunosuppression. Different studies have suggested that COX-2 overexpression is not related to the clinicopathological characteristics of gastric cancer patients but is related to tumour node metastasis clinical stage, depth of invasion and metastasis [17, 18]. Furthermore, it seems that COX-2 protein expression is associated with the intestinal histological subtype, tumour size, proximal location, advanced clinical stage and lymph node involvement. Thus, it seems likely that COX-2 plays a role in early gastric carcinogenesis [19, 20]. *Helicobacter pylori* infection, tumour sup-

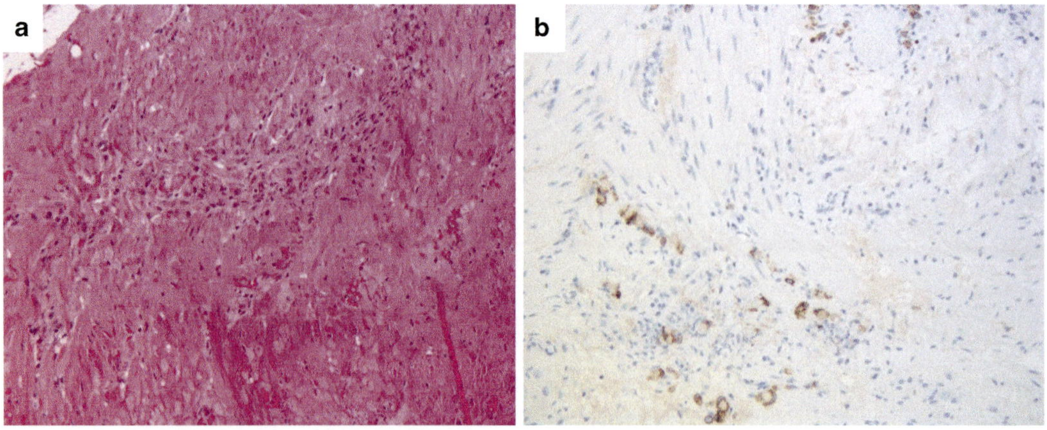

Fig. 5.9 (**a**) Diffuse-type adenocarcinoma (H&E), expressing; (**b**) MUC1, original magnification 200× (haematoxylin counterstain)

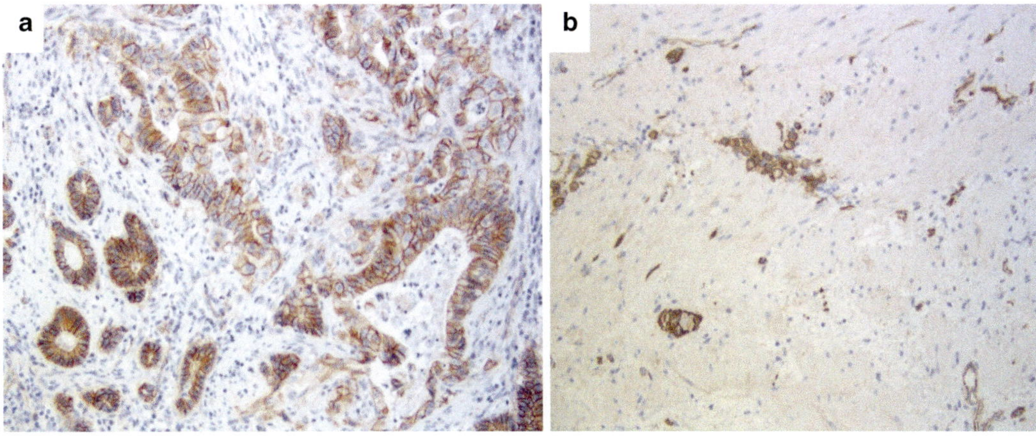

Fig. 5.10 (**a**) Immunohistochemical expression of β-catenin in a gastric tubular-papillary adenocarcinoma, original magnification 200× (haematoxylin counterstain); (**b**) immunohistochemical expression of β-catenin in diffuse-type gastric adenocarcinoma, original magnification 200× (haematoxylin counterstain)

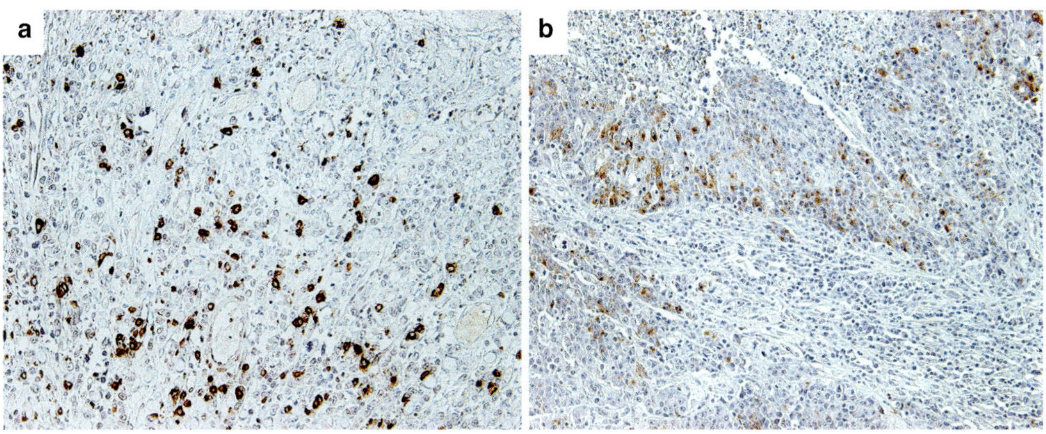

Fig. 5.11 (**a**) Immunohistochemical expression of chromogranin A in a gastric tubular-papillary adenocarcinoma, original magnification 200× (haematoxylin counterstain). (**b**) Immunohistochemical expression of synaptophysin in a gastric tubular-papillary adenocarcinoma, original magnification 200× (haematoxylin counterstain)

pressor gene mutation and activation of nuclear factor-kappa B may be responsible for the elevated expression of COX-2 in gastric cancer [21].

Carcinoembryonic Antigen (CEA)

In adults, CEA is expressed only in cancer cells, primarily adenocarcinomas, and may be used for diagnostic purposes. It is a set of highly related glycoproteins that are involved in cell adhesion. CEA is usually produced in the gastrointestinal tissue during the development of the foetus and terminates before birth. In gastric cancer, CEA has been used to distinguish between this and other similar types of cancers. Because of the possibility of cross-reactivity, false-positive results are observed, and this assay is typically used in combination with other analyses.

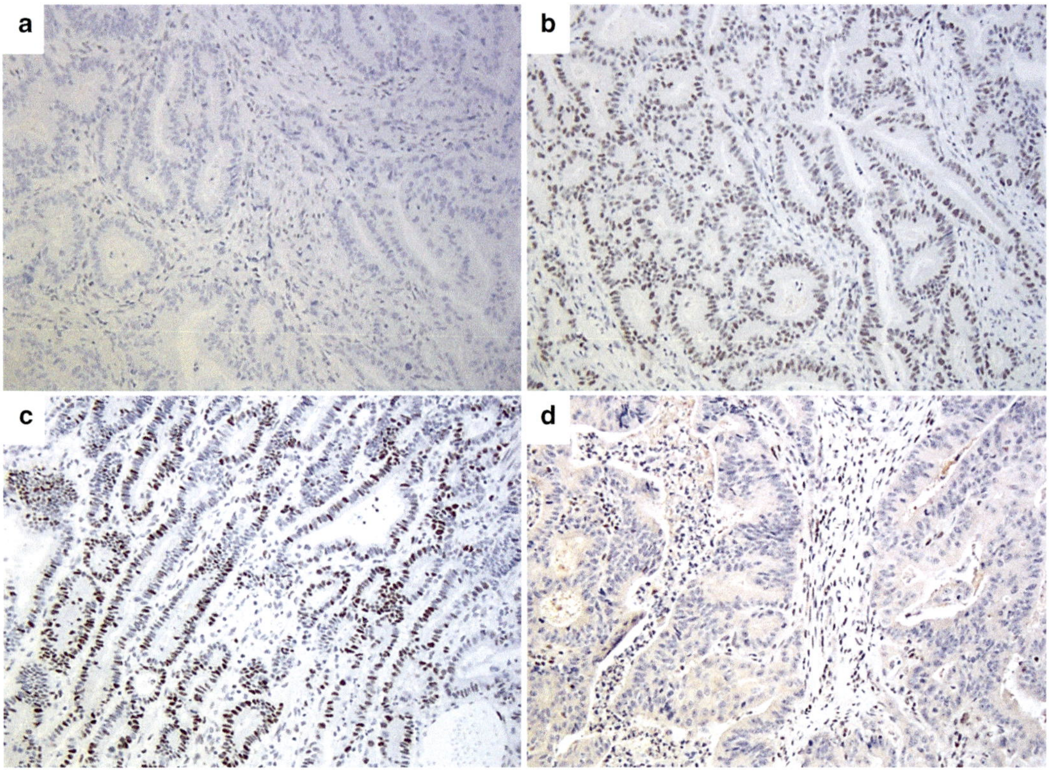

Fig. 5.12 (**a**) Immunohistochemical expression of MLH1 in a gastric tubular-papillary adenocarcinoma, negative case original magnification 200× (haematoxylin counterstain); (**b**) immunohistochemical expression of MSH2 in gastric tubular-papillary adenocarcinoma, original magnification 200× (haematoxylin counterstain); (**c**) immunohistochemical expression of MSH6 in a gastric tubular-papillary adenocarcinoma, original magnification 200× (haematoxylin counterstain); (**d**) immunohistochemical expression of PMS2 in a gastric tubular-papillary adenocarcinoma, negative case, original magnification 200× (haematoxylin counterstain)

DNA Mismatch Repair Proteins MLH1, MSH2, MSH6 and PMS2

DNA mismatch repair (MMR) genes encode proteins that detect and repair DNA mismatches that can occur during cell replication. Mutations in any of the MMR genes MSH2, MLH1, MSH6 or PMS2 increase the risk of different types of gastric cancer. These proteins function as heterodimers; MLH1 associates with PMS2, and MSH2 associates with MSH6 [22] (Fig. 5.12).

Prognostic Tissue Biomarkers

P53 Protein

P53 is a nuclear protein that functions as a transcriptional factor whose duty is to maintain genomic stability. When DNA damage occurs, p53 binds to the DNA and activates the transcription of genes responsible for stopping the cellular cycle and causing apoptosis of the cell. p53 is encoded by the gene TP53 located on chromosome 17p13.1. It is a tumour suppressor gene that is inactivated in the development of many malignancies, including gastric cancer. The expression rate of p53 detected by immunohistochemistry is reported to be 13–54% in gastric cancer [23].

Mutations in TP53 lead to nuclear staining due to the accumulation of mutant p53, which is resistant to degradation. A cell without the mutation does not show immunohistochemical staining of p53 because there is no such accumulation in the cell [24].

The prognostic role of p53 expression in gastric cancer has been searched in many studies, but it is controversial. In some studies, it has been suggested that patients without p53 expression have a longer survival, and p53 is a bad prognostic factor [25, 26].

Other studies report a correlation between p53 overexpression and the size of the gastric tumour [27].

The association between p53 overexpression with lymph nodes, metastasis and shorter survival remains controversial because it has been reported in some studies but not in others. Therefore, to date, p53's role as a prognostic marker needs to be confirmed [28] (Fig. 5.13).

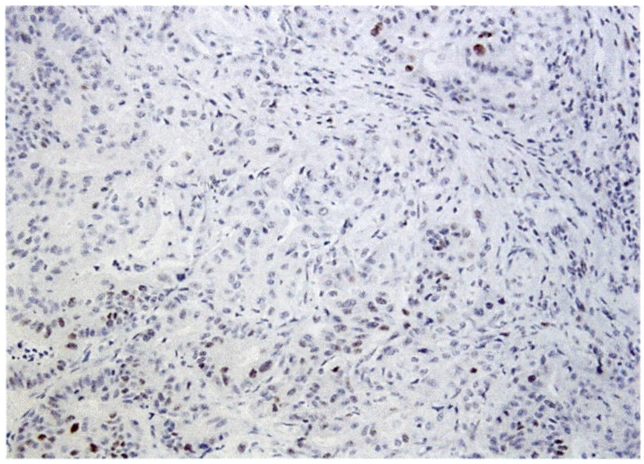

Fig. 5.13 Immunohistochemical expression of P53 in a gastric tubular-papillary adenocarcinoma, original magnification 200× (haematoxylin counterstain)

Carcinoembryonic Antigen (CEA)

In most cases, the CEA level is low in the blood of healthy individuals. Serum and tissue CEA is a representative tumour marker that has been known to be elevated in almost all solid tumours, mostly colorectal cancers, but also in gastric cancers and other neoplastic tissues. Therefore, it can be considered a negative prognostic factor [29].

Many studies have shown that increased preoperative serum CEA levels are associated with an increased risk of recurrence and a poor prognosis, and the prognostic effect of the serum CEA level is independent of the tumour-node-metastasis stage; thus, it can be considered a prognostic marker of gastric cancer. Otherwise, the expression of CEA in tissues is unclear and still under study. It is likely related to the serum expression of CEA, but is not correlated with the size or location of the primary tumour [30] (Fig. 5.14).

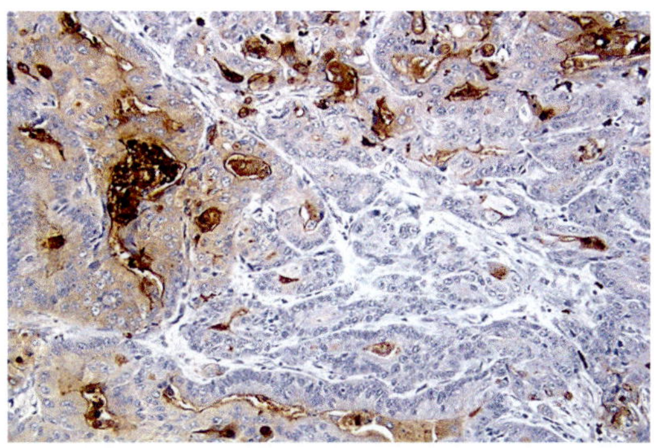

Fig. 5.14 Immunohistochemical expression of CEA in a gastric tubular-papillary adenocarcinoma, original magnification 200× (haematoxylin counterstain)

E-Cadherin

E-cadherin (epithelial-cadherin) is a transmembrane glycoprotein encoded by the CDH1 gene located on chromosome 16 (q22.1). It plays a crucial role in calcium-mediated adhesion, the differentiation of epithelial gastric cells and the prevention of neoplastic transformation. CHD1 has been reported to be one of the most important suppressor genes in gastric cancer, and its inactivation leads to an increase in the proliferation, invasion and metastasis of tumour cells. Different mechanisms can lead to the downregulation of E-cadherin, including mutations in the CDH1 gene, loss of heterozygosis (LOH), silencing by a suppressor that binds the gene promoter or hypermethylation and microRNAs that control E-cadherin expression. Furthermore, germline mutations in the CDH1 gene can cause hereditary diffuse gastric cancer (HDGC) [31].

It seems that different alterations lead to various clinical manifestations and histotypes, and there is an association between abnormal protein expression, tumour grade and metastases to regional lymph nodes. Therefore, E-cadherin can be considered a prognostic biomarker, associated with a worse prognosis and lower survival rate.

It can also be considered a predictive biomarker of the sensitivity to a specific therapy. In particular, its impairment reduces the response to

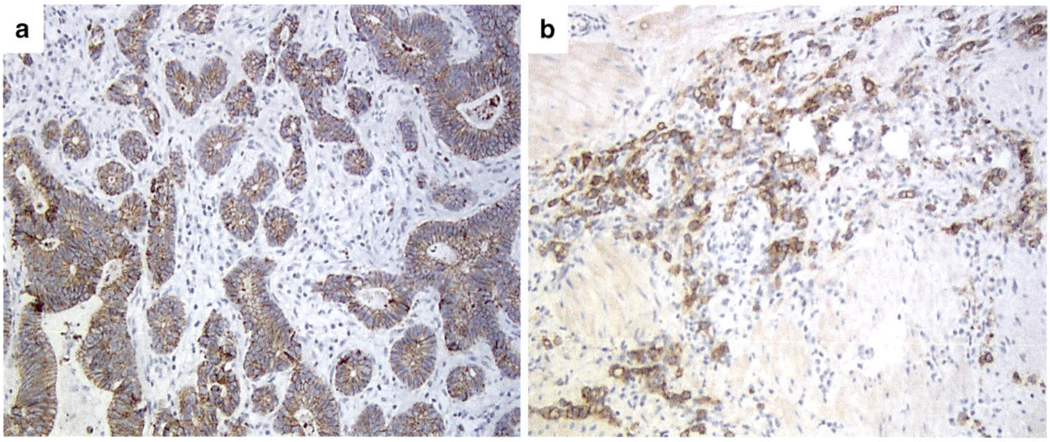

Fig. 5.15 (**a**) Immunohistochemical expression of E-cadherin in a gastric of tubular-papillary adenocarcinoma original magnification 200× (haematoxylin counterstain). (**b**) Immunohistochemical expression of E-cadherin in a gastric diffuse-type adenocarcinoma original magnification 200× (haematoxylin counterstain)

both conventional and targeted therapies. Therefore, it could be important to identify CDH1 mutations at the moment of the diagnosis to predict whether that cancer is going to be responsive to therapy so it could help in choosing a more suitable therapy for a specific patient [32] (Fig. 5.15).

EGFR

EGFR belongs to the family of tyrosine kinase receptors. EGFR overexpression, which is observed in 27–44% of gastric cancer patients, has been generally reported to be a poor prognostic factor. It is probably related to a cancer histology of slight differentiation, low survival and high stage, but there are still many doubts about this correlation [33, 34]. EGFR seems to have no predictive value. Indeed, the use of anti-EGFR (cetuximab and panitumumab) associated with chemotherapy does not show any improvement in clinical outcome.

FGFR

The FGFR/FGF cascade is a complex intracellular pathway that controls cellular proliferation and tumour growth, angiogenesis and dissemination. Four members of the FGFR family, FGFR1, FGFR2, FGFR3 and FGFR4, have been identified. These receptors are different depending on their ligand, binding affinity and tissue distribution [35].

Genetic modification or overexpression of FGFRs has been associated with the initiation and progression of several tumour types due to gene amplification, translocation and mutations, leading to enhanced kinase activity. *FGFR* gene abnormalities have been reported in various cancers, including stomach cancer. In particular, in gastric cancer, *FGFR2* amplification is reported to occur in 2–9% of patients. FGFR2 gene amplification is described as an independent poor prognostic factor in GC patients and is associated with higher pT and pN, lymphovascular invasion and distant metastasis. FGFR could also be a promising predictive marker; thus, different inhibitory molecules of the receptor are being tested [36].

MET

MET is a tyrosine kinase receptor (RKT) belonging to the family of hepatocyte growth factor receptors (HGFRs). It binds HGF/SF (hepatocyte growth factor/scatter factor) and plays a central role in the process of embryonic development, wound healing and organ regeneration. Autophosphorylation of MET leads to the activation of several downstream pathways (PI3K, Akt and RAS-MAPK) responsible for cancer cell survival, proliferation, invasion and metastasis. It is overexpressed in approximately 50% of advanced gastric cancer cases. It can be considered a negative prognostic factor. In fact, MET gene overexpression is related to a poor prognosis, and it is associated with a more aggressive disease and a shorter OS and disease-free survival than MET-negative gastric cancers. Furthermore, MET can be considered a predictive biomarker. The monoclonal antibody rilotumumab can prevent binding of the MET receptor with its ligand HGF; this targeted therapy, in association with chemotherapy, improves the survival of patients [37].

VEGF

Vascular endothelial growth factor (VEGF) is one of the most important factors driving tumour angiogenesis. The VEGF family consists of seven members: VEGF-A, VEGF-B, VEGF-C, VEGF-D, VEGF-E, VEGF-F and placental growth factor (PlGF). These proteins act through specific tyrosine kinase receptors (VEGFR1, VEGFR2 and VEGFR3), expressed primarily on endothelial cells. High levels of angiogenic factors in serum and tumours are associated with worse outcomes in patients with gastric carcinomas. In particular, VEGF-A, the most extensively studied angiogenic factor, could be a useful biomarker for disease progression and remission but not for diagnosis [38].

PIK3/mTOR

The phosphoinositide-3 kinase (PI3K)-protein kinase (PKB/AKT)-mammalian target of rapamycin (mTOR) pathway is a canonical pathway involved in anti-apoptosis and prosurvival and regulates several normal cellular activities, such as cell proliferation, survival and migration. Mutations in the PI3KCA gene, which encodes the alpha p110 catalytic subunit of PI3K, lead to constitutive activation of the PI3K/mTOR pathway. The PIK3CA mutation has been associated with a worse prognosis, reduced survival and increased lymph node metastasis. Therefore, it can be considered a negative prognostic factor [39].

In the last few years, targeted therapies have been tested to inhibit the PI3K/mTOR pathway, such as the one with everolimus, an mTOR inhibitor that seems to promise an improvement in survival in patients with gastric carcinoma. Thus, mTOR can probably also be used as a predictive marker [40].

Microsatellite Instability (MSI)

Microsatellite DNAs are widespread, short and repetitive DNA sequences that are randomly distributed in the human genome. When mismatch repair genes, including *hMLH1* and *hMSH2*, are inactivated, replication errors, such as insertions or deletions of bases within microsatellite regions, cannot be repaired. These phenomena are known as microsatellite instability (MSI). Alternatively, MSI can also be caused by epigenetic promoter methylation. Based on the frequency of mutation, MSI is categorized as low level (MSI-L), high level (MSI-H) and microsatellite stable (MSS). MSI has been used in the prognosis of numerous types of cancer. In gastric cancer, MSI is mainly related to hereditary type that occurs because of mutations during DNA replication. Patients with gastric cancer and MSI-H tend to be older and female and have a distally located tumour, with a well-differentiated adenocarcinoma type and in lower tumour stages [41].

The association between MSI-H and gastric cancer prognosis remains ambiguous. Certain studies support that MSI-H is associated with a good prognosis, while others are conflicting [42].

PLK1

Polo-like kinase 1 (PLK1), also known as serine/threonine-protein kinase 13 (STPK13), is a regulator protein of the cell cycle. Its aberrant expression is a driver of cancerous transformation and progression in various neoplasms, including GC.

Different studies have suggested that GC patients with a high expression of PLK1 had an inferior survival outcome [43].

High expression of PLK1 promotes GC cell metastasis rates and epithelial-mesenchymal transition by regulating the activation of the protein kinase B pathway [44].

Thus, an in-depth understanding of the molecular mechanism of PLK1 in tumour metastasis and in the inferior prognosis may lead to the discovery of new prognostic models. PLK1 could be a valid prognostic marker, and it could play a significant role in future clinical trials.

Predictive Tissue Biomarkers

HER2

HER2 (encoded by the proto-oncogene ERBB2 located on chromosome 17) is one of the four members of the human EGFR family (EGFR or HER1, HER2, HER3 and HER4) in the receptor tyrosine kinase (RTK) superfamily. It is located in the nucleus, and it is involved in the regulation of cell proliferation, differentiation, motility and apoptosis. Amplification of the ERBB2 gene results in the overexpression of HER2 protein, leading to cancer cell survival, growth and proliferation through the PI3K-AKT and MAPK pathways. HER2 overexpression, identified previously in breast cancer, has become a very important predictive biomarker in GC that allows clinicians to identify patients who would have a survival benefit from biological therapy.

Accurate identification of patient candidates for treatment with HER2-targeted therapy is now a fundamental step to optimize the therapeutic strategies in gastric carcinoma and breast cancer. Immunohistochemical (IHC) examination of the state of HER2 is recommended in all patients with advanced or metastatic carcinoma. This analysis allows the definition of the expression of HER2 at the membrane level, defined as 0 (negative), 1+ (negative), 2+ (equivocal) or 3+ (positive) (Figs. 5.16 and 5.17).

Tumours with IHC 3+ positivity are eligible for treatment with specific agents, whereas equivocal cases (IHC 2+) should be tested with in situ hybridization (ISH) techniques to evaluate the amplification status of HER2. Although both fluorescence in situ hybridization (FISH) and silver in situ hybridization (SISH) are approved by the European Medicines Agency to retest immunohistochemistry 2+ HER2 samples, it is widely accepted that SISH is a more suitable methodology than FISH for gastric cancer because it uses bright-field methodology and, therefore, can rapidly detect HER2-positive tumour foci within a heterogeneous sample [45].

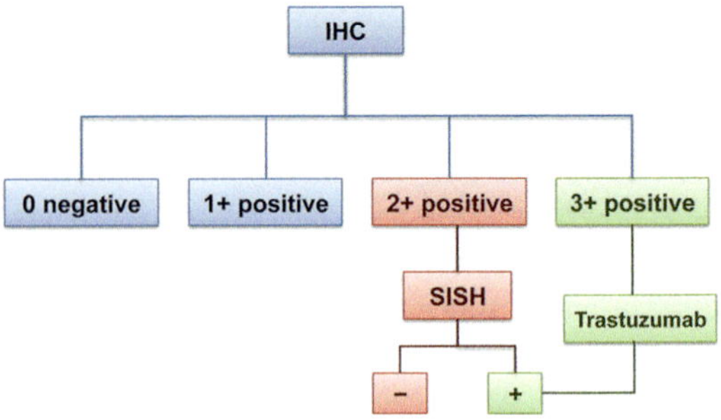

Fig. 5.16 Algorithm for the evaluation of HER2 in gastric carcinoma

The SISH "dual-colour" method, which uses two fluorochromes or two different chromogenes to visualize the same chromosome preparation on the same chromosome region 17 (CEP 17 probe) and the number of copies of the HER2 gene, is the most used and advisable approach (Fig. 5.18).

The definition of gene amplification is based on the evaluation of the relationship between HER2 gene signals and the centromeric signals of chromosome 17. The criteria for the definition are described in Fig. 5.19.

Currently, trastuzumab is the only targeted therapy permitted for advanced gastric cancer. Other drugs against HER2, such as lapatinib, pertuzumab and trastuzumab emtansine, are now being studied in clinical trials. Instead, the role of HER2 as a prognostic biomarker remains doubtful; indeed, some studies show an association of HER2 with a worse prognosis and a more aggressive disease, while others do not show a significant difference in the prognosis between HER2-positive and HER2-negative cancers. Some studies have suggested an association of ERBB2 amplification with tumour size, lymph node metastasis, local invasion and cancer stage; other studies have found no link between them [46, 47].

PD-1 and PD-L1

Programmed death 1 (PD-1) and its ligand programmed death ligand 1 and 2 (PD-L1 and

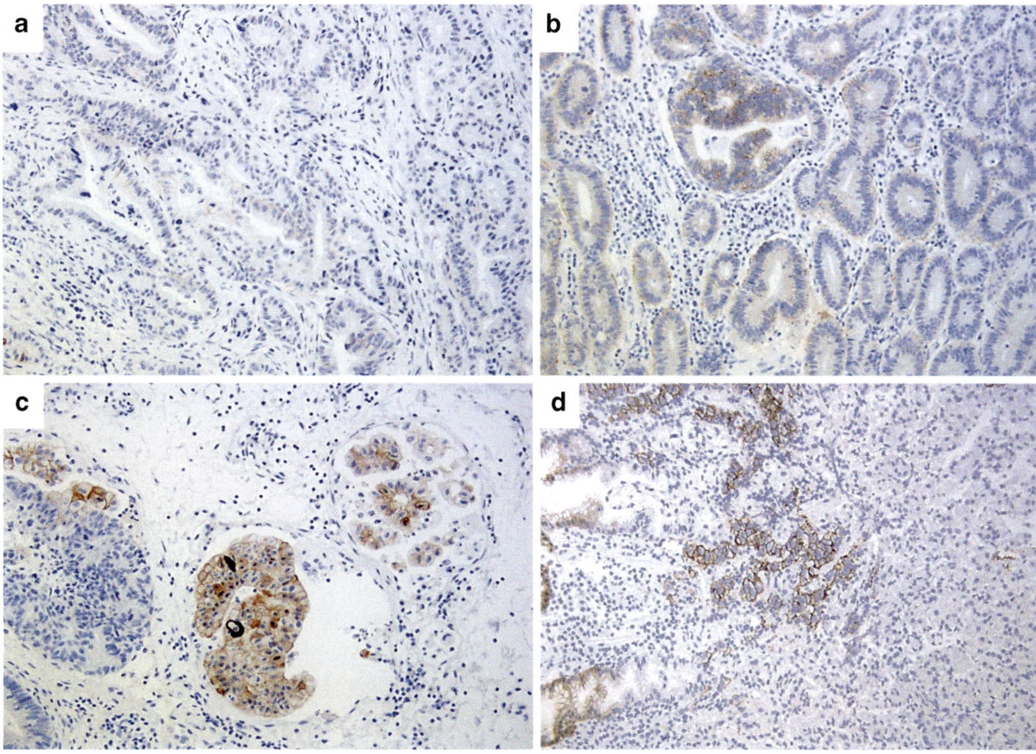

Fig. 5.17 (**a**) Immunohistochemical expression of HER2 (score 1+) in a gastric tubular-papillary adenocarcinoma, original magnification 200× (haematoxylin counterstain). (**b**) Immunohistochemical expression of HER2 (score 2+) in a gastric tubular-papillary adenocarcinoma original magnification 200× (haematoxylin counterstain). (**c**) Immunohistochemical expression of HER2 with vascular invasion in a gastric tubular-papillary adenocarcinoma original magnification 200× (haematoxylin counterstain). (**d**) Immunohistochemical expression of HER2 (score 3+) in gastric tubular-papillary adenocarcinoma, original magnification 200× (haematoxylin counterstain)

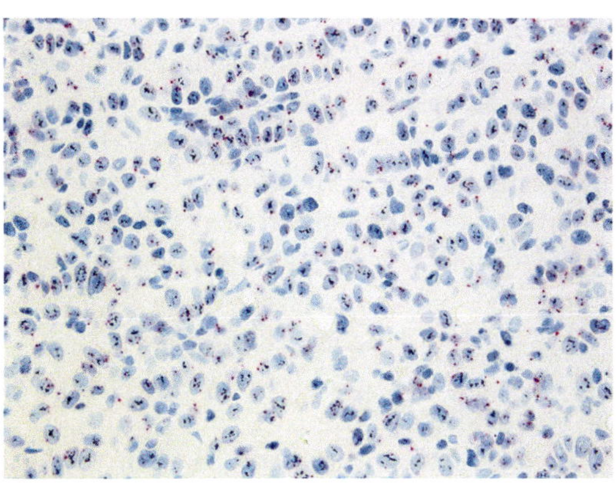

Fig. 5.18 Dual-colour SISH HER2 amplification in a gastric cancer, original magnification 200× (haematoxylin counterstain)

PD-L2) are a group of negative co-stimulatory molecules that can suppress T-cell proliferation in carcinoma. Neoplastic cells express the PD-1/PD-L1 pathway to escape the immune surveillance of T cells and the immune system response to the cancer [48].

The clinical efficacy of PD-1/PD-L1 inhibition has been observed for various malignancies, such as melanoma and non-small cell lung cancer (NSCLC), and it could be a promising way even in the treatment of gastric cancer. Types of cancers that show positive expression of PD-L1 are associated with a higher response rate to anti-PD-1/PD-L1 treatment. A monoclonal antibody anti-PD-1 pembrolizumab has manifested effi-

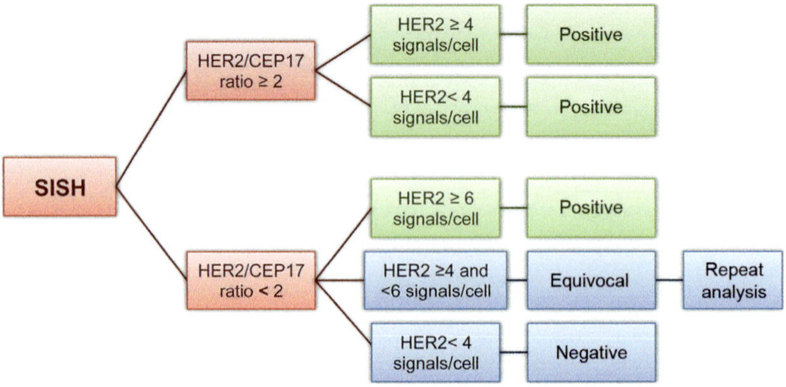

Fig. 5.19 Criteria for definition of HER2 amplification with SISH method

cacy in patients affected by advanced gastric cancer in the phase IB KEYNOTE-012 trial, a multicentre, open-label, phase 1b trial that included cohorts of patients with advanced gastric cancer and other cancer types [49]. Pembrolizumab is a selective, humanized, high-affinity IgG4-κ monoclonal antibody designed to bind to PD-1 and thus block the interaction between PD-1 and its ligand. It seems to have an acceptable safety profile and has shown promising antitumour activity in several types of advanced solid tumours [50].

Therefore, overexpression of PD-L1 can then be considered a predictive biomarker of the response to a targeted therapy. Targeting the PD1/PD-L1 pathway represents a promising strategy for the treatment of GC [51].

Correlation of GC and Tissue Biomarkers

Tissue Biomarkers in Precancerous Lesions

Immunohistochemistry and in situ hybridization may assist in the assessment of metaplasia and dysplasia. Most cases of GIM show CK7 and CK20 in the superficial and deep crypt cells [52] and are also positive for CDX2 [53].

The complete type of GIM is negative for MUC1, MUC5AC and MUC6 but positive for MUC2, while incomplete GIM is universally positive. *H. pylori* infection has been found in over 80% of patients with GIM and can then be identified using the Das-1 antibody, which stains *H. pylori* in gastric-associated GIM [54]. Interestingly, cells at the base of metaplastic glands are positive for LGR5+ and other intestinal stem cell (ISC) markers (OLFM4 and EPHB2). Because of the GI–I transition, this intestinal-like stem cell phenotype can be targeted to reverse IM and potentially prevent their progression into gastric cancers [55]. Otherwise, GEDs are often positive for p53 expression and Ki-67, and their expression increases according to the grading of dysplasia.

Tissue Biomarkers of GA

GA shows variable expression of CK7, CK20, CDX2, MUC2 and MUC5AC.

CK7 expression is an important marker of committed gastric epithelial cells and GA. Approximately 50% of GC are strongly positive for CK7. However, approximately 40% of GC show CK20 expression in a patchy or diffuse distribution. The positivity/negativity of both or one of the two markers seems to have the following percentages: approximately 35% of GC are CK7+ and CK20+, 25% are CK7− and CK20+, 25% are CK7+ and CK20–, and 15% are both CK7 and CK20−.

Several studies examined CDX2 in GC. Its expression seems to be variable and heterogeneous in the different types of GC.

Additionally, the various mucins in GC have different expression levels. GC can show the expression of MUC2 and MUC5AC, but it is almost always negative for MUC1 [56, 57].

Some variants of epithelial GA have been described. For example, recently, a new histological type of gastric adenocarcinoma called gastric adenocarcinoma with chief cell differentiation (GA-CCD) was described by Tsukamoto et al. [58]. Immunohistochemical evaluation of GA-CCD revealed diffuse positivity for MUC6 and negative staining for MUC5AC and MUC2 [59, 60].

As already stated, HER2 expression is evident in one out of five cases of stomach cancers often with a heterogeneous staining pattern [61].

Cases of poorly differentiated adenocarcinoma with prominent lymphoplasmacytic stroma may also be positive for the Epstein-Barr virus (EBV). Tumours of the upper gastrointestinal tract such as Barrett's oesophagus, oesophageal adenocarcinoma and gastric adenocarcinoma may show similar immunohistochemical findings.

In addition, it seems that 15–70% of common gastric carcinomas show expression of the neuroendocrine markers chromogranin A and synaptophysin.

In general, endocrine differentiation may be important for pathologic classification and could also be clinically relevant. In a particular study, the presence of endocrine differentiation detected with a cut-off of 20% of CgA+ and/or Syn+ tumour cells was significantly correlated with a higher relapse rate and higher disease-specific mortality than conventional tumours and tumours expressing CgA and/or Syn in 1–20% of cells [62].

A list of the most promising tissue biomarkers in gastric cancer is reported in Table 5.1.

Table 5.1 Emerging diagnostic, prognostic and predictive biomarkers and their targeted drug development

Biomarker characteristics	Diagnostic value	Prognostic value	Predictive value
Cytokeratins (*CK7; CK18; CK20; CDX2*): component of intermediate filaments involved in the fixation of the nucleus and maintenance of cell morphology	Important role for the diagnosis of GA	–	–
Mucin (*MUC1, MUC2 MUC5AC and MUC6*): mucosal protection and function	Has been used to evaluate the mucin phenotypes of gastric cancer	–	–
β-catenin: constituents of the cytoskeleton	Important role in the diagnosis of GA	–	–
Chromogranin A: neuroendocrine secretory protein	Diagnostic role in neuroendocrine carcinoma (NEC)	–	–
Synaptophysin: integral membrane glycoprotein	Diagnostic role in neuroendocrine carcinoma (NEC)	–	–
Cyclooxygenase 2 (*COX2*): conversion of arachidonic acid to prostaglandin H2	Useful in the diagnosis of GC	–	–
MLH1, MSH2, MSH6 and PMS2: detect and repair DNA mismatches that can occur during cell replication	Useful in the diagnosis of GC	–	–
P53: transcriptional factor whose function is to maintain genomic stability	Useful in the diagnosis of GC	Doubtful prognostic value	–
CEA: set of highly related glycoproteins that are involved in cell adhesion	–	It is associated with an increased risk of recurrence and a poor prognosis	–

(continued)

Table 5.1 (continued)

Biomarker characteristics	Diagnostic value	Prognostic value	Predictive value
E-cadherin: role in calcium-mediated adhesion and cell differentiation	–	It is associated with a worse prognosis and a lower survival rate	It is associated with a reduced response to conventional and targeted therapy
EGFR: tyrosine kinase receptors	–	It is associated with slightly differentiated to high-stage tumours and a low survival	–
FGFR: controls cellular proliferation and tumour growth, angiogenesis and dissemination	–	It is associated with a poor prognosis in GC patients	Probable predictive value
MET: role in the process of embryonic development, wound healing and organ regeneration	–	It is associated with more aggressive disease, a shorter OS and disease-free survival	It is a predictive biomarker of the response to rilotumumab
VEGF: the most important factors driving tumour angiogenesis	–	It is associated with worse outcomes in patients with gastric carcinomas	–
PIK3/mTOR: involved in anti-apoptosis and prosurvival	–	It is associated with a worse prognosis, reduced survival and increase lymph node metastasis	It is a predictive biomarker of the response to everolimus
Microsatellite instability (*MSI*): short and repetitive DNA sequences that are randomly distributed in the human genome	–	It is probably associated with well-differentiated adenocarcinoma	–
PLK1: is a multifaceted regulator of the cell cycle	–	It is associated with an inferior survival outcome	–
HER2: it is involved in cell proliferation, differentiation, motility and apoptosis	–	Still controversial prognostic value	It is a predictive biomarker of the response to trastuzumab
PD-1/ *PD-L1*: negative co-stimulatory molecules that can suppress T-cell proliferation in carcinoma	–	–	Overexpression is a predictive biomarker of the response to pembrolizumab

Promising New Biomarkers for Gastric Carcinoma

Matrix Metalloproteinase (MMP)

Matrix metalloproteinases (MMPs) are proteins that belong to a family of zinc-dependent endoproteinases, and their functions are to degrade elements of the extracellular matrix. They are involved in many physiological and pathological processes. MMPs are upregulated in gastric cancer, and they have been associated with specific disease characteristics of cancer. Different studies conducted on this topic require that MMP and TIMP, as well as their inhibitors, can be used as markers of invasion depth, peritoneal dissemination and metastasis. Unfortunately, currently, MMP inhibitors have not demonstrated a significant clinical benefit as therapy. However, their therapeutic role will be clarified in the future [63].

MicroRNA

MicroRNAs (miRNA) are 20- to 22-nucleotide noncoding RNA fragments whose functions are to bind the 3'UTR regions of their target genes and regulate their expression by modulating translation. MicroRNAs are involved in the regulation of different processes of the cell, such as proliferation, differentiation, migration and invasion [64]. It seems that they play a very important role in the carcinogenesis of gastric cancer; they can increase the expression of oncogenes or reduce the expression of tumour suppressor genes. Therefore, they may have prognostic significance and be associated with a worse prognosis.

Hepatocyte Nuclear Factor 4 Alpha (HNF4A)

HNF4A is a nuclear transcription factor that binds DNA as a homodimer. It is involved in different mechanisms such as invasion, metastasis and the epithelial-to-mesenchymal transition. Different studies have shown that HNF4A is a very good marker to discriminate between primary and metastatic gastric and breast carcinomas [65].

Other studies have suggested that HNF4α is a potential direct or indirect target for pharmacological drugs that act on the intestinal epithelium, and it seems that one HNF4α isoform was shown to correlate with Epstein-Barr viral infection in GC tumours [66].

FBXO2

FBXO2 belongs to the F-box family of proteins and is a cytoplasmic protein and ubiquitin ligase F-box protein with specificity for high-mannose glycoproteins. These proteins are classified into three different families based on the presence of specific recognition domains. Members of this family are important in cell cycle regulation, play key roles in tumourigenesis and have oncogenic or tumour-suppressive activities. A recent study has suggested that FBOX2 has clinical relevance in GC, and it demonstrates that FBXO2 levels are positively associated with lymph node metastasis, suggesting that high expression of FBXO2 could play an important role in the prediction of metastasis development in gastric cancer. Likely, the future role of FBXO2 in gastric cancer will provide promising new diagnostic biomarkers and therapeutic targets [67].

AURKA

Aurora kinase A (AURKA) is a protein belonging to a family of molecules that consists of highly conserved serine-threonine kinases that play critical roles in the regulation of mitotic events such as spindle assembly, function of centrosomes and cytoskeleton and cytokinesis. AURKA has been implicated in the regulation of cell cycle progression, mitosis and a key number of oncogenic signalling pathways in various malignancies. Several studies have shown that the overexpression of AURKA has been observed in early preneoplastic stages of gastric cancer in mouse models and humans [68].

Others have reported that AURKA promotes activation of the AKT prosurvival signalling pathway [69]. Furthermore, it was shown that AURKA can regulate and suppress GSK3β kinase activity in gastric cancer cell lines [70]. The interaction between AURKA and GSK3β causes the activation of β-catenin/TCF transcription complex, which leads to increased mRNA expression of different oncogenic proteins such as CCND1, c-MYC, c-MYC-binding protein, CLDN1, FGF18 and VEGF. However, little is known about its role in gastric cancer prognosis.

Thus, it seems that overexpression of AURKA mediates several pro-tumorigenic functions in addition to mitosis, thereby suggesting AURKA as a potential therapeutic target [71].

CDH17

Cadherin-17 (CDH17), which is also called liver-intestine (LI) cadherin, is a member of the cadherin superfamily of cell adhesion molecules, but its biological function remains unknown. CDH17 is expressed in mice and humans almost exclusively in the epithelial cells of both the embryonic and adult small intestines and colons, and it has no detectable expression in the liver or stomach [72]. Nevertheless, it seems that the protein is overexpressed in some GC cases. After the first study based on CDH17 as an intestinal metaplasia marker by Grotzinger et al. [73], several studies have evaluated CDH17 expression in gastric cancer. CDH17 was expressed in 50–78% of GC tissues with intestinal-type predominance [74, 75], suggesting that LI-cadherin is likely a marker for the intestinal phenotype [76].

REG4

Regenerating islet-derived family, member 4 (REG4) is a small secretory protein belonging to the group VII C-type lectin family, and its function may be related to proliferation and regeneration under physiological conditions [77].

Different studies have reported that REG4 is significantly overexpressed in GC tissues (especially in signet-ring cell carcinoma) compared with healthy tissue, and high expression of REG4 is positively related to lymph node metastasis [78].

Furthermore, it was reported that REG4 induces the expression of a series of anti-apoptosis genes (Bcl-2, Bcl-xl and survivin) by activating the epidermal growth factor receptor (EGFR)/protein kinase B (AKT)/activator protein 1 (AP-1) signalling pathway [79].

In the non-neoplastic stomach, foveolar epithelial cells do not express Reg 4, whereas goblet cells of intestinal metaplasia and neuroendocrine cells at the base of intestinal metaplasia express Reg 4, suggesting that Reg 4 is a marker for the intestinal phenotype [76, 80].

OLFM4

OLFM4 encodes olfactomedin 4 protein (also known as hGC-1 or GW112) and was originally cloned from human myeloblasts. Olfactomedin 4 expression is evident in crypt base columnar cells, which are intestinal stem cells in the intestinal metaplasia of the stomach; however, in the non-neoplastic stomach, it is not detected. Thus, this protein is useful to detect intestinal stem cells [81].

Some studies on well-differentiated adenocarcinomas have suggested that GC patients with positive expression of OLFM4 have a better survival rate than those with OLFM4-negative GC. The expression of olfactomedin 4 is frequently observed in the gastric phenotype so it likely plays an important role in the gastric phenotype of GC [82].

Both Reg4 and OLFM4 are secreted proteins, and serum Reg4 and OLFM4 serve as tumour markers for GC. The data suggest that serum OLFM4 combined with Reg4 is likely to be suitable for the screening of GC [76, 81].

HOXA10

Homeobox A10 (HOXA10) is a member of the homeobox gene family, which is evolutionarily well conserved and participates in several biological processes, such as the regulation of embryonic morphogenesis and differentiation and the control of normal development patterning along the anteroposterior axis [83].

It controls the organogenesis of the uterus during embryonic development and endometrial differentiation in adults. The deregulation of HOXA10 is correlated with the progression of endometrial carcinoma [84] but also promotes cell proliferation in other cancer types. The understanding of the role of HOXA10 in GC remains controversial, but HOXA10 appears to be expressed in the intestinal metaplasia of the stomach and may be a marker for the intestinal phenotype. Furthermore, the prognosis of patients with positive expression of HoxA10 is significantly better than that of patients with negative expression of HoxA10 [76, 85].

TSPAN8

TSPAN8 encodes tetraspanin 8 protein, which is a member of the tetraspanin family of proteins that span the membrane four times and is involved in numerous biological processes [86]. In human cancers, overexpression of tetraspanin 8 has been shown to be related to hepatocellular carcinoma, pancreatic cancer, colon cancer and oesophageal cancer. It was also reported that TSPAN8 mRNA is upregulated in GC tissues compared to normal gastric tissues by microarray analysis. One study reported that TSPAN8 is not specific to gastric or intestinal GC but plays a crucial role in both phenotypes of GC [76].

Conclusion

Gastric cancer is a noteworthy disease due to its heterogeneous properties. Although the molecular alterations of this neoplasm have been under study for several years and despite the many advances in the diagnostic and prognostic fields, identifying new biomarkers and improving knowledge regarding known biomarkers are fundamental steps.

With the development of modern technologies, such as genome and exome sequencing and the use of miRNA microarrays, several new biomarkers have been identified with diagnostic, prognostic and predictive value.

Importantly, experimental trials are needed to screen new serum and tissue biomarkers before their clinical use and, thus far, promising results are expected in this field in the next future.

References

1. Saberi Anvara M, Minuchehra Z, Shahlaeib M, Kheitana S. Gastric cancer biomarkers; A systems biology approach. Biochem Biophys Rep. 2018;13:141–6; 2405–5808/© 2018 Published by Elsevier B.V. https://doi.org/10.1016/j.bbrep.2018.01.001.
2. Lee J, Kim K-M. Biomarkers for gastric cancer: molecular classification revisited. Precision Future Med. 2017;1(2):59–68. https://doi.org/10.23838/pfm.2017.00079.
3. Wroblewski LE, Peek RM, Wilson KT. Helicobacter pylori and gastric cancer: factors that modulate disease risk. Clin Microbiol Rev. 2010;23:713–39. https://doi.org/10.1128/CMR.00011-10.
4. Song X, Xin N, Wang W, Zhao C. Wnt/β-catenin, an oncogenic pathway targeted by H. pylori in gastric carcinogenesis. Oncotarget. 2015;6:35579–88. https://doi.org/10.18632/oncotarget.5758.
5. Tatematsu M, Tsukamoto T, Inada K. Stem cells and gastric cancer: role of gastric and intestinal mixed intestinal metaplasia. Cancer Sci. 2003;94(2):135–41. https://doi.org/10.1111/j.1349-7006.2003.tb01409.x.
6. Baek DH, Kim GH, Park DY, Lee BE, Jeon HK, Lim W, Song GA. Gastric epithelial dysplasia: characteristics and long-term follow-up results after endoscopic resection according to morphological categorization. BMC Gastroenterol. 2015;15:17. https://doi.org/10.1186/s12876-015-0249-7.
7. Bosman FT, Carneiro F, Hruban RH, Theise ND. WHO classification of tumours of the digestive system. 4th ed. Lyon: International Agency for Research on Cancer (IARC); 2010.
8. Peleteiro B, Lopes C, Figueiredo C, Lunet N. Salt intake and gastric cancer risk according to Helicobacter pylori infection, smoking, tumour site and histological type. Br J Cancer. 2011;104(1):198–207. https://doi.org/10.1038/sj.bjc.6605993.
9. Paredes J, Figueiredo J, Albergaria A, et al. Epithelial E- and P-cadherins: role and clinical significance in cancer. Biochim Biophys Acta. 2012;1826(2):297–311. https://doi.org/10.1016/j.bbcan.2012.05.002.
10. Ajani JA, Lee J, Sano T, Janjigian YY, Fan D, Song S. Gastric adenocarcinoma. Nat Rev Dis Primers. 2017;3:17036. https://doi.org/10.1038/nrdp.2017.36.
11. Oyama K, Fushida S, Kinoshita J, Okamoto K, Makino I, Nakamura K, Hayashi H, Inokuchi M, Nakagawara H, Tajima H, Fujita H, Takamura H, Ninomiya I, Kitagawa H, Fujimura T, Ohta T. Serum cytokeratin 18 as a biomarker for gastric cancer. Clin Exp Med. 2013;13:289–95. https://doi.org/10.1007/s10238-012-0202-9.
12. Kim MA, Lee HS, Yang HK, Kim WH. Cytokeratin expression profile in gastric carcinomas. Hum Pathol. 2004;35(5):576–81. https://doi.org/10.1016/j.humpath.2003.12.007.
13. Altree-Tacha D, Tyrrell J, Haas T. CDH17 is a more sensitive marker for gastric adenocarcinoma than CK20 and CDX2. Arch Pathol Lab Med. 2017;141(1):144–150. https://doi.org/10.5858/arpa.2015-0404-OAR.
14. Boltin D, Niv Y. Mucins in gastric cancer – an update. J Gastrointest Dig Syst. 2013;3(123):15519. https://doi.org/10.4172/2161-069X.1000123.
15. Chiurillo MA. Role of the Wnt/β-catenin pathway in gastric cancer: an in-depth literature review. World J Exp Med. 2015;5(2):84–102. https://doi.org/10.5493/wjem.v5.i2.84.
16. Kim JJ, Kim JY, Hur H, Cho YK, Han S-U. Clinicopathologic significance of gastric adenocarcinoma with neuroendocrine features. J Gastric Cancer. 2011;11(4):195–9. https://doi.org/10.5230/jgc.2011.11.4.195.
17. Mao XY, Wang XG, Lv XJ, Xu L, Han CB. COX-2 expression in gastric cancer and its relationship with angiogenesis using tissue microarray. World J Gastroenterol. 2007;13:3466–71. https://doi.org/10.3748/wjg.v13.i25.3466.
18. Murata H, Kawano S, Tsuji S, Tsuji M, Sawaoka H, Kimura Y, Shiozaki H, Hori M. Cyclooxygenase-2 overexpression enhances lymphatic invasion and metastasis in human gastric carcinoma.

Am J Gastroenterol. 1999;94:451–5. https://doi.org/10.1111/j.1572-0241.1999.876_e.x.
19. Mrena J, Wiksten JP, Thiel A, Kokkola A, Pohjola L, Lundin J, Nordling S, Ristimäki A, Haglund C. Cyclooxygenase-2 is an independent prognostic factor in gastric cancer and its expression is regulated by the messenger RNA stability factor HuR. Clin Cancer Res. 2005;11:7362–8. https://doi.org/10.1158/1078-0432.ccr-05-0764.
20. Al-Moundhri MS, Al-Hadabi I, Al-Mawaly K, Kumar S, Al-Lawati FA, Bhatnager G, Kuruvila S, Al-Hamdani A, El-Sayed SM, Al-Bahrani B. Prognostic significance of cyclooxygenase-2, epidermal growth factor receptor 1, and microvascular density in gastric cancer. Med Oncol. 2012;29:1739–47. https://doi.org/10.1007/s12032-011-0098-3.
21. Cheng J, Fan X-M. Role of cyclooxygenase-2 in gastric cancer development and progression. World J Gastroenterol. 2013;19(42):7361–8. https://doi.org/10.3748/wjg.v19.i42.7361.
22. Dowty JG, Win AK, et al. Cancer risks for *MLH1* and *MSH2* mutation carriers. Hum Mutat. 2013;34(3):490. https://doi.org/10.1002/humu.22262.doi:10.1002/humu.22262.
23. Karim S. Clinicopathological and p53 gene alteration comparison between young and older patients with gastric cancer. Asian Pac J Cancer Prev. 2014;15:1375–9. https://doi.org/10.7314/APJCP.2014.15.3.1375.
24. Pietrantonio F, De Braud F, Da Prat V, et al. A review on biomarkers for prediction of treatment outcome in gastric cancer. Anticancer Res. 2013;33:1257–66. Available from: http://ar.iiarjournals.org/content/33/4/1257.full.pdf.
25. Gonçalves AR, Carneiro AJ, Martins I, et al. Prognostic significance of p53 protein expression in early gastric cancer. Pathol Oncol Res. 2011;17:349. https://doi.org/10.1007/s12253-010-9333-z.
26. Yıldırım M, Kaya V, Demirpence O, Gunduz S, Bozcuk H. Prognostic significance of p53 in gastric cancer: a meta analysis. Asian Pac J Cancer Prev. 2015;16(1):327–32. https://doi.org/10.7314/APJCP.2015.16.1.327.
27. Lu HZ, Wu JP, Luo W, et al. Correlation between aneuploidy of chromosome 17, over- expression of TP53 and TOP-II alpha and the clinicophatological features and diagnosis of adenocarcinoma. ZhonghuaZhong Liu ZaZhi. 2009;31(10):754–8. https://doi.org/10.3760/cma.j.issn.0253-3766.2009.10.009.
28. Carlomagno N, Incollingo P, Tammaro V, et al. Diagnostic, predictive, prognostic, and therapeutic molecular biomarkers in third millennium: a breakthrough in gastric cancer. BioMed Res Int. 2017;2017:7869802, 11 pages. https://doi.org/10.1155/2017/7869802.
29. Sisik A, Kaya M, Bas G, Basak F, Alimoglu O. CEA and CA 19-9 are still valuable markers for the prognosis of colorectal and gastric cancer patients. Asian Pac J Cancer Prev. 2013;14(7):4289–94. https://doi.org/10.7314/APJCP.2013.14.7.4289.
30. Saito G, Sadahiro S, Okada K, Tanaka A, Suzuki T, Kamijo A. Relation between carcinoembryonic antigen levels in colon cancer tissue and serum carcinoembryonic antigen levels at initial surgery and recurrence. Oncology. 2016;91:85–9. https://doi.org/10.1159/000447062.
31. Liu X, Chu K-M. E-cadherin and gastric cancer: cause, consequence, and applications. BioMed Res Int. 2014;2014:637308, 9 pages. https://doi.org/10.1155/2014/637308.
32. Corso G, Carvalho J, Marrelli D, et al. Somatic mutations and deletions of the e-cadherin gene predict poor survival of patients with gastric cancer. J Clin Oncol. 2013;31(7):868–75. https://doi.org/10.1200/JCO.2012.44.4612. Epub 2013 Jan 22.
33. Fuse N, Kuboki Y, et al. Prognostic impact of HER2, EGFR, and c-MET status on overall survival of advanced gastric cancer patients. Gastric Cancer. 2016;19(1):183–91. https://doi.org/10.1007/s10120-015-0471-6. Epub2015Feb 15.
34. Kim MA, Lee HS, Lee HE, Jeon YK, Yang HK, Kim WH. EGFR in gastric carcinomas: prognostic significance of protein overexpression and high gene copy number. Histopathology. 2008;52(6):738–46. https://doi.org/10.1111/j.1365-2559.2008.03021.x. Epub 2008 Apr 5.
35. Yashiro M, Matsuoka T. Fibroblast growth factor receptor signaling as therapeutic targets in gastric cancer. World J Gastroenterol. 2016;22(8):2415–23. https://doi.org/10.3748/wjg.v22.i8.2415.
36. Hierro C, Alsina M, Sánchez M, Serra V, Rodon J, Tabernero J. Targeting the fibroblast growth factor receptor 2 in gastric cancer: promise or pitfall? Ann Oncol. 2017;28(6):1207–16. https://doi.org/10.1093/annonc/mdx081.
37. Zhu M, Tang R, Doshi S, et al. Exposure-response analysis of rilotumumab in gastric cancer: the role of tumour MET expression. Br J Cancer. 2015;112(3):429–37. https://doi.org/10.1038/bjc.2014.649. Epub 2015 Jan 13.
38. Macedo F, Ladeira K, Longatto-Filho A, Martins SF. Gastric cancer and angiogenesis: is VEGF a useful biomarker to assess progression and remission? J Gastric Cancer. 2017;17(1):1–10. https://doi.org/10.5230/jgc.2017.17.e1.
39. Ying J, Xu Q, Liu B, Zhang G, Chen L, Pan H. The expression of the PI3K/AKT/mTOR pathway in gastric cancer and its role in gastric cancer prognosis. Onco Targets Ther. 2015;8:2427–33. https://doi.org/10.2147/OTT.S88592. eCollection 2015.
40. Ohtsu A, Ajani JA, Bai YX, Bang YJ, Chung HC, Pan HM, Sahmoud T, Shen L, Yeh KH, Chin K, Muro K, Kim YH, Ferry D, Tebbutt NC, Al-Batran SE, Smith H, Costantini C, Rizvi S, Lebwohl D, Van Cutsem E. Everolimus for previously treated advanced gastric cancer: results of the randomized, double-blind, phase III GRANITE-1 study. J ClinOncol. 2013;31(31):3935–43. https://doi.org/10.1200/JCO.2012.48.3552. Epub 2013 Sep 16.

41. Zhu L, Li Z, Wang Y, Zhang C, Liu Y, Qu X. Microsatellite instability and survival in gastric cancer: a systematic review and meta-analysis. Mol Clin Oncol. 2015;3(3):699–705. https://doi.org/10.3892/mco.2015.506.
42. Fang WL, Chang SC, Lan YT, et al. Microsatellite instability is associated with a better prognosis for gastric cancer patients after curative surgery. World J Surg. 2012;36:2131–8. https://doi.org/10.1007/s00268-012-1652-7.
43. Otsu H, Iimori M, Ando K, Saeki H, Aishima S, Oda Y, Morita M, Matsuo K, Kitao H, Oki E, Maehara Y. Gastric cancer patients with high PLK1 expression and DNA aneuploidy correlate with poor prognosis. Oncology. 2016;91:31–40. https://doi.org/10.1159/000445952.
44. Cai XP, Chen LD, Song HB, Zhang CX, Yuan ZW, Xiang ZX. PLK1 promotes epithelial-mesenchymal transition and metastasis of gastric carcinoma cells. Am J Transl Res. 2016;8:4172–83. Available from: https://www.ncbi.nlm.nih.gov/pmc/articles/PMC5095310/pdf/ajtr0008-4172.pdf
45. Rüschoff J, Hanna W, Bilous M, Hofmann M, Osamura RY, Penault-Llorca F, van de Vijver M, Viale G. HER2 testing in gastric cancer: a practical approach. Mod Pathol. 2012;25:637–50. https://doi.org/10.1038/modpathol.2011.198.
46. Kimura Y, Oki E, Yoshida A, et al. Significance of accurate human epidermal growth factor receptor-2 (HER2) evaluation as a new biomarker in gastric cancer. Anticancer Res. 2014;34(8):4207–12. Available from: http://ar.iiarjournals.org/content/34/8/4207.full.pdf.
47. Kim MA, Jung EJ, Lee HS, et al. Evaluation of HER-2 gene status in gastric carcinoma using immunohistochemistry, fluorescence in situ hybridization, and real-time quantitative polymerase chain reaction. Hum Pathol. 2007;38(9):1386–93. https://doi.org/10.1016/j.humpath.2007.02.005.
48. Fife BT, Pauken KE. The role of the PD-1 pathway in autoimmunity and peripheral tolerance. Ann N Y Acad Sci. 2011;1217(1):45–59. https://doi.org/10.1111/j.1749-6632.2010.05919.x.
49. Muro K, Chung HC, Shankaran V, Geva R, Catenacci D, Gupta S, Eder JP, Golan T, Le DT, Burtness B, Mc Ree AJ, Lin C-C, Pathiraja K, Lunceford J, Emancipator K, Juco J, Koshiji M, Bang Y-J. Pembrolizumab for patients with PD-L1-positive advanced gastric cancer (KEYNOTE-012): a multicentre, open-label, phase 1b trial. Lancet Oncol. 2016;17:717–26. https://doi.org/10.1016/S1470-2045(16)00175-3.
50. Patnaik A, Kang SP, Rasco D, et al. Phase I study of pembrolizumab (MK-3475; anti-PD-1 monoclonal antibody) in patients with advanced solid tumors. Clin Cancer Res. 2015;21:4286–93. https://doi.org/10.1158/1078-0432.CCR-14-2607.
51. Wu Y, Cao D, Qu L, Cao X, Jia Z, Zhao T, Wang Q, Jiang J. PD-1 and PD-L1 co-expression predicts favorable prognosis in gastric cancer. Oncotarget. 2017;8(38):64066–82. https://doi.org/10.18632/oncotarget.19318.
52. Shen B, Ormsby AH, Shen C, et al. Cytokeratin expression patterns in noncardia, intestinal metaplasia-associated gastric adenocarcinoma: implication for the evaluation of intestinal metaplasia and tumors at the esophagogastric junction. Cancer. 2002;94:820–31. https://doi.org/10.1002/cncr.10215.
53. Kim HS, Lee JS, Freund JN, et al. CDX-2 homeobox gene expression in human gastric carcinoma and precursor lesions. J Gastroenterol Hepatol. 2006;21:438–42. https://doi.org/10.1111/j.1440-1746.2005.03933.x.
54. Wong HH, Chu P. Immunohistochemical features of the gastrointestinal tract tumors. J Gastrointest Oncol. 2012;3(3):262–84. https://doi.org/10.3978/j.issn.2078-6891.2012.019.
55. Jang BG, Lee BL, Kim WH. Intestinal stem cell markers in the intestinal metaplasia of stomach and Barrett's esophagus. PLoS One. 2015;10(5):e0127300. https://doi.org/10.1371/journal.pone.0127300.
56. Flucke U, Steinborn E, Dries V, et al. Immunoreactivity of cytokeratins (CK7, CK20) and mucin peptide core antigens (MUC1, MUC2, MUC5AC) in adenocarcinomas, normal and metaplastic tissues of the distal oesophagus, oesophago-gastric junction and proximal stomach. Histopathology. 2003;43:127–34. https://doi.org/10.1046/j.1365-2559.2003.01680.x.
57. Lau SK, Weiss LM, Chu PG. Differential expression of MUC1, MUC2, and MUC5AC in carcinomas of various sites: an immunohistochemical study. Am J Clin Pathol. 2004;122:61–9. https://doi.org/10.1309/9R66-73QE-C06D-86Y4.
58. Tsukamoto T, Yokoi T, Maruta S, et al. Gastric adenocarcinoma with chief cell differentiation. Pathol Int. 2007;57(8):517–22. https://doi.org/10.1111/j.1440-1827.2007.02134.x.
59. Singhi AD, Lazenby AJ, Montgomery EA. Gastric adenocarcinoma with chief cell differentiation. A proposal for reclassification as oxyntic gland polyp/adenoma. Am J Surg Pathol. 2012;36(7):1030–5. https://doi.org/10.1097/PAS.0b013e31825033e7.
60. Chan K, Brown IS, Kyle T, Lauwers GY, Kumarasinghe MP. Chief cell predominant gastric polyps: a series of 12 cases with literature review. Histopathology. 2016;68(6):825–33. https://doi.org/10.1111/his.12859.
61. Abrahao-Machado LF, Scapulatempo-Neto C. HER2 testing in gastric cancer: an update. World J Gastroenterol. 2016;22(19):4619–25. https://doi.org/10.3748/wjg.v22.i19.4619.
62. Vincenzo Canzonieri MD, et al. Exocrine and endocrine modulation in common gastric carcinoma. Am J Clin Pathol. 2012;137:712–21. https://doi.org/10.1309/AJCPM13KVNCZQBUV.
63. Sampieri CL, León-Córdoba K, Remes-Troche JM. Matrix metalloproteinases and their tissue inhibitors in gastric cancer as molecular markers. J Cancer Res Ther. 2013;9(3):356–63. https://doi.org/10.4103/0973-1482.119302.

64. Han T-S, Hur K, Xu G, et al. MicroRNA-29c mediates initiation of gastric carcinogenesis by directly targeting ITGB1. Gut. 2015;64(2):203–14. https://doi.org/10.1136/gutjnl-2013-306640.
65. Bult P, Vogelaar IP, Ligtenberg MJL, Hoogerbrugge N, van Krieken JH. HNF4A immunohistochemistry facilitates distinction between primary and metastatic breast and gastric carcinoma. Virchows Arch. 2014;464(6):673–9. https://doi.org/10.1007/s00428-014-1574-x.
66. Uozaki H, Barua RR, Minhua S, et al. Transcriptional factor typing with SOX2, HNF4aP1, and CDX2 closely relates to tumor invasion and Epstein-Barr virus status in gastric cancer. Int J Clin Exp Pathol. 2011;4:230–40. Available from: https://www.ncbi.nlm.nih.gov/pmc/articles/PMC3071656/pdf/ijcep0004-0230.pdf.
67. Sun X, Wang T, Guan Z-R, Zhang C, Chen Y, Jin J, Hua D. FBXO2, a novel marker for metastasis in human gastric cancer. Biochem Biophys Res Commun. 2018;495:2158–64. https://doi.org/10.1016/j.bbrc.2017.12.097.
68. Katsha A, Soutto M, Sehdev V, Peng D, Washington MK, Piazuelo MB, et al. Aurora kinase A promotes inflammation and tumorigenesis in mice and human gastric neoplasia. Gastroenterology. 2013;145:1312–22. https://doi.org/10.1053/j.gastro.2013.08.050.
69. Dar AA, Zaika A, Piazuelo MB, Correa P, Koyama T, Belkhiri A, et al. Frequent overexpression of Aurora kinase A in upper gastrointestinal adenocarcinomas correlates with potent antiapoptotic functions. Cancer. 2008;112:1688–98. https://doi.org/10.1002/cncr.23371.
70. Dar AA, Belkhiri A, El-Rifai W. The aurora kinase A regulates GSK-3beta in gastric cancer cells. Oncogene. 2009;28:866–75. https://doi.org/10.1038/onc.2008.434.
71. Katsha A, Belkhiri A, Goff L, El-Rifai W. Aurora kinase A in gastrointestinal cancers: time to target. Mol Cancer. 2015;14:106. https://doi.org/10.1186/s12943-015-0375-4.
72. Gessner R, Tauber R. Intestinal cell adhesion molecules. Liver-intestine cadherin. Ann N Y Acad Sci. 2000;915:136–43. https://doi.org/10.1111/j.1749-6632.2000.tb05236.x.
73. Grotzinger C, Kneifel J, Patschan D, Schnoy N, Anagnostopoulos I, et al. LI-cadherin: a marker of gastric metaplasia and neoplasia. Gut. 2001;49:73–81.
74. Ito R, Oue N, Yoshida K, Kunimitsu K, Nakayama H, Nakachi K, Yasui W. Clinicopathological significant and prognostic influence of cadherin-17 expression in gastric cancer. J Pathol. 2005;205(5):615–22. https://doi.org/10.1007/s00428-005-0015-2.
75. Sakamoto N, Oue N, Sentani K, et al. Liver-intestine cadherin induction by epidermal growth factor receptor is associated with intestinal differentiation of gastric cancer. Cancer Sci. 2012;103:1744–50.
76. Oue N, Sentani K, Sakamoto N, Yasui W. Clinicopathologic and molecular characteristics of gastric cancer showing gastric and intestinal mucin phenotype. Cancer Sci. 2015;106:951–8. https://doi.org/10.1111/cas.12706.
77. Li FY, Ren XB, Xu EP, Huang Q, Sheng HQ, Lv BJ, Lai MD. RegIV expression showing specificity to gastrointestinal tract and its potential role in diagnosing digestive tract neuroendocrine tumor. J Zhejiang Univ Sci B. 2010;11:258–66. https://doi.org/10.1631/jzus.B0900383.
78. Duan Y, Hu L, Liu B, Yu B, Li J, Yan M, Yu Y, Li C, Su L, Zhu Z, Xiang M, Liu B, Yang Q. Tumor suppressor miR-24 restrains gastric cancer progression by downregulating RegIV. Mol Cancer. 2014;13:127–39. https://doi.org/10.1186/1476-4598-13-127.
79. Bishnupuri KS, Luo Q, Murmu N, Houchen CW, Anant S, Dieckgraefe BK. Reg IV activates the epidermal growth factor receptor/Akt/AP-1 signaling pathway in colon adenocarcinomas. Gastroenterology. 2006;130:137–49. https://doi.org/10.1053/j.gastro.2005.10.001.
80. Nakata K, Nagai E, Ohuchida K, et al. REG4 is associated with carcinogenesis in the ‘intestinal’ pathway of intraductal papillary mucinous neoplasms. Mod Pathol. 2009;22:460–8. https://doi.org/10.1038/modpathol.2008.205.
81. Oue N, Sentani K, Noguchi T, et al. Serum olfactomedin 4 (GW112, hGC-1) in combination with Reg IV is a highly sensitive biomarker for gastric cancer patients. Int J Cancer. 2009;125:2383–92. https://doi.org/10.1002/ijc.24624.
82. Seko N, Oue N, Noguchi T, et al. Olfactomedin 4 (GW112, hGC-1) is an independent prognostic marker for survival in patients with colorectal cancer. Exp Ther Med. 2010;1:73–8. https://doi.org/10.3892/etm_00000013.
83. McGinnis W, Krumlauf R. Homeobox genes and axial patterning. Cell. 1992;68:283–302. https://doi.org/10.1016/0092-8674(92)90471-N.
84. Yoshida H, et al. Deregulation of HOXA10 homeoglobal gene in endometrial carcinoma: role in epithelial-mesenchymal transition. Cancer Res. 2006;66:889–97. https://doi.org/10.1158/0008-5472.CAN-05-2828.
85. Sentani K, Oue N, Naito Y, et al. Upregulation of HOXA10 in gastric cancer with the intestinal mucin phenotype: reduction during tumor progression and favorable prognosis. Carcinogenesis. 2012;33(5):1081–8. https://doi.org/10.1093/carcin/bgs121.
86. Zöller M. Tetraspanins: push and pull in suppressing and promoting metastasis. Nat Rev Cancer. 2009;9:40–55. https://doi.org/10.1038/nrc2543.

Serum Biomarkers in Gastric Cancer

6

Agostino Steffan, Silvia Cervo, Valentina Fanotto, and Fabio Puglisi

Acronyms

AG Atrophic gastritis
AUC Area under the curve
CA 19-9 Carbohydrate antigen 19-9
CA 72-4 Carbohydrate antigen 72-4
CA 125 Carbohydrate antigen 125
CEA Carcinoembryonic antigen
cfDNA Cell-free DNA
CI Confidence interval
CTCs Circulating tumor cells
DSS Disease-specific survival
DFS Disease-free survival
G-17 Gastrin-17
GC Gastric cancer
HP *Helicobacter pylori*
HR Hazard ratio
IgG Immunoglobulin G
IM Intestinal metaplasia
NCA Nonspecific cross-reacting antigen
OR Odds ratio
OS Overall survival
PG Pepsinogen
TAG-72 Tumor-associated glycoprotein 72

Introduction

Circulating tumor biomarkers are defined as those substances produced by the tumor itself or by the organism in response to the presence of a neoplasia, which can be measured in the blood or in other biological fluids.

Serum tumor markers are blood-based biomarkers that are potentially useful in cancers detection, surveillance following curative surgery, prediction of drug response or resistance, and monitoring therapy in advance setting.

Irrespective of its application, the ideal tumor marker is represented by a biochemical indicator selectively secreted by cancer cells alone, which should theoretically allow an accurate and relatively

A. Steffan · S. Cervo
Immunopathology and Cancer Biomarkers, IRCCS, CRO Aviano, National Cancer Institute, Aviano, PN, Italy

CRO-Biobank, IRCCS, CRO Aviano, National Cancer Institute, Aviano, PN, Italy

V. Fanotto
Medical Oncology Department, IRCCS, CRO Aviano, National Cancer Institute, Aviano, PN, Italy

Department of Clinical Oncology, IRCCS, CRO Aviano, National Cancer Institute, Aviano, PN, Italy

Department of Medicine (DAME), University of Udine, Udine, Italy

F. Puglisi (✉)
Department of Clinical Oncology, IRCCS, CRO Aviano, National Cancer Institute, Aviano, PN, Italy

Department of Medicine (DAME), University of Udine, Udine, Italy
e-mail: fabio.puglisi@cro.it

© Springer Nature Switzerland AG 2019
V. Canzonieri, A. Giordano (eds.), *Gastric Cancer In The Precision Medicine Era*, Current Clinical Pathology, https://doi.org/10.1007/978-3-030-04861-7_6

simple diagnosis of neoplasia; it should therefore exhibit a high positive and negative predictive value. Actually, the commonly used tumor biomarkers are neither specific nor sensitive; moreover, normal levels were set using the Gaussian function.

Another element of complexity in the interpretation of the clinical value of a given marker is certainly represented by the lack of homogeneity of the available data, which often derive from retrospective analyses with low statistical power. In order to standardize and increase the quality of the data reported in the studies that analyze potential prognostic factors in patients with cancer, the National Cancer Institute-European Organization for Research and Treatment of Cancer working group on cancer diagnostics, in 2005, set out specific methodological recommendations (Reporting Recommendations for Tumor Marker Prognostic Studies) [1]. However, the problem of the almost complete lack of prospectively validated data remains; this step would represent the confirmation of biological assumptions and retrospective analyses of many tumor markers.

Some tumor markers found in serum, such as carcinoembryonic antigen (CEA) and carbohydrate antigen 19-9 (CA 19-9), can be elevated in 30–40% of gastric cancer (GC).

In addition to these commonly used markers, carbohydrate antigen 125 (CA 125) and carbohydrate antigen 72-4 (CA 72-4) have been reported to be elevated in advanced GC [2]. In 2010, the National Academy Clinical Biochemistry reiterated that no biomarker is recommended for routine clinical use during the diagnostic phase, while its use may be more useful in the course of the post-surgery follow-up and to monitor the response to antineoplastic treatment [3]. In line with these recommendations, international guidelines do not accept tumor markers in the process of GC diagnosis [4].

Their usefulness in GC can be acknowledged in:

- monitoring the effectiveness of antineoplastic therapy, but radiological assessment remains the gold standard [4];
- the surveillance period, but their role is controversial because an early detection of relapse does not necessarily translate into prognostic advantages [4].

The main characteristics of the classic tumor markers in GC are shown in Table 6.1.

Specific gastric biomarkers, i.e., pepsinogen (PG) I, PGII, gastrin-17 (G-17), and anti-*Helicobacter pylori* (HP) antibodies, are being used to identify patients at risk for development of GC, particularly combined in a panel test (GastroPanel) which provides comprehensive information on both the structure and the function of the entire stomach mucosa [5, 6].

CEA

CEA was initially isolated from fetal colon and colon cancer tissue in 1965 [7]; it is localized mainly to epithelial cell membranes facing the lumen in normal adult intestine, whereas it is found on adjacent cell membranes in both embryonic intestine and colon tumors [8]. CEA consists of a large family of related cell surface glycoproteins of which the major proteins are CEA and nonspecific cross-reacting antigen (NCA) [9]. Since the domain structures of CEA, NCA 50, and the heavy chain of immunoglobulin G (IgG) are very similar, CEA belongs to the immunoglobulin gene "superfamily". CEA is a glycoprotein with a molecular weight of 150 to 300 kDa; it is a single polypeptide chain consisting of 641 amino acids and containing 45–55% carbohydrate. It displays a cell adhesion activity and signal-regulatory properties [10].

CEA is normally present in the serum during the fetal period and then disappears in most adult individuals. The CEA concentration is elevated in a variety of cancers, such as colorectal (70%), lung (45%), gastric (50%), breast (40%), pancreatic (55%), ovarian (25%), and uterine (40%) carcinomas [11]. Therefore, it is not organ specific; in addition, its elevation could be associated with benign conditions, such as cirrhosis (45%), pulmonary emphysema (30%), rectal polyps (5%), benign breast disease (15%), and ulcerative colitis (15%) [11]. This, together with the number of tumors that do not produce CEA, does not recommend its testing for screening [12]. The half-life of CEA is 6–8 days; it has a hepatic metabolism [13]. Most assays use the immunometric format for determination of serum CEA; they use polyclonal

Table 6.1 Classic Tumor Markers in Gastric Cancer

	Chemical nature	Molecular weight	Half-life	Causes of elevated circulating level		
				Neoplastic	Benign	Other
CEA	Glycoprotein	200 kD	6–8 days	Colorectal carcinoma Potentially elevated in all types of adenocarcinoma	Chronic hepatopathy Cirrhosis Jaundice Pulmonary benign diseases Chronic renal failure Chronic respiratory diseases	Smoking Alcohol abuse
CA 19-9	Glycoprotein (mucin)	210 kD (purified form)	4–8 days	Pancreas and biliary tract carcinoma Other malignant tumors (stomach, colon, ovary, fallopian tubes, lung, breast, bladder)	Acute and chronic pancreatitis Cholelithiasis Jaundice Rheumatic and autoimmune diseases Diabetes Diabetic nephropathy Chronic hepatopathy Cirrhosis Acute hepatitis Benign pulmonary disease Cystic fibrosis	
CA 72.4	Glycoprotein (mucin)	220–400 kD	3–7 days	Gastric carcinoma Other malignant tumors: ovary, colon	Gastrointestinal diseases Heart disease Pancreatitis Hepatopathies Benign gynecologic disease (above all ovarian cysts) Renal failure Pneumonia Pulmonary fibrosis Rheumatic diseases Familial Mediterranean fever	Pregnancy Ibuprofen-treated pericardial effusion Steroids Omeprazole NSAIs

(continued)

Table 6.1 (continued)

	Chemical nature	Molecular weight	Half-life	Causes of elevated circulating level		
				Neoplastic	Benign	Other
CA 125	Glycoprotein (mucin)	500 kD	5–6 days	Ovary, fallopian tube, and endometrial carcinoma Other malignant tumors	Endometriosis Pelvic inflammation Hepatopathy Jaundice Leiomyoma of the uterus Systemic lupus erythematosus Inflammatory bowel diseases Serositis Congestive heart failure Pneumonia Pleurisy Acute pancreatitis Cirrhosis Acute hepatitis Autoimmune diseases Chronic renal failure Ascites Peritoneal inflammation	Pregnancy Menstruation Recent laparotomy Interferon

Analytic causes of variation of serum biomarker levels

Human antibodies directed against murine IgG used for the assay

False-positive mechanism: bridge between monoclonal antibodies; remedy: addition of murine serum or Ig

False-negative mechanism: steric interference with binding site; remedy: two incubation doses and monoclonal antibodies or a combination of the two types. Normal values are of <3 ng/mL in nonsmokers or of <5 ng/mL in smokers. Since the concentration of CEA measured is method dependent, values should always be compared using the same method; if methods change, all patients who are being monitored should be tested in parallel using both old and new methods [11].

In 2015, a meta-analysis supported the association of elevated pretreatment serum CEA levels with a poor prognosis for GC patients in terms of overall survival (OS) [hazard ratio (HR) 1.716, 95% confidence interval (CI) 1.594–1.848)], disease-specific survival (DSS) (HR 1.940, 95% CI 1.563–2.408), and disease-free survival (DFS) (HR 2.275, 95% CI 1.836–2.818) [14]. The independent prognostic value of pretreatment serum CEA levels remains in patients with GC after adjustment for covariates (i.e., age, Borrmann type, CA 19-9, depth of invasion, sex, histology, liver metastasis, location, nodal involvement, TNM stage, tumor size, lymphatic invasion, and peritoneal metastases). Measurement during the postoperative follow-up would then be particularly important for those patients who had elevated preoperative values, although one cannot deny the relevance of measuring tumor markers among patients who did not have an elevated preoperative value [15]. In fact, more than 90% of patients with elevated preoperative levels of CEA had increased CEA levels again at the time of recurrence, whereas CEA levels increased for the first time at recurrence in 54.7% of cases; sensitivity for CEA for indicating recurrence was 65.8% [16].

Monitoring changing patterns in CEA to determine the relationship between changes in the serum levels and the response assessment in imaging studies throughout the treatment course revealed a significant correlation between the assessment of response by tumor markers and by imaging studies during systemic chemotherapy. However, although increases in serum tumor markers after chemotherapy were general indicators of tumor progression, an initial rise in the CEA levels after the start of chemotherapy should not be an indicator of progressive disease in some cases [15].

CA 19-9

Also known as the sialylated form of the Lewis A blood group antigen, this carbohydrate antigen is a glycolipid, denoted as Le^{xa}. Its expression requires the Lewis gene product, 1,4-fucosyl transferase; therefore patients who are genotypically Le^{a-b-} (~5%) do not express CA 19-9 [11].

CA 19-9 is generally produced by normal human pancreatic and biliary ductal cells and by gastric, colon, endometrial, and salivary epithelia. Most of the CA 19-9 secreted by these cells is metabolized in serum, resulting in very low serum concentration in healthy people. On the contrary, in cases of pancreatobiliary carcinoma, epithelial cells of the tumor can produce a notable quantity of CA 19-9, resulting in an increased serum CA 19-9 level [17]. The antigen is found in serum as a mucin, which is a high molecular weight glycoprotein complex (200–1000 kDa).

The monoclonal antibody against CA 19-9 was developed from a human colon carcinoma cell line, SW-116 [18], and several immunoassays have been produced, with considerable differences among them, which make the results non-interchangeable for individual patients [19].

The CA 19-9 upper reference limit is 37 U/mL, as determined from the 99th percentile of normal subjects; this is the cutoff value able to discriminate between pancreatic cancer and benign pancreatic disease with clinical sensitivities of 69% and 93% and clinical specificities of 76–99% [11]. However, this value is often used for the diagnosis of GC, and it is unknown whether this cutoff is appropriate as a prognostic value [20]. CA 19-9 level >37 U/mL is found in patients with pancreatic (80%), hepatobiliary (67%), gastric (40–50%), hepatocellular (30–50%), colorectal (30%), breast (15%), and bladder cancers. However, 10–20% of patients with pancreatitis and other benign gastrointestinal conditions have elevated concentrations up to 120 U/mL [11].

In 2015, a meta-analysis including thirty-eight studies evaluated the relationship between CA 19-9 and clinicopathologic characteristics and the prognostic value of CA 19-9 in GC [20]. Results showed that there were significant differences in the incidence of high CA 19-9 levels according to stage (III/IV vs. I/II, odds ratio (OR) 3.36; 95% CI 2.34–4.84), pT classification (pT3/

T4 vs. pT1/T2, OR 2.40; 95% CI 1.60–3.59), nodal status (positive vs. negative, OR 2.91; 95% CI 2.21–3.84), distant metastases (yes vs. no, OR 2.76; 95% CI 1.12–6.82), and vascular invasion (yes vs. no, OR 1.66; 95% CI 1.11–2.48). In addition, CA 19-9 was significantly associated with poor OS (HR 1.83; 95% CI 1.56–2.15), DFS (HR 1.85; 95% CI 1.16–2.95), and DSS (HR 1.33; 95% CI 1.10–1.60) in GC.

Similar to CEA, dosing CA 19-9 during the postoperative follow-up seems to be particularly important for those patients who had elevated preoperative values; likewise, an initial rise in the CA 19-9 levels after the start of chemotherapy should not be an indicator of progressive disease in some cases [15].

CA 72-4

Initially called tumor-associated glycoprotein 72 (TAG-72), CA 72-4 is a mucin-like glycoprotein found on the surface of tumor cells, with a molecular weight of 200–420 kDa [2]. It was identified by the use of the monoclonal antibody B72.3, developed from the membrane-enriched fraction of breast carcinoma in a patient with liver metastases [11, 13]. CA 72-4 is not expressed by normal adult tissues, except for secretory phase endometrium and transitional mucosa of the colon; on the contrary, it could be expressed by tumors of epithelial origin (colorectal, gastric, ovarian, pancreatic, endometrial, and breast carcinomas) [13]. CA 72-4 is assayed in peripheral blood, but there are studies that compared serum levels to peritoneal lavage fluid levels [21]. Serum normal value (depending on the laboratory technique) is <6.9 U/mL, with a detection limit of 0.2 U/mL [22]. The overall sensitivity of this test is estimated to be of 40% in GC, with an overall specificity of 95% [23]. According to a review published in 2009, CA 72-4 is considered the major marker for GC, although it can also be associated with other carcinoma (e.g., colorectal cancer, pancreatic carcinoma, and lung cancer) [24]. In GC the positive rate of CA 72-4 is higher respect to those of CEA and CA 19-9 (30%, 21.1%, and 27.8%, respectively). Similarly to the other two biomarkers, CA 72-4 positive rate is higher in more advanced stages than in earlier ones. The positive rates for the three serum biomarkers were similar in detecting major tumors; however, CA 72-4 had the highest positive rate in patients with nodal involvement or serosal invasion. Therefore, CA 72-4 could be the most useful marker for detecting advanced GC [15]. In 2012, a meta-analysis of Chinese studies posed CA 72-4 as the most highly correlated serum tumor biomarker for GC in the Chinese population [25]. Elevated CA 72-4 was associated with tumor depth, nodal involvement, peritoneal and distant metastases, as well as stage [15, 26]. In a longitudinal study, Aloe and colleagues showed that the median presurgical serum CA 72-4 levels were significantly elevated in relapsing patients; moreover, positive presurgical serum CA 72-4 levels had an independent prognostic value in predicting recurrence [27].

CA 125

In 1981, Bast and colleagues identified the CA 125 glycoprotein antigen through the development of the OC 125 murine monoclonal antibody against cell line OVCA 433, which was developed from a patient with a serous papillary cystadenocarcinoma [28]. Subsequently, the CA 125 molecule has been cloned by the use of a partial cDNA sequence originating from the peptide core of the molecule identified. This new mucin molecule has been designated as CA 125/MUC16 [mucin 16, cell surface-associated (MUC16) gene] and consists of a 156-amino-acid tandem-repeat region in the N-terminus and a possible transmembrane region and tyrosine phosphorylation site in the C-terminus [29]. The first immunoassay for CA 125 used the OC 125 antibody for both capture and detection; afterward, a second-generation assay (CA 125 II) was developed, incorporating M11 and OC 125 antibodies, which have distinct nonoverlapping epitopes. Concentration of CA 125 may vary among manufacturers owing to differences in calibration, assay design, and reagent specificities. Values from different methods are not interchangeable, so patients who are serially monitored should be reassessed if there is a change in methodology [30]. The cutoff of 35 U/mL for the CA 125 and CA 125 II assays was determined from the distribution of values in healthy population so as to include 99% of normal individuals [31]. As in other immunoassays, assay interferences may be observed if heterophilic antibodies are present in the serum, particularly following therapeutic or diagnostic use of monoclonal antibodies [30].

CA 125 is a differentiation antigen expressed by amniotic and coelomic epithelium during fetal development. In adults, it is found in the structures derived from coelomic epithelium (the mesothelial cells of the pleura, pericardium, and peritoneum) and in tubal, endometrial, and endocervical epithelium. The surface epithelium of normal fetal and adult ovaries does not express the determinant, except in inclusion cysts, area of metaplasia, and papillary excrescences [32].

Elevated serum CA 125 levels are associated with a variety of benign and malignant causes of pelvic mass; in fact, this marker could be increased in serum not only if gynecologic malignancies are present but also in endometriosis with endometriomas, salpingo-oophoritis with tubo-ovarian abscess, adenomyosis, leiomyomata uteri, and benign epithelial ovarian neoplasms [12]. In addition, increased CA 125 levels were found in conditions able to damage the peritoneal, pleural, and cardiac serosa, in renal failure, in hepatic and pulmonary diseases, as well as during pregnancy and during the menstrual cycle. Elevated levels of CA 125 were also observed in peritoneal carcinomatosis of ovarian or gastric origin [13]. Elevated serum CA 125 levels have been associated with peritoneal metastasis of GC [23, 33, 34].

Pepsinogen I and II

Pepsinogen (PG) is a precursor of the digestive enzyme pepsin. In humans, there are two isozymogens, PGI and PGII, with different biochemical and immunological properties [35, 36]. While PGI is synthesized by the oxyntic glands of the gastric mucosa, specifically by the chief cells and the mucous neck cells of the gastric corpus, PGII is also produced in the cardiac, pyloric, and duodenal Brunner gland cells [36]. Most of the PG is secreted into the gastric lumen, but a small amount (about 1%) can be found in the blood. Blood PG levels reflect the morphology and function of the gastric mucosa and other pathological conditions such as inflammation, HP infection, atrophic gastritis (AG), and intestinal metaplasia (IM) [37]. In the clinical practice, PGI levels and PGI/PGII ratio are often used for diagnosis; the ratio in normal subjects is about 4:1. Patients affected by AG are at increased risk of GC: the risk being even 5-fold in patients with advanced AG in the corpus and even 90-fold in advanced atrophic pangastritis (both corpus and antrum affected) compared to subjects with normal gastric mucosa [38].

The serum or plasma PGI assay seems to be a reliable test for detecting patients with advanced corpus AG [39]. PGI levels in the blood correlate with the number of chief cells in the gastric corpus mucosa. Since AG results in the loss of chief cells, it can be revealed by a linear decrease in blood PGI levels.

During the process of chronic AG, mucosal atrophy advances from the pyloric gland toward the oral side, and the PGI/PGII ratio decreases with the advancement of the disease [40]. The ratio is <3 when AG is advanced (moderate or severe) in the gastric corpus. The risk of GC is fivefold increased when PGI/PGII ratio is low [39].

The potential utility of PG as a diagnostic biomarker for AG and GC has been shown by numerous studies (it has been included in cancer screening programs in Japan as noninvasive test) [40]. In 2015 a meta-analysis, which included 31 studies involving 1520 GC patients and 2265 AG patients, identified a moderate capacity for serum PG to detect GC and AG [40]. The summary sensitivity and specificity for GC diagnosis were 0.69 (95% CI: 0.60–0.76) and 0.73 (95% CI: 0.62–0.82), respectively, with an area under the curve (AUC) of 0.76 (95% CI: 0.72–0.80). The summary sensitivity and specificity for AG diagnosis were 0.69 (95% CI: 0.55–0.80) and 0.88 (95% CI: 0.77–0.94), respectively, with an AUC of 0.85 (95% CI: 0.82–0.88). It has to be noted that the between-study heterogeneity is dramatically marked, with sensitivity varying between 5.8% and 98.6% and specificity between 64.0% and 100%. Moreover, PG tests alone, which have been used for some time for screening of GC risk groups [41], have given only a modest impact on global GC mortality [42].

Gastrin-17

Gastrin is a gastrointestinal hormone which stimulates gastric acid secretion, promotes growth of gastrointestinal epithelial cells, and inhibits their apoptosis [43]. The gastrin gene is located on human chromosome 17q21 and encodes a 101-amino-acid polypeptide [44]. As a result of the post-translational maturation process of progastrin, the G-cells in the antrum release a mixture of acid stimulatory gastrins into the circulation. The dominant (80–90%) gastrin form in blood of healthy subjects is gastrin-17 (G-17), which is almost exclusively produced by the antrum G-cells [45], followed by gastrin-34 (5–10%). Fasting serum G-17 is considered as a noninvasive biomarker reflecting the structure and functional status of gastric mucosa. G-17 concentration, in fact, depends on intragastric acidity, on the number of antrum G-cells, and normally increases after food stimulation. Secretion of gastrin is regulated by pH level in gastric cavity: gastrin level decreases along with increase of gastric acid and considerably increases after eating [46]. In antrum AG, mucous antrum membrane is atrophied, and, as a consequence, the number of G-cells decreases, resulting in a reduction of G-17 secreted into circulation. Conversely, when gastric body is atrophied, gastric acid reduces, and then the secretion of G-17 increases together with its concentration in blood [47].

Since the 1990s [48], several studies of G-17 as a biomarker of GC screening have been conducted; anyway its clinical utility remains unclear, and the cutoff points for different gastric diseases are not established [49]. In 2016, two different meta-analyses evidenced that G-17 is able to detect AG with 48% sensitivity and 79% specificity [50], in particular AG of the antrum with 53.8% pooled sensitivity and 84.1% pooled specificity [5].

GastroPanel

GastroPanel test was designed by the Finn Biohit Oyj in the late 1990s to meet the increasing demand of noninvasive test for screening of GC risk. This ELISA-based panel includes three markers of mucosal atrophy (PGI and PGII for the corpus, G-17 for the antrum) and a HP IgG antibody assay. The added value of using this panel instead of the single biomarkers lies in the fact that it provides comprehensive information on both the structure and the function of the entire stomach mucosa, not restricted to either corpus or antrum alone [5, 6].

Since GC develops in a stepwise manner, subjects presenting precancerous lesions (AG, IM, and dysplasia) are at risk of developing carcinoma. HP, as a causative etiological agent of AG, is a well-established precursor of non-cardiac GC [51, 52]. It has been estimated that up to 1.8%, 10%, and 73% of patients affected by AG, IM, and dysplasia, respectively, progress to GC [53]. It is then crucial to identify the high-risk subjects in order to improve the GC diagnosis.

The rationale of GastroPanel test is based on the differential site of production of the biomarkers:

- PGI is only secreted by the corpus mucosa;
- PGII is also produced in the gastric antrum and duodenum;
- G-17 is only secreted by the antral mucosa;

and then: [6, 54]

- patients affected by corpus AG show lower blood PGI or PGI/PGII ratio;
- patients affected by antrum AG show low blood G-17 combined with positive anti-HP antibodies.

Even if GastroPanel has been designed for screening of patients at risk for GC and not for invasive GC, it has been tested in different settings, also including first-degree relatives of GC patients and autoimmune chronic AG [55]; moreover, GC and gastric precancerous lesion occurrence show a significant geographic variation [5]. For this reason its sensitivity and specificity in AG and GC diagnosis show high variability among studies [5]. Moreover, studies from different geographic regions use different cutoff values for the single biomarkers, representing a critical source of bias [5].

In 2016, a meta-analysis covering all previous published studies on GastroPanel applied to AG diagnosis reported a better performance in diagnosing corpus AG (pooled sensitivity, 70.2%; pooled specificity, 93.9%) than antrum AG (pooled sensitivity, 53.8%; pooled specificity, 84.1%) [5]. A more recent meta-analysis (2017) found similar results for the diagnosis of corpus AG (sensitivity, 70.4%; specificity, 98.4%) but a higher performance for the diagnosis of antrum AG (sensitivity, 64.5%; specificity, 95.1%) [6]. Overall, the reported performance of the GastroPanel test for AG at any grade of severity and location is 74.7% sensitivity, 95–6% specificity, and 91% negative predictive value [6]. It has to be noted that, in both cases, most studies were conducted in Europe, so the test performance should be better explored in other populations.These findings would support the use of this test for diagnosis and screening of AG, to identify subjects to refer to endoscopy, as advocated by an international panel of expert [54]. Due to its high specificity, this assay represents an effective test for stomach health [5, 6, 54, 56] with high longitudinal negative predictive value for GC [49, 57].

Recent Advances and Future Perspectives

In the era of precision medicine, an extremely intriguing tool is represented by the so-called liquid biopsy, which can be generically considered a sample of any body fluid that may potentially contain material derived from a tumor. In the peripheral blood of cancer patients, it could be retrieved intact circulating tumor cells (CTCs), cell-derived vesicles (i.e., exosomes), and cell-free RNA and DNA (cfDNA) from the tumor. The most widely accepted hypothesis is that tumor cells release DNA in the bloodstream via apoptosis, necrosis, or cell secretion in tumor microenvironment [58].

Blood tests detecting somatic mutations provide high specificity as they search for driver gene mutations which are expected to be present only in abnormal clonal proliferations of cells [59–61]. Also in gastrointestinal cancers, liquid biopsy may represent a prognostic or predictive biomarker and a noninvasive tool for monitoring disease in terms of evaluation of response to systemic therapy as well as in monitoring clonal evolution [62]. Another purpose of liquid biopsy is that of screening and earlier detection. However, mutation-based liquid biopsy was principally used in patients with advanced cancers, since patients with early stage disease can harbor a plasma concentration of mutant template molecules which is often beyond the limit of detection of the most diffuse technologies [63]. Recently, a new multi-analyte blood test called CancerSEEK was developed; it combined eight protein biomarkers (CEA, CA 125, CA 19-9, prolactin, hepatocyte growth factor, osteopontin, myeloperoxidase, and tissue inhibitor of metalloproteinases 1) with genetic biomarkers, thus increasing sensitivity without decreasing specificity. Regarding patients with diagnosis of non-metastatic clinically detected GC, the sensitivity of CancerSEEK was almost 70%; moreover, this test, without any clinical information about the patients, was able to localize the source of the positive test to a single organ in a median of 63% of patients [64]. The combination of a multi-analyte test with other non-blood-based screening test could provide more information in order to get to an earlier detection of malignancy, which is crucial to reducing cancer deaths.

References

1. McShane LM, et al. Reporting recommendations for tumor marker prognostic studies. J Clin Oncol. 2005;23:9067–72.
2. Sun Z, Zhang N. Clinical evaluation of CEA, CA19-9, CA72-4 and CA125 in gastric cancer patients with neoadjuvant chemotherapy. World J Surg Oncol. 2014;12:397.

3. Sturgeon CM, et al. National Academy of Clinical Biochemistry Laboratory Medicine Practice Guidelines for use of tumor markers in liver, bladder, cervical, and gastric cancers. Clin Chem. 2010;56:e1–48.
4. Smyth EC, et al. Gastric cancer: ESMO Clinical Practice Guidelines for diagnosis, treatment and follow-up. Ann Oncol. 2016;27:v38–49.
5. SyrjäNen K. A panel of serum biomarkers (GastroPanel®) in non-invasive diagnosis of atrophic gastritis. Systematic review and meta-analysis. Anticancer Res. 2016;36:5133–44.
6. Zagari RM, et al. Systematic review with meta-analysis: diagnostic performance of the combination of pepsinogen, gastrin-17 and anti-*Helicobacter pylori* antibodies serum assays for the diagnosis of atrophic gastritis. Aliment Pharmacol Ther. 2017;46:657–67.
7. Gold P, Freedman SO. Specific carcinoembryonic antigens of the human digestive system. J Exp Med. 1965;122:467–81.
8. Benchimol S, et al. Carcinoembryonic antigen, a human tumor marker, functions as an intercellular adhesion molecule. Cell. 1989;57:327–34.
9. Hammarström S. The carcinoembryonic antigen (CEA) family: structures, suggested functions and expression in normal and malignant tissues. Semin Cancer Biol. 1999;9:67–81.
10. Öbrink B. CEA adhesion molecules: multifunctional proteins with signal-regulatory properties. Curr Opin Cell Biol. 1997;9:616–26.
11. Burtis CA, Ashwood ER, Bruns DE. Tietz textbook of clinical chemistry and molecular diagnostics – E-book. St. Louis: Elsevier Health Sciences; 2012.
12. Sell S. Serological cancer markers. New York: Springer Science & Business Media; 2012.
13. Cascinu S, Labianca R. La Medicina Oncologica: Diagnosi, Terapia e gestione clinica. Milano: Edra Masson; 2015.
14. Deng K, et al. The prognostic significance of pretreatment serum CEA levels in gastric cancer: a meta-analysis including 14651 patients. PLoS One. 2015;10(4):e0124151.
15. Shimada H, Noie T, Ohashi M, Oba K, Takahashi Y. Clinical significance of serum tumor markers for gastric cancer: a systematic review of literature by the Task Force of the Japanese Gastric Cancer Association. Gastric Cancer. 2014;17:26–33.
16. Takahashi Y, et al. The usefulness of CEA and/or CA19-9 in monitoring for recurrence in gastric cancer patients: a prospective clinical study. Gastric Cancer. 2003;6:142–5.
17. Wang T, et al. Carbohydrate antigen 19-9-positive gastric adenocarcinoma: autopsy findings and review of the literature. Case Rep Gastroenterol. 2017;11:545–53.
18. Koprowski H, et al. Colorectal carcinoma antigens detected by hybridoma antibodies. Somatic Cell Genet. 1979;5:957–71.
19. Hotakainen K, Tanner P, Alfthan H, Haglund C, Stenman U-H. Comparison of three immunoassays for CA 19-9. Clin Chim Acta. 2009;400:123–7.
20. Song Y, et al. Clinicopathologic and prognostic value of serum carbohydrate antigen 19-9 in gastric cancer: a meta-analysis. Dis Markers. 2015;2015:549843. https://doi.org/10.1155/2015/549843.
21. Fernandes LL, et al. CA72-4 antigen levels in serum and peritoneal washing in gastric cancer: correlation with morphological aspects of neoplasia. Arq Gastroenterol. 2007;44:235–9.
22. Căinap C, et al. Classic tumor markers in gastric cancer. Current standards and limitations. Clujul Med. 2015;88:111–5.
23. Emoto S, et al. Clinical significance of CA125 and CA72-4 in gastric cancer with peritoneal dissemination. Gastric Cancer. 2012;15:154–61.
24. Sharma S. Tumor markers in clinical practice: general principles and guidelines. Indian J Med Paediatr Oncol. 2009;30:1–8.
25. Chen X-Z, et al. Correlation between serum CA724 and gastric cancer: multiple analyses based on Chinese population. Mol Biol Rep. 2012;39:9031–9.
26. Abbas M, et al. The relevance of gastric cancer biomarkers in prognosis and pre- and post- chemotherapy in clinical practice. Biomed Pharmacother. 2017;95:1082–90.
27. Aloe S, et al. Prognostic value of serum and tumor tissue CA 72-4 content in gastric cancer. Int J Biol Markers. 2008;18:21–7.
28. Bast RC, et al. Reactivity of a monoclonal antibody with human ovarian carcinoma. J Clin Invest. 1981;68:1331–7.
29. Yin BWT, Lloyd KO. Molecular cloning of the CA125 ovarian cancer antigen: identification as a new mucin, MUC16. J Biol Chem. 2001;276:27371–5.
30. Sturgeon CM, et al. National Academy of Clinical Biochemistry Laboratory Medicine Practice Guidelines for use of tumor markers in testicular, prostate, colorectal, breast, and ovarian cancers. Clin Chem. 2008;54:e11–79.
31. Diamandis EP. Tumor markers: physiology, pathobiology, technology, and clinical applications. Washington, DC: American Association for Clinical Chemistry; 2002.
32. Kabawat SE, et al. Tissue distribution of a coelomic-epithelium-related antigen recognized by the monoclonal antibody OC125. Int J Gynecol Pathol. 1983;2:275–85.
33. Hwang GI, et al. Predictive value of preoperative serum CEA, CA19-9 and CA125 levels for peritoneal metastasis in patients with gastric carcinoma. Cancer Res Treat. 2004;36:178–81.
34. Nakata B, et al. Serum CA 125 level as a predictor of peritoneal dissemination in patients with gastric carcinoma. Cancer. 1998;83:2488–92.
35. Samloff IM. Immunologic studies of human group I pepsinogens. J Immunol. 1971;1950(106):962–8.
36. Nasrollahzadeh D, et al. Accuracy and cut-off values of pepsinogens I, II and gastrin 17 for diagnosis of

gastric fundic atrophy: influence of gastritis. PLoS One. 2011;6:e26957.
37. Samloff IM, Varis K, Ihamaki T, Siurala M, Rotter JI. Relationships among serum pepsinogen I, serum pepsinogen II, and gastric mucosal histology. A study in relatives of patients with pernicious anemia. Gastroenterology. 1982;83:204–9.
38. Slpponen P, Kekki M, Haapakoski J, Ihamäki T, Siurala M. Gastric cancer risk in chronic atrophic gastritis: statistical calculations of cross-sectional data. Int J Cancer. 1985;35:173–7.
39. Dinis-Ribeiro M, et al. Meta-analysis on the validity of pepsinogen test for gastric carcinoma, dysplasia or chronic atrophic gastritis screening. J Med Screen. 2004;11:141–7.
40. Huang Y, et al. Significance of serum pepsinogens as a biomarker for gastric cancer and atrophic gastritis screening: a systematic review and meta-analysis. PLoS One. 2015;10:e0142080.
41. Miki K. Gastric cancer screening by combined assay for serum anti-Helicobacter pylori IgG antibody and serum pepsinogen levels – 'ABC method'. Proc Jpn Acad Ser B Phys Biol Sci. 2011;87:405–14.
42. Lomba-Viana R, et al. Serum pepsinogen test for early detection of gastric cancer in a European Country. Eur J Gastroenterol Hepatol. 2012;24:37–41.
43. Farias CB, et al. Stimulation of proliferation of U138-MG glioblastoma cells by gastrin-releasing peptide in combination with agents that enhance cAMP signaling. Oncology. 2008;75:27–31.
44. Sawada M, Dickinson CJ. The G cell. Annu Rev Physiol. 1997;59:273–98.
45. Dockray GJ, Varro A, Dimaline R, Wang T. The gastrins: their production and biological activities. Annu Rev Physiol. 2001;63:119–39.
46. The EUROGAST Study Group. An international association between Helicobacter pylori infection and gastric cancer. Lancet. 1993;341:1359–63.
47. Yamada T. Helicobacter pylori in peptic ulcer disease. JAMA J Am Med Assoc. 1994;272:65.
48. Hallissey MT, Dunn JA, Fielding JW. Evaluation of pepsinogen A and gastrin-17 as markers of gastric cancer and high-risk pathologic conditions. Scand J Gastroenterol. 1994;29:1129–34.
49. Sun L, et al. A comprehensive evaluation of fasting serum gastrin-17 as a predictor of diseased stomach in Chinese population. Scand J Gastroenterol. 2014;49:1164–72.
50. Wang X, et al. The diagnostic value of gastrin-17 detection in atrophic gastritis: a meta-analysis. Medicine (Baltimore). 2016;95:e3599.
51. Correa P. Chronic gastritis: a clinico-pathological classification. Am J Gastroenterol. 1988;83:504–9.
52. Correa P. Human gastric carcinogenesis: a multistep and multifactorial process – First American Cancer Society Award Lecture on Cancer Epidemiology and Prevention. Cancer Res. 1992;52:6735–40.
53. de Vries AC, Haringsma J, Kuipers EJ. The detection surveillance and treatment of premalignant gastric lesions related to Helicobacter pylori infection. Helicobacter. 2007;12(1):1–15.
54. Agréus L, et al. Rationale in diagnosis and screening of atrophic gastritis with stomach-specific plasma biomarkers. Scand J Gastroenterol. 2012;47:136–47.
55. De Re V, et al. Pepsinogens to distinguish patients with gastric intestinal metaplasia and Helicobacter pylori infection among populations at risk for gastric cancer. Clin Transl Gastroenterol. 2016;7:e183.
56. Syrjänen KJ, Sipponen P, Härkönen M, Peetsalu A, Korpela S. Accuracy of the GastroPanel test in the detection of atrophic gastritis. Eur J Gastroenterol Hepatol. 2015;27:102–4.
57. Kurilovich S, et al. Stomach-specific Biomarkers (GastroPanel) can predict the development of gastric cancer in a Caucasian population: a longitudinal nested case-control study in Siberia. Anticancer Res. 2016;36:247–53.
58. Perakis S, Speicher MR. Emerging concepts in liquid biopsies. BMC Med. 2017;15(1):75.
59. Haber DA, Velculescu VE. Blood-based analyses of cancer: circulating tumor cells and circulating tumor DNA. Cancer Discov. 2014;4:650–61.
60. Bettegowda C, et al. Detection of circulating tumor DNA in early- and late-stage human malignancies. Sci Transl Med. 2014;6:224ra24.
61. Butler TM, Spellman PT, Gray J. Circulating-tumor DNA as an early detection and diagnostic tool. Curr Opin Genet Dev. 2017;42:14–21.
62. Nordgård O, Tjensvoll K, Gilje B, Søreide K. Circulating tumour cells and DNA as liquid biopsies in gastrointestinal cancer. Br J Surg. 2018;105:e110–20.
63. Bardelli A, Pantel K. Liquid Biopsies, What We Do Not Know (Yet). Cancer Cell. 2017;31:172–9.
64. Cohen JD, et al. Detection and localization of surgically resectable cancers with a multi-analyte blood test. Science. 2018;359(6378):926–30. https://doi.org/10.1126/science.aar3247.

Part III

Gastric Cancer Therapy: Multimodal Treatment Approach

New Agents in the Treatment of Advanced Gastric Cancer: Targeted Therapy and Immunotherapy

7

Angela Buonadonna, Gian Maria Miolo, Valentina Fanotto, Federico Navarria, Elisa Palazzari, Claudio Belluco, Stefania Maiero, Vincenzo Canzonieri, Giulio Bertola, and Antonino De Paoli

Abbreviations

ASCO	American Society of Clinical Oncology
ATM	Ataxia telangiectasia
BSC	Best supportive care
CDH-1	Cadherin-1
CIN	Chromosomal instability
CTLA-4	Cytotoxic T-lymphocyte-associated protein 4
EBV	Epstein-Barr virus
EGFR	Epidermal growth factor receptor
EGJ	Esophagogastric junction
ERK	Extracellular signal-regulated kinases
FGFR2	Fibroblast growth factor receptor 2
GATA6	GATA-binding protein 6
GC	Gastric cancer
GS	Genomically stable
HER2	Human epidermal growth factor receptor 2
HR	Hazard ratio
JAK2	Janus kinase 2
KLF5	Kruppel-like factor 5
KRAS	Kirsten rat sarcoma viral oncogene homolog
MET	Mesenchymal-epithelial transition

A. Buonadonna (✉) · G. M. Miolo
Medical Oncology Department, IRCCS, CRO Aviano, National Cancer Institute, Aviano, PN, Italy
e-mail: abuonadonna@cro.it

V. Fanotto
Medical Oncology Department, IRCCS, CRO Aviano, National Cancer Institute, Aviano, PN, Italy

Department of Clinical Oncology, IRCCS, CRO Aviano, National Cancer Institute, Aviano, PN, Italy

Department of Medicine (DAME), University of Udine, Udine, UD, Italy

F. Navarria · E. Palazzari · A. De Paoli
Radiation Oncology Department, IRCCS, CRO Aviano, National Cancer Institute, Aviano, PN, Italy

C. Belluco · G. Bertola
Surgical Oncology Department, IRCCS, CRO Aviano, National Cancer Institute, Aviano, PN, Italy

S. Maiero
Oncological Gastroenterology Department, IRCCS, CRO Aviano, National Cancer Institute, Aviano, PN, Italy

V. Canzonieri
Pathology Department, IRCCS, CRO Aviano, National Cancer Institute, Aviano, PN, Italy

Department of Medical, Surgical and Health Sciences, University of Trieste, Trieste, TS, Italy

CRO Biobank, IRCCS, CRO Aviano, National Cancer Institute, Aviano, PN, Italy

Department of Biology, Temple University, Philadelphia, PA, USA

© Springer Nature Switzerland AG 2019

V. Canzonieri, A. Giordano (eds.), *Gastric Cancer In The Precision Medicine Era*, Current Clinical Pathology, https://doi.org/10.1007/978-3-030-04861-7_7

MS	Microsatellite unstable
mTOR	Mechanistic target of rapamycin
OS	Overall survival
PARP	Poly-ADP ribose polymerase
PD-1	The programmed cell death 1 protein
PD-L1	Programmed death-ligand 1
PD-L2	Programmed death-ligand 2
PFS	Progression-free survival
PIK3CA	Phosphatidylinositol-4,5-bisphosphate 3-kinase catalytic subunit alpha
RHOA	Ras homolog gene family, member A
RR	Response rate
RTK	Receptor tyrosine kinase
TCGA	The Cancer Genome Atlas
T-DM1	Trastuzumab emtansine
TKI	Tyrosine kinase inhibitors
VEGFR	Vascular endothelial growth factor receptor

Introduction

Gastric cancer is the third leading cause of cancer mortality and the fifth most commonly diagnosed malignant disease [1]. The prognosis of GC is poor, especially for patients with metastatic disease, for whom the 5-year overall survival (OS) rate is approximately 5% [2]. For these patients, systemic therapy is the mainstay of treatment, and the goals of this therapy include palliation of symptoms and prolongation of survival. Systemic treatment with chemotherapy was the first to show a survival benefit over best supportive care (BSC) [3]. Despite some benefits from chemotherapy regimens, including docetaxel, fluoropyrimidines, irinotecan, cisplatin, and oxaliplatin, metastatic disease has a dismal prognosis, with a median OS of approximately 11 months for patients not harboring human epidermal growth factor receptor 2 (HER2) overexpression [4]. Conventional cytotoxic chemotherapy has been the backbone of advanced gastric cancer (GC) treatment for decades and still represents a key element of the therapeutic armamentarium. However, only small increments in survival outcomes have been reached.

For locally advanced GC, perioperative chemotherapy in the West and adjuvant chemotherapy in the East are standard. In stage IV chemotherapy prolongs survival and controls cancer-related symptoms [5]. Oxaliplatin and cisplatin plus fluoropyrimidine (5-fluorouracil, capecitabine, or S-1) are standard in a first-line setting. The addition of a third drug increases response rates and survival outcomes but leads to significant increases in toxicity [6, 7]. Patients for triplet chemotherapy should therefore be selected carefully. Responses to chemotherapy are often of short duration, and median overall survival (OS) in advanced GC is no longer than 8–11 months median in the West and 13–17 months in East Asia/Japan.

Over the past several decades, we have witnessed the advent of precision medicine, and remarkable advancements in the fields of targeted therapy and immunotherapy have recently been achieved. Precision medicine involves characterizing the molecular pathways of carcinogenesis and pharmaceutical development of monoclonal antibodies and small molecule inhibitors that interfere with crucial molecular targets.

A better understanding of genetic alterations and molecular signatures of gastric cancer has been reached in the last years. It will serve as a roadmap for better treatment stratification and future drug development. GC has numerous somatic genetic alterations, some of them contributing to chemotherapeutic resistance [8].

The molecular characterization of GC is rapidly evolving. Genes related to RTK/RAS signaling, in particular FGFR2, KRAS, ERBB2, EGFR, and MET, can be amplified in GC. These amplifications are frequently but not universally mutually exclusive [9, 10].

The Cancer Genome Atlas (TCGA) Project (Table 7.1) performed a comprehensive molecular evaluation of 295 gastric adenocarcinomas and has proposed a molecular classification scheme by which GC is categorized into four subtypes: Epstein-Barr virus (EBV)-positive tumors, microsatellite unstable (MSI) tumors, genomically stable (GS) tumors, and tumors with chromosomal instability (CIN) [11]. EBV-positive tumors represent 9% of gastric adenocarcinomas and display recurrent phosphatidylinositol 3-kinase CA

Table 7.1 The new molecularly based classification of GC according to the Cancer Genome Atlas (TCGA) 2014

Subtype	Epstein-Barr virus (EBV)-infected tumors	Microsatellite instability (MSI) tumors	Genomically stable (GS) tumors	Tumors with chromosomal instability (CIN)
Typical molecular features	EBV positive Profound hypermethylation CDKN2A silencing 80% PIK3CA mutation PD-L1/PD-L2 overexpression	DNA hypermethylation Silencing of MLH1 Elevated somatic mutations (PIK3CA 42% and ERBB3 26%)	Tumors lacking aneuploidy and elevated rates of mutation or hypermethylation Somatic RHOA and CDH-1 mutations CLDN18-ARHGAP6 or ARHGAP26 fusions	Marked aneuploidy TP53 mutations Recurrent amplifications of receptor tyrosine kinases (HER2 24%)
Association with anatomy or traditional subtypes	Fundus and body	Fundus, body, and antrum	Mostly diffuse subtype	Majority of tumors at the esophagogastric junction

(PIK3CA) mutations and amplification of HER2, JAK2, and programmed cell death-ligands 1 and 2 (PD-L1 and PD-L2). The MSI subtype represents 22% of GCs and is prevalent in women and older adults. These tumors are strongly associated with MLH1 promoter hypermethylation and show elevated mutation rates, elevated levels of microsatellite instability, and recurrent mutations in PIK3CA, HER3, and HER2. GS tumors are observed in 20% of GC patients, are enriched for the diffuse-type adenocarcinoma, and have frequent mutations in RHOA and CDH-1. Fusions involving RHO-family GTPase-activating proteins (CLDN18 and ARHGAP26) are also enriched in this subtype, and their fusion products impact RHOA function, which is involved in cell contractility and cellular motility. Finally, the CIN subtype accounts for 50% of gastric adenocarcinomas, is enriched by intestinal histology, and shows frequent TP53 mutations and receptor tyrosine kinase (RTK)/RAS amplifications [11, 12].

Another notable study sought to identify the most prevalent molecular alterations in GC. The authors identified 22 recurrent focal somatic copy number alterations including known targets such as fibroblast growth factor receptors 2 (FGFR2) and HER2 and also novel genes such as KLF5 and GATA6. Interestingly, RTK/RAS amplifications were frequent and occurred in approximately 37% of GCs, and KRAS amplifications were also frequent and associated with an adverse prognosis [9]. The design of future GC trials, particularly in molecularly targeted and immune therapy, should consider genetic and immunity differences, as they may impact treatment response and clinical outcomes.

Targeted Agents

Data from systematic profiling studies has revealed numerous molecular alterations in GC. This increased knowledge has significantly improved pharmaceutical development to design and clinically test selective inhibitors against proteins and lipid kinases that play crucial roles in carcinogenesis.

Anti-HER2 Agents

HER2 is a tyrosine kinase member of the epidermal growth factor receptor (EGFR) family. HER2 is involved in the carcinogenesis of many types of cancer, and its overexpression can be identified in up to 30% of GCs with some differences regarding histological and location characteristics. The overexpression is more common in the intestinal type (34%) than in the diffuse type (6%) and more prevalent in esophagogastric junction (GEJ) tumors (32%) than other locations of the stomach (18%) [13, 14].

Trastuzumab, a recombinant humanized monoclonal antibody against HER2, was the first targeted agent to be approved for GC in 2010. The approval was based on a phase 3 trial (ToGA) that evaluated 594 patients with HER2-positive advanced gastric or EGJ cancer. Trastuzumab (8 mg/kg loading dose, then 6 mg/kg every 3 weeks) was investigated as a first-line treatment in association with chemotherapy consisting of capecitabine plus cisplatin or fluorouracil plus cisplatin administered every 3 weeks for six cycles. The median OS was 13.8 months for the trastuzumab plus chemotherapy arm and 11.1 months for patients in the chemotherapy-alone arm (hazard ratio (HR) 0.74; 95% CI 0.60–0.91; $P = 0.0046$). The response rate (RR) was also higher in the experimental arm (47% versus 35%), as was the median progression-free survival (PFS) (6.7 months versus 5.5 months; HR 0.71; $P = 0.0002$) [14].

Other HER2 blockade drugs were not as successful as trastuzumab. The phase 3 LOGIC trial evaluated the efficacy of lapatinib, a tyrosine kinase inhibitor of EGFR and HER2, as a first-line treatment in combination with chemotherapy (capecitabine plus oxaliplatin). The median OS of the experimental arm was not significantly different from that of the control arm of chemotherapy alone (12.2 versus 10.5 months; HR 0.91; $P = 0.3492$) (check Table 7.2 for details) [15]. The TYTAN trial evaluated lapatinib in the second-line setting with paclitaxel. Similar to the LOGIC trial, the median OS was not significantly different (11.0 months for lapatinib and paclitaxel versus 8.9 months for paclitaxel alone; $P = 0.1044$) [16] (Table 7.2). Trastuzumab emtansine (T-DM1) also failed to show survival advantage over standard chemotherapy. The phase 3 GATSBY trial investigated the efficacy of T-DM1 in patients previously treated for HER2-positive GCs. The median OS was 7.9 months with T-DM1 and 8.6 months with taxane (HR 1.15; one-sided $P = 0.86$) [17] (Table 7.2). Currently, the phase 3 JACOB trial (NCT01774786) is ongoing and will evaluate the efficacy and safety of pertuzumab in combination with trastuzumab, fluoropyrimidine, and cisplatin as a first-line treatment in participants with HER2-positive metastatic GCs.

Anti-vascular Endothelial Growth Factor Receptor (VEGF) Agents

Ramucirumab, a recombinant monoclonal antibody that binds to VEGFR-2, is approved alone and in combination with paclitaxel as a second-line treatment based on two randomized phase 3 trials. The REGARD trial randomized 355 patients, who showed disease progression during first-line platinum-containing or fluoropyrimidine-containing treatment to ramucirumab alone (8 mg/kg IV every 2 weeks) or placebo. The median OS was 5.2 months for the ramucirumab arm and 3.8 months for the placebo arm (HR 0.776; $P = 0.047$). Median progression-free survival was 2.1 months in patients receiving ramucirumab and 1.3 months in those receiving placebo (HR 0.483; $P < 0.0001$). The RR was 3% in both arms [18]. The RAINBOW study compared weekly paclitaxel (80 mg/m^2 on days 1, 8, and 15 of each 28-day cycle) plus ramucirumab (8 mg/kg IV every 2 weeks) to a placebo arm using 665 patients with metastatic GC or EGJ cancer after first-line platinum- and fluoropyrimidine-based combination therapy. The median OS was significantly longer in the ramucirumab arm versus that in the placebo arm (9.6 months versus 7.4 months; HR 0.807; $P = 0.017$) as well as the median PFS (4.4 months versus 2.9 months; HR 0.635; $P < 0.0001$). The RR was also greater in the ramucirumab plus paclitaxel arm (28% versus 16%; $P = 0.0001$) [19].

The benefit of bevacizumab, a monoclonal antibody that binds to soluble VEGF and prevents binding to VEGFR, is uncertain. The AVAGAST trial investigated bevacizumab as a first-line treatment with capecitabine plus cisplatin every 21 days for a maximum of six cycles. Thereafter, capecitabine plus either bevacizumab or placebo was continued until disease progression. There was no significant survival benefit for the experimental arm over the control arm (median OS of 12.1 versus 10.1 months, HR 0.87; $P = 0.1002$), but the median PFS (6.7 versus 5.3 months; HR 0.80; $P = 0.0037$) and overall RR (46.0% versus 37.4%; $P = 0.0315$) were significantly improved [20] (Table 7.2). The AVATAR

Table 7.2 Gastric cancer-targeted therapy—negative trials

Study	Phase	Line	No.	Investigational arm	Control arm	RR	PFS	OS
LOGIC	3	First	545	Lapatinib + capecitabine and oxaliplatin	Capecitabine + oxaliplatin	53% vs 39%; $P = 0.0031$	6.0 vs 5.4 months; $P = 0.0381$	12.2 vs 10.5 months; $P = 0.3492$
TYTAN	3	Second	261	Lapatinib + paclitaxel	Paclitaxel	27% vs 9%; $P < 0.001$	5.5 vs 4.4 months; $P = 0.244$	11.0 vs 8.9 months; $P = 0.1044$
GATSBY	3	Second	345	T-DM1	Taxane	20.6% vs 19.6%; $P = 0.8406$	2.7 vs 2.9 months; $P = 0.31$	7.9 vs 8.6 months; $p = 0.86$
AVAGAST	3	First	774	Bevacizumab + capecitabine+ cisplatin	Capecitabine + cisplatin	46.0% vs 37.4%; $P = 0.0315$	6.7 vs 5.3 months; $P = 0.0037$	12.1 vs 10.1 months; $P = 0.1002$
AVATAR	3	First	202	Bevacizumab + capecitabine+ cisplatin	Capecitabine + cisplatin	41% vs 34%; $P = 0.35$	6.3 vs 6.0 months; $P = 0.47$	10.5 vs 11.4 months; $P = 0.56$
Lee et al.	2	Second	107	Sunitinib + docetaxel	Docetaxel	41.1% vs 14.3%; $P = 0.002$	3.9 vs 2.6 months; $P = 0.206$	8.0 vs 6.6 months; $P = 0.802$
EXPAND	3	First	904	Cetuximab + capecitabine + cisplatin	Capecitabine + cisplatin	30% vs 29%; $P = 0.77$	4.4 vs 5.6 months; $P = 0.32$	9.4 vs 10.7 months; $P = 0.95$
REAL3	3	First	553	Panitumumab + epirubicin, oxaliplatin, and capecitabine	Epirubicin + oxaliplatin+ capecitabine	46% vs 42%; $P = 0.42$	6.0 vs 7.4 months; $P = 0.068$	8.8 vs 11.3 months; $P = 0.013$
GRANITE-1	3	Second or third	656	Everolimus	Placebo	4.5% vs 2.1%	1.7 vs 1.4 months; $P < 0.001$	5.4 vs 4.3 months; $P = 0.124$

trial was a phase 3 study, similar to the AVAGAST trial, which was conducted only in Chinese patients. Similar to AVAGAST, the AVATAR trial showed that, compared with the placebo plus chemotherapy, addition of bevacizumab to capecitabine-cisplatin chemotherapy did not improve the median OS (10.5 versus 11.4 months, HR 1.11; $P = 0.56$) [21] (Table 7.2).

Apatinib, an orally active VEGFR-2 inhibitor, was evaluated in a phase 3 Chinese trial that randomized 267 patients with advanced GC or EGJ adenocarcinoma who had progressed through two or more prior lines of chemotherapy. Patients received 850 mg oral apatinib or placebo once daily. The median OS was modestly, but significantly, prolonged (6.5 versus 4.7 months; HR 0.709; $P = 0.0156$), and the median PFS was also improved (2.6 versus 1.8 months; HR 0.444; $P < 0.001$) [22]. Apatinib is approved in China for treatment of advanced GC but is not available in the United States or Europe.

Sunitinib and sorafenib are tyrosine kinase inhibitors (TKIs) that inhibit VEGFR-1, VEGFR-2, and VEGFR-3, as well as other tyrosine kinases. Sunitinib was investigated in a randomized phase 2 trial as a second-line therapy in combination with docetaxel. The primary time-to-progression endpoint was not significantly prolonged with the combination therapy compared with docetaxel alone (3.9 months versus 2.6 months, HR 0.77; $P = 0.206$) [23] (Table 7.2). Sorafenib was evaluated in a phase 2 trial in combination with docetaxel and cisplatin as a first-line treatment for metastatic GC or EGJ adenocarcinoma. The median OS was 13.6 months, the median PFS was 5.8 months, and the objective RR was noted in 41% of patients [24].

Anti-EGFR Agents

EGFR overexpression occurs in 2.3–40% of GCs, depending on the study and the methodology used to investigate the overexpression (immunohistochemistry or fluorescence in situ hybridization) [10]. However, targeted agents against EGFR have had disappointing clinical outcomes. The phase 3 EXPAND trial evaluated cetuximab, a chimeric monoclonal antibody against EGFR, in a first-line setting with chemotherapy (capecitabine and cisplatin). The median PFS (primary endpoint) was 4.4 months for chemotherapy plus cetuximab and 5.6 months for patients in the chemotherapy-alone arm (HR 1.09; $P = 0.32$) [25] (Table 7.2). Similarly, the REAL3 trial enrolled patients in a first-line setting for chemotherapy (epirubicin, oxaliplatin, and capecitabine) with or without panitumumab (a fully human monoclonal antibody against EGFR). The median OS, which was the primary endpoint, was 8.8 months for chemotherapy plus panitumumab versus 11.3 months for the chemotherapy-alone arm (HR 1.37; 95%; $P = 0.013$) [26] (Table 7.2).

PI3K/AKT/mTOR Pathway Inhibition

PI3K/AKT/mTOR is one of the most frequently activated pathways in human cancer and is activated in up to 60% of GCs [27]. Everolimus, a mechanistic (formerly known as mammalian) target of rapamycin (mTOR) inhibitor, was investigated in a phase 3 trial (GRANITE-1) in which 656 patients were randomized to the everolimus (10 mg daily) or placebo group after progression to one or two lines of systemic chemotherapy. The median OS was not significantly different (5.4 months for the everolimus arm versus 4.3 months for the placebo arm, HR 0.90; $P = 0.124$), and the median PFS was modestly improved (1.7 months for the everolimus arm versus 1.4 months for the placebo arm, HR 0.66; $P < 0.001$) [28] (Table 7.2). Currently, another phase 3 trial is investigating everolimus in a second-line setting in association with paclitaxel (NCT01248403).

Several other drugs that target the PI3K/AKT/mTOR pathway are under investigation. AZD5363, an AKT inhibitor, is being investigated in two phase 2 trials in combination with paclitaxel as a second-line treatment for patients with GC harboring a PIK3CA mutation (NCT02451956) and in biomarker-negative (PIK3CA/MEK/RAS/TP53/MET) patients

(NCT02449655). Another randomized phase 2 trial is investigating the efficacy of GDC-0068, another AKT inhibitor, in combination with modified FOLFOX6 in a first-line scenario (NCT01896531). Finally, a phase IB dose-escalation study is evaluating the PI3K inhibitor BYL719 in patients with GCs harboring a PIK3CA mutation or HER2 amplification (NCT01613950).

c-MET Inhibitors

Mesenchymal-epithelial transition (MET) receptor amplification or overexpression occurs in 0–23% of GCs [29]. c-MET inhibitors have been tested in GC patients with disappointing results. Two phase 3 trials investigated the safety and efficacy of rilotumumab, a monoclonal antibody against c-Met. RILOMET-1 and RILOMET-2 were designed to test rilotumumab in combination with chemotherapy as a first-line treatment. Both trials were closed in November 2014 based on an increase in the number of deaths in the rilotumumab and chemotherapy arms [29]. METGastric was another phase 3 trial that evaluated onartuzumab, a monovalent anti-MET antibody; enrollment was halted early due to the negative results in a phase 2 trial. The analysis of the 592 patients enrolled failed to show the benefit of onartuzumab associated with mFOLFOX6 in the first-line scenario [8]. Foretinib and tivantinib, TKIs against c-MET, also failed to show sustained activity in GC patients in phase 2 trials [11].

Fibroblast Growth Factor Receptor Blockade

Fibroblast growth factor receptors (FGFR1–FGFR4) are transmembrane tyrosine kinase receptors that play important roles in carcinogenesis by regulating angiogenesis and cell proliferation, migration, and differentiation. FGFR2 amplification is evident in approximately 5–10% of GC tumors and is associated with a poor prognosis [30, 31].

AZD4547 is a selective FGFR1–FGFR3 inhibitor that has been evaluated in comparison with paclitaxel in a randomized phase 2 trial (the SHINE study) as a second-line treatment for GC patients with FGFR2 polysomy or gene amplification. The PFS analysis did not show any statistically significant differences between the two arms [32]. Dovitinib is an oral multi-targeted TKI that targets FGFR1–FGFR3. A phase 2 trial is ongoing and evaluating dovitinib monotherapy as a salvage treatment in patients with metastatic GC harboring FGFR2 amplifications (NCT01719549). Another phase I/II study is evaluating dovitinib in association with docetaxel as a second-line treatment (NCT01921673).

Poly-ADP Ribose Polymerase (PARP) Inhibition

PARP, together with the ataxia telangiectasia (ATM) protein, plays an essential role in the DNA damage response [33]. Low ATM protein expression is evident in approximately 13–22% of tumors from patients with GC and is correlated with sensitivity to PARP inhibition [33, 34]. Olaparib is a PARP inhibitor that was investigated in a randomized phase 2 trial in which olaparib plus paclitaxel was compared with paclitaxel alone in a population of recurrent or metastatic GC patients whose disease had progressed after first-line chemotherapy; the population was enriched with patients with low or undetectable ATM levels. A total of 124 patients were enrolled, and the median PFS (primary endpoint) was not significantly different between the two arms (3.91 months for olaparib and paclitaxel arm and 3.55 months for paclitaxel alone arm; $P = 0.131$). However, the median OS was significantly improved in the overall population of the study in favor of the combination arm (13.1 versus 8.3 months, HR 0.56; $P = 0.005$), and the results were even more pronounced in the population with low ATM levels (not reached versus 8.2 months, HR 0.35; $P = 0.002$) [35]. A phase 3 trial is ongoing to evaluate this combination in the second-line setting (NCT01924533).

Claudin-18.2

Claudins constitute a family of proteins that participate in controlling the flow of molecules between cellular tight junctions. Isoform 2 of the tight junction molecule claudin-18 (CLDN18.2) is frequently expressed in GCs and is involved in carcinogenesis [36]. Claudiximab is a chimeric monoclonal antibody against CLDN18.2 [37]. The FAST trial, a phase 2b trial, evaluated the role of claudiximab in association with chemotherapy in the first-line scenario. A total of 161 patients with GC and EGJ tumors who were claudin-18.2 positive by immunohistochemistry were randomized to receive the EOX regimen (epirubicin 50 mg/m^2, oxaliplatin 130 mg/m^2 d1, and capecitabine 625 mg/m^2 bid, d1–d21, every 21 days) with or without claudiximab (loading dose 800 mg/m^2, then 600 mg/m^2 d1, every 21 days). The study met its primary endpoint with a median PFS of 7.9 months for the experimental arm versus 4.8 months for the chemotherapy-alone arm (HR 0.47; $P = 0.0001$). The median OS was also significantly higher for the claudiximab arm (13.3 versus 8.4 months; HR 0.51; $P < 0.001$) [37]. Future phase 3 trials evaluating the role claudiximab for GC patients are expected.

Immunotherapy Agents

Immunotherapy is already a reality in oncology and has achieved outstanding results in many cancer types [38–40]. The mechanisms involved in the immune suppression by the tumor are complex. The programmed cell death 1 protein (PD-1) and its ligands (PD-L1 and PD-L2) are key factors that control the ability of tumors to evade the immune surveillance [41]. Similarly, cytotoxic T-lymphocyte-associated protein 4 (CTLA-4) negatively regulates T-cell effector responses and is implicated in tumor immunological evasion signature [42]. Currently, several immunotherapy agents that address this mechanism are being tested as treatments for GC patients.

Pembrolizumab

Pembrolizumab is an anti-PD-1 monoclonal antibody. The phase 1b KEYNOTE 012 trial has evaluated 39 patients with PD-L1-positive gastric or EGJ tumors who received pembrolizumab (10 mg/kg every 2 weeks). This trial has shown manageable toxicities and promising results with 22% of patients achieving an overall response [43]. Early results of the KEYNOTE-059 trial were presented at the 2017 annual meeting of the American Society of Clinical Oncology (ASCO). Cohort 1 comprised 259 patients (not selected by PD-L1 status) who had progressed on ≥2 prior chemotherapy regimens and received pembrolizumab 200 mg every 3 weeks. The RR was 11.2% in the entire cohort and 15.5% for patients with PD-L1-positive tumors. Grade 3–5 treatment-related adverse events (AEs) occurred in 17% of patients [44]. In cohort 2, the safety and efficacy of pembrolizumab (200 mg every 3 weeks) plus chemotherapy (cisplatin 80 mg/m^2 + 5-FU 800 mg/m^2 or capecitabine 1000 mg/m^2 every 3 weeks) as a first-line treatment was evaluated. A total of 25 patients were enrolled with an RR of 60%, a median PFS of 6.6 months, and a median OS of 13.8 months. Grade 3–4 treatment-related AEs occurred in 76% of patients in this cohort [45]. Future trials will further clarify the role of pembrolizumab in the treatment of metastatic GC patients. The ongoing phase 3 KEYNOTE-061 trial is evaluating pembrolizumab versus paclitaxel as a second-line treatment (NCT02370498), and the phase 3 KEYNOTE-062 is evaluating pembrolizumab associated with cisplatin plus 5-FU as a first-line treatment (NCT02494583).

Nivolumab

Nivolumab is another anti-PD-1 monoclonal antibody with promising results in GC. The phase 1/2 CheckMate 032 study evaluated nivolumab with or without ipilimumab in heavily pretreated patients with gastric, esophageal, or EGJ cancers. Updated results were presented at the 2017 ASCO Annual Meeting. The study evaluated three cohorts: 59 patients received

3 mg/kg nivolumab every 2 weeks, 49 patients received 1 mg/kg nivolumab plus 3 mg/kg ipilimumab every 3 weeks (N1 + I3), and 52 patients received 3 mg/kg nivolumab plus 1 mg/kg ipilimumab (N3 + I1). In the nivolumab-alone cohort, the RR was 12%, and the median OS was 6.2 months [46].

The results from a phase 3 trial that evaluated nivolumab as a salvage treatment in 493 patients with gastric and EGJ cancers were presented at the 2017 ASCO Gastrointestinal Cancer Symposium. All patients had failed two or more previous chemotherapy regimens and were randomized to receive nivolumab 3 mg/kg or placebo every 2 weeks. The median OS was 5.32 months for the nivolumab arm versus 4.14 months for the placebo arm (HR 0.63; $P < 0.0001$). The RR was also significantly better for the nivolumab arm (11.2% versus 0%; $P < 0.0001$), as was the median PFS (1.61 months versus 1.45 months, HR 0.60; $P < 0.0001$). Grade 3 or higher treatment-related AEs occurred in 11.5% of patients in the nivolumab arm [47].

Ipilimumab

Ipilimumab is a monoclonal antibody that targets CTLA-4. A phase 2 study evaluated the safety and efficacy of ipilimumab versus BSC for patients with advanced gastric or EGJ cancers as a second-line treatment. Fifty-seven patients were randomized to 10 mg/kg ipilimumab every 3 weeks for four doses versus BSC. Immune-related PFS, the primary endpoint, was not improved (2.92 months for ipilimumab versus 4.90 months for BSC, HR 1.44; $P = 0.09$) [48].

As described above, the CheckMate 032 trial investigated the efficacy of nivolumab plus ipilimumab. The RR was 24% in the N1 + I3 cohort and 8% in the N3 + I1 cohort. The median OS was 6.9 months for the N1 + I3 patients and 4.8 months for the N3 + I1 patients. Grade 3–4 treatment-related AEs were higher for the N1 + I3 cohort than those for the nivolumab-alone patients and N3 + I1 patients. For example, grade 3–4 diarrhea was observed in 14% of patients in the N1 + I3 cohort and in only 2% of patients in the other two cohorts [43]. The phase 3 CheckMate 649 trial is currently recruiting metastatic gastric or EGJ cancer patients with or without PD-L1 expression to evaluate the efficacy of nivolumab plus versus oxaliplatin plus fluoropyrimidine as a first-line treatment (NCT02872116).

Avelumab

Avelumab is a monoclonal antibody against PD-L1. The phase 1b JAVELIN trial analyzed a cohort of patients with gastric and EGJ tumors. Patients received avelumab as first-line maintenance or a second-line treatment. A total of 151 patients received avelumab (10 mg/kg IV every 2 weeks). An unconfirmed response was observed in 9.0% of patients in the maintenance group and in 9.7% of patients who received the medication as a second-line treatment. The disease control rate was 57.3% and 29.0%, and the median PFS was 12 weeks and 6 weeks for the first-line maintenance and second-line treatment groups, respectively. Grade 3 or higher treatment-related AEs were observed in 9.7% of patients [49]. These results led to the development of phase 3 trials addressing avelumab as a first-line maintenance therapy (NCT02625610) and as a third-line treatment (NCT02625623) for metastatic gastric and EGJ cancers.

Novel Cytotoxic Drugs

Nab-paclitaxel (Nab-PTX) is a nanoparticle albumin-bound PTX which does not contain cremophor or ethanol as a formulation vehicle used for poorly water-soluble drugs. As a result, nab-PTX has a smaller risk of hypersensitivity reactions, and high doses can be administered over a short infusion time. ABSOLUTE is a Japanese phase 3 trial that showed non-inferiority of weekly nab-PTX to soluble-based PTX as second-line chemotherapy for advanced GC in terms of OS [50]. In contrast, non-inferiority of nab-PTX every 3 weeks to soluble-based PTX in OS was not confirmed with lower QoL scores.

DHP107 is a novel oral lipid formulation of paclitaxel. DREAM is a randomized phase 3 study for advanced GC after failure of first-line therapy to compare DHP107 and paclitaxel [51]. Non-inferiority regarding PFS was confirmed, although higher gastrointestinal toxicities are reported. A randomized phase 2 trial of S-1 plus leucovorin (TAS-118) versus S-1 plus leucovorin and oxaliplatin (SOL) versus S-1 plus cisplatin in advanced GC patients showed a higher response rate of SOL with a longer OS [52]. Currently, the phase 3 SOLAR study comparing TAS-118 plus oxaliplatin with S-1 plus cisplatin is ongoing in Asian countries.

TAS-102 is a novel oral nucleoside antitumor agent containing trifluridine and tipiracil hydrochloride, which prevents the degradation of trifluridine. Based on a phase 2 trial of TAS-102 for pretreated advanced GC with a disease control rate of 65.5% [53], the ongoing global phase 3 trial is investigating the efficacy and safety of TAS-102 in patients with advanced GC refractory to standard treatments.

Conclusions and Future Prospects

After years of stagnation in the medical treatment of GC, including numerous negative phase 3 trials investigating molecularly targeted drugs, eventually, some progress is emerging. This development is linked to our increasing knowledge of genetic alterations and molecular signatures in GC, as elaborated by The Cancer Genome Atlas consortium and other networks. A major limitation, however, is the biological heterogeneity, which is inherent to GC [54]. A major step forward is expected from immunotherapy. Anti-PD-1- and anti-PD-L1-directed agents, alone or in combination with anti-CTLA-4, show a promising activity. Appropriate molecular stratification of the population for targeted treatment remains challenging. Progress achieved with antiangiogenic agents, namely, with the VEGFR-2-directed antibody ramucirumab in second-line treatment of advanced GC, was rather small. Now, first-line data are awaited, and the integration of ramucirumab in multimodal treatment concepts as well as combination with novel targeted agents like immune checkpoint inhibitors remains interesting. Other emerging therapeutic options comprise targeting of the tight junction protein Claudin-18.2, STAT-3-dependent gene expression as a cancer stemness-related pathway, and tumor stroma modification via inhibition of MMP-9.

Acknowledgments The authors thank Silvia Flora for manuscript editing assistance.

References

1. Torre LA, Bray F, Siegel RL, Ferlay J, Lortet-Tieulent J, Jemal A. Global cancer statistics, 2012. CA Cancer J Clin. 2015;65(2):87–108.
2. Reim D, Loos M, Vogl F, Novotny A, Schuster T, Langer R, et al. Prognostic implications of the seventh edition of the international union against cancer classification for patients with gastric cancer: the Western experience of patients treated in a single-center European institution. J Clin Oncol. 2013;31(2):263–71.
3. Wagner AD, Unverzagt S, Grothe W, Kleber G, Grothey A, Haerting J, et al. Chemotherapy for advanced gastric cancer. Cochrane Database Syst Rev. 2010;17(3):CD004064.
4. Bilici A. Treatment options in patients with metastatic gastric cancer: current status and future perspectives. World J Gastroenterol. 2014;20(14):3905–15.
5. Smyth EC, Verheij M, Allum W, Cunningham D, Cervantes A, Arnold D, et al. Gastric cancer: ESMO Clinical Practice Guidelines for diagnosis, treatment and follow-up. Ann Oncol. 2016;27(Suppl 5):v38–49.
6. Frustaci S, Buonadonna A, Turchet E, Corona G, Tabaro G, Miolo G, et al. Phase I trial of docetaxel, oxaliplatin, and capecitabine (DOC) in untreated gastric cancer patients. Int J Clin Oncol. 2013;18(3):510–6.
7. Mohammad NH, ter Veer E, Ngai L, Mali R, van Oijen MG, van Laarhoven HW. Optimal first-line chemotherapeutic treatment in patients with locally advanced or metastatic esophagogastric carcinoma: triplet versus doublet chemotherapy: a systematic literature review and meta-analysis. Cancer Metastasis Rev. 2015;34:429–41.
8. Lawrence MS, Stojanov P, Polak P, Kryukov GV, Cibulskis K, Sivachenko A, et al. Mutational heterogeneity in cancer and the search for new cancer-associated genes. Nature. 2013;499:214–8.
9. Deng N, Goh LK, Wang H, Das K, Tao J, Tan IB, et al. A comprehensive survey of genomic alterations in gastric cancer reveals systematic patterns of molecular exclusivity and co-occurrence among distinct therapeutic targets. Gut. 2012;61:673–84.

10. Kwak EL, Ahronian LG, Siravegna G, Mussolin B, Godfrey JT, Clark JW, et al. Molecular heterogeneity and receptor coamplification drive resistance to targeted therapy in MET-amplified esophagogastric cancer. Cancer Discov. 2015;5:1271–81.
11. Bass AJ, Thorsson V, Shmulevich I, Reynolds SM, Miller M, Bernard B, et al. Comprehensive molecular characterization of gastric adenocarcinoma. Nature. 2014;513(7517):202–9.
12. Farran B, Muller S, Montenegro RC. Gastric cancer management: kinases as a target therapy. Clin Exp Pharmacol Physiol. 2017;44(6):613–22.
13. Ang YL, Yong WP, Tan P. Translating gastric cancer genomics into targeted therapies. Crit Rev Oncol Hematol. 2016;100:141–6.
14. Bang YJ, Van Cutsem E, Feyereislova A, Chung HC, Shen L, Sawaki A, et al. Trastuzumab in combination with chemotherapy versus chemotherapy alone for treatment of HER2-positive advanced gastric or gastro-oesophageal junction cancer (ToGA): a phase 3, open-label, randomised controlled trial. Lancet (London, England). 2010;376(9742):687–97.
15. Hecht JR, Bang Y-J, Qin SK, Chung HC, Xu JM, Park JO, et al. Lapatinib in combination with capecitabine plus oxaliplatin in human epidermal growth factor receptor 2–positive advanced or metastatic gastric, esophageal, or gastroesophageal adenocarcinoma: TRIO-013/LOGiC—a randomized phase III trial. J Clin Oncol. 2016;34(5):443–51.
16. Satoh T, Xu RH, Chung HC, Sun GP, Doi T, Xu JM, et al. Lapatinib plus paclitaxel versus paclitaxel alone in the second-line treatment of HER2-amplified advanced gastric cancer in Asian populations: TyTAN – a randomized, phase III study. J Clin Oncol. 2014;32(19):2039–49.
17. Thuss-Patience PC, Shah MA, Ohtsu A, Van Cutsem E, Ajani JA, Castro H, et al. Trastuzumab emtansine versus taxane use for previously treated HER2-positive locally advanced or metastatic gastric or gastro-oesophageal junction adenocarcinoma (GATSBY): an international randomised, open-label, adaptive, phase 2/3 study. Lancet Oncol. 2017;18(5):640–53.
18. Fuchs CS, Tomasek J, Yong CJ, Dumitru F, Passalacqua R, Goswami C, et al. Ramucirumab monotherapy for previously treated advanced gastric or gastro-oesophageal junction adenocarcinoma (REGARD): an international, randomised, multicentre, placebo-controlled, phase 3 trial. Lancet (London, England). 2014;383(9911):31–9.
19. Wilke H, Muro K, Van Cutsem E, Oh SC, Bodoky G, Shimada Y, et al. Ramucirumab plus paclitaxel versus placebo plus paclitaxel in patients with previously treated advanced gastric or gastro-oesophageal junction adenocarcinoma (RAINBOW): a double-blind, randomised phase 3 trial. Lancet Oncol. 2014;15(11):1224–35.
20. Ohtsu A, Shah MA, Van Cutsem E, Rha SY, Sawaki A, Park SR, et al. Bevacizumab in combination with chemotherapy as first-line therapy in advanced gastric cancer: a randomized, double-blind, placebo-controlled phase III study. J Clin Oncol. 2011;29(30):3968–76.
21. Shen L, Li J, Xu J, Pan H, Dai G, Qin S, et al. Bevacizumab plus capecitabine and cisplatin in Chinese patients with inoperable locally advanced or metastatic gastric or gastroesophageal junction cancer: randomized, double-blind, phase III study (AVATAR study). Gastric Cancer. 2015;18(1):168–1676.
22. Li J, Qin S, Xu J, Xiong J, Wu C, Bai Y, et al. Randomized, double-blind, placebo-controlled phase III trial of apatinib in patients with chemotherapy-refractory advanced or metastatic adenocarcinoma of the stomach or gastroesophageal junction. J Clin Oncol. 2016;34(13):1448–54.
23. Yi JH, Lee J, Lee J, Park SH, Park JO, Yim DS, et al. Randomised phase II trial of docetaxel and sunitinib in patients with metastatic gastric cancer who were previously treated with fluoropyrimidine and platinum. Br J Cancer. 2012;106(9):1469–74.
24. Sun W, Powell M, O'Dwyer PJ, Catalano P, Ansari RH, Benson AB 3rd. Phase II study of sorafenib in combination with docetaxel and cisplatin in the treatment of metastatic or advanced gastric and gastroesophageal junction adenocarcinoma: ECOG 5203. J Clin Oncol. 2010;28(18):2947–51.
25. Lordick F, Kang YK, Chung HC, Salman P, Oh SC, Bodoky G, et al. Capecitabine and cisplatin with or without cetuximab for patients with previously untreated advanced gastric cancer (EXPAND): a randomised, open-label phase 3 trial. Lancet Oncol. 2013;14(6):490–9.
26. Waddell T, Chau I, Cunningham D, Gonzalez D, Okines AF, Okines C, et al. Epirubicin, oxaliplatin, and capecitabine with or without panitumumab for patients with previously untreated advanced oesophagogastric cancer (REAL3): a randomised, open-label phase 3 trial. Lancet Oncol. 2013;14(6):481–9.
27. Lang SA, Gaumann A, Koehl GE, Seidel U, Bataille F, Klein D, et al. Mammalian target of rapamycin is activated in human gastric cancer and serves as a target for therapy in an experimental model. Int J Cancer. 2007;120(8):1803–10.
28. Ohtsu A, Ajani JA, Bai YX, Bang YJ, Chung HC, Pan HM, et al. Everolimus for previously treated advanced gastric cancer: results of the randomized, double-blind, phase III GRANITE-1 study. J Clin Oncol. 2013;31(31):3935–43.
29. Marano L, Chiari R, Fabozzi A, De Vita F, Boccardi V, Roviello G, et al. c-Met targeting in advanced gastric cancer: an open challenge. Cancer Lett. 2015;365(1):30–6.
30. Su X, Zhan P, Gavine PR, Morgan S, Womack C, Ni X, et al. FGFR2 amplification has prognostic significance in gastric cancer: results from a large international multicentre study. Br J Cancer. 2014;110(4):967–75.
31. Inokuchi M, Fujimori Y, Otsuki S, Sato Y, Nakagawa M, Kojima K. Therapeutic targeting of fibroblast growth factor receptors in gastric cancer. Gastroenterol Res Pract. 2015;2015:796380.

32. Jacome AA, Coutinho AK, Lima EM, Andrade AC, Dos Santos JS. Personalized medicine in gastric cancer: where are we and where are we going? World J Gastroenterol. 2016;22:1160–71.
33. Kubota E, Williamson CT, Ye R, Elegbede A, Peterson L, Lees-Miller SP, et al. Low ATM protein expression and depletion of p53 correlates with olaparib sensitivity in gastric cancer cell lines. Cell Cycle (Georgetown, Tex). 2014;13(13):2129–37.
34. Kim HS, Kim MA, Hodgson D, Harbron C, Wellings R, O'Connor MJ, et al. Concordance of ATM (ataxia telangiectasia mutated) immunohistochemistry between biopsy or metastatic tumor samples and primary tumors in gastric cancer patients. Pathobiology. 2013;80(3):127–37.
35. Bang YJ, Im SA, Lee KW, Cho JY, Song EK, Lee KH, et al. Randomized, double-blind phase II trial with prospective classification by ATM protein level to evaluate the efficacy and tolerability of olaparib plus paclitaxel in patients with recurrent or metastatic gastric cancer. J Clin Oncol. 2015;33(33):3858–65.
36. Iravani O, Tay BW, Chua PJ, Yip GW, Bay BH. Claudins and gastric carcinogenesis. Exp Biol Med (Maywood). 2013;238(4):344–9.
37. Singh P, Toom S, Huang Y. Anti-claudin 18.2 antibody as new targeted therapy for advanced gastric cancer. J Hematol Oncol. 2017;10(1):105.
38. Reck M, Rodríguez-Abreu D, Robinson AG, Hui R, Csőszi T, Fülöp A, et al. Pembrolizumab versus chemotherapy for PD-L1–Positive Non–Small-Cell Lung Cancer. N Engl J Med. 2016;375(19):1823–33.
39. Larkin J, Chiarion-Sileni V, Gonzalez R, Grob JJ, Cowey CL, Lao CD, et al. Combined nivolumab and ipilimumab or monotherapy in untreated melanoma. N Engl J Med. 2015;373(1):23–34.
40. Motzer RJ, Escudier B, McDermott DF, George S, Hammers HJ, Srinivas S, et al. Nivolumab versus everolimus in advanced renal-cell carcinoma. N Engl J Med. 2015;373(19):1803–13.
41. Topalian SL, Hodi FS, Brahmer JR, Gettinger SN, Smith DC, McDermott DF, et al. Safety, activity, and immune correlates of anti-PD-1 antibody in cancer. N Engl J Med. 2012;366(26):2443–54.
42. Walker LS, Sansom DM. The emerging role of CTLA4 as a cell-extrinsic regulator of T cell responses. Nat Rev Immunol. 2011;11(12):852–63.
43. Muro K, Chung HC, Shankaran V, Geva R, Catenacci D, Gupta S, et al. Pembrolizumab for patients with PD-L1-positive advanced gastric cancer (KEYNOTE-012): a multicentre, open-label, phase 1b trial. Lancet Oncol. 2016;17(6):717–26.
44. Fuchs CS, Doi T, Jang RWJ, Muro K, Satoh T, Machado M, et al. KEYNOTE-059 cohort 1: efficacy and safety of pembrolizumab (pembro) monotherapy in patients with previously treated advanced gastric cancer. J Clin Oncol. 2017;35(15_suppl):abstr 4003.
45. Bang YJ, Muro K, Fuchs CS, Golan T, Geva R, Hara H, et al. KEYNOTE-059 cohort 2: safety and efficacy of pembrolizumab (pembro) plus 5-fluorouracil (5-FU) and cisplatin for first-line (1L) treatment of advanced gastric cancer. J Clin Oncol. 2017;35(15_suppl):abstr 4012.
46. Janjigian YY, Ott PA, Calvo E, Kim JW, Ascierto PA, Sharma P, et al. Nivolumab ± ipilimumab in pts with advanced (adv)/metastatic chemotherapy-refractory (CTx-R) gastric (G), esophageal (E), or gastroesophageal junction (GEJ) cancer: CheckMate 032 study. J Clin Oncol. 2017;35(15_suppl):abstr 4014.
47. Kang YK, Satoh T, Ryu MH, Chao Y, Kato K, Chung HC, et al. Nivolumab (ONO-4538/BMS-936558) as salvage treatment after second or later-line chemotherapy for advanced gastric or gastro-esophageal junction cancer (AGC): a double-blinded, randomized, phase III trial. J Clin Oncol. 2017;35(suppl 4S):abstract 2.
48. Bang YJ, Cho JY, Kim YH, Kim JW, Di Bartolomeo M, Ajani JA, et al. Efficacy of sequential ipilimumab monotherapy vs best supportive care for unresectable locally advanced/metastatic gastric or gastroesophageal junction cancer. Clin Cancer Res. 2017;23(19):5671–8.
49. Chung HC, Arkenau HT, Wyrwicz L, Oh DY, Lee KW, Infante JR, et al. Avelumab (MSB0010718C; anti-PD-L1) in patients with advanced gastric or gastroesophageal junction cancer from JAVELIN solid tumor phase Ib trial: analysis of safety and clinical activity. J Clin Oncol. 2016;34(15_suppl):4009.
50. Shitara K, Takashima A, Fujitami K, Koeda K, Hara H, Nakayama N, et al. Nab-paclitaxel versus solvent based paclitaxel in patients with previously treated advanced gastric cancer: an open-label, randomised phase III trial (ABSOLUTE Trial). Lancet Gastroenterol. 2017;2(4):277–87.
51. Kang YK, Ryu MH, Park SH, Kim JG, Kim JW, Cho SH, et al. Efficacy and safety findings from DREAM: a phase III study of DHP107 (oral paclitaxel) versus i.v. paclitaxel in patients with advanced gastric cancer after failure of first-line chemotherapy. Ann Oncol. 2018;29(5):1220–6.
52. Hironaka S, Sugimoto N, Yamaguchi K, Moriwaki T, Komatsu Y, Nishina T, et al. S-1 plus leucovorin versus S-1 plus leucovorin and oxaliplatin versus S-1 plus cisplatin in patients with advanced gastric cancer: a randomised, multicentre, open label, phase 2 trial. Lancet Oncol. 2016;17:99–108.
53. Bando H, Doi T, Muro K, Yasui H, Nishina T, Yamaguchi K, et al. A multicenter phase II study of TAS-102 monotherapy in patients with pre-treated advanced gastric cancer (EPOC1201). Eur J Cancer. 2016;62:46–53.
54. Lordick F, Janjigian YY. Clinical impact of tumour biology in the management of gastroesophageal cancer. Nat Rev Clin Oncol. 2016;13:348–60.

Combined Modality Treatment for Locally Advanced Gastric Cancer: Current Evidences and New Perspectives

8

Antonino De Paoli, Federico Navarria, Elisa Palazzari, Matteo Olivieri, Claudio Belluco, Michela Guardascione, Renato Cannizzaro, Vincenzo Canzonieri, Giulio Bertola, Roberto Innocente, and Angela Buonadonna

Introduction

Gastric cancer still represents a major global health problem. In spite of a decrease in incidence and mortality rates during the last decades in Western countries, gastric cancer remains a common malignancy in regions such as Eastern Asia, Eastern Europe, and parts of South America making it the second leading cause of cancer death in the world [1]. Significant changes in the epidemiology of gastric cancer have also occurred. Compared to Eastern countries, the incidence of both proximal gastric and distal esophageal adenocarcinomas has risen in Western countries during the past two decades, with related diagnostic, prognostic, and treatment implications [2].

Apart from Japan, where mass screening programs have been developed for an early detection of this disease, most patients have advanced or unresectable tumor at diagnosis, and only less than half of them are likely candidates for curative surgery [3]. However, even when curative resection can be performed, the reported 5-year survival rate of 20–40% for stage II–III disease is still disappointing [4]. Locoregional recurrences are common after curative resection, remaining a substantial problem also in the modern surgical series; in addition, distant metastases occur, as a component of failure, in a significant part of recurred patients [5–7]. Extended D2 lymph node dissection has the advantage of accurate nodal staging, and it has demonstrated to improve cancer-specific survival but also to increase

A. De Paoli (✉) · F. Navarria · E. Palazzari
R. Innocente
Radiation Oncology Department, IRCCS, CRO Aviano, National Cancer Institute, Aviano, PN, Italy
e-mail: adepaoli@cro.it

M. Olivieri · C. Belluco · G. Bertola
Surgical Oncology Department, IRCCS, CRO Aviano, National Cancer Institute, Aviano, PN, Italy

M. Guardascione · A. Buonadonna
Medical Oncology Department, IRCCS, CRO Aviano, National Cancer Institute, Aviano, PN, Italy

R. Cannizzaro
Oncological Gastroenterology Department, IRCCS, CRO Aviano, National Cancer Institute, Aviano, PN, Italy

V. Canzonieri
Pathology Department, IRCCS, CRO Aviano, National Cancer Institute, Aviano, PN, Italy

Department of Medical, Surgical and Health Sciences, University of Trieste, Trieste, TS, Italy

CRO Biobank, IRCCS, CRO Aviano, National Cancer Institute, Aviano, PN, Italy

Department of Biology, Temple University Philadelphia, PA, USA

© Springer Nature Switzerland AG 2019

V. Canzonieri, A. Giordano (eds.), *Gastric Cancer In The Precision Medicine Era*, Current Clinical Pathology, https://doi.org/10.1007/978-3-030-04861-7_8

surgical morbidity and mortality [8–10]. Because of the increased postoperative (postop) mortality, which has been related to splenic and pancreatic resections, several authors suggested D2 dissection without splenopancreasectomy for these patients [11], and a more recent Cochrane systematic review and meta-analysis support the non-inferiority of spleen preservation versus splenectomy, in terms of survival, in patients with proximal gastric cancer [12].

Despite years of randomized trials, the results of adjuvant chemotherapy (CT) still remain disappointing, and the more recent meta-analysis indications for survival benefit await confirmation by further trials using modern and potentially more active drug combinations [13, 14]. A major interest has emerged during the past few years in other adjunctive treatment modalities, resulting in different but beneficial approaches including postop chemoradiotherapy (CT-RT), perioperative (periop) CT, and preoperative (preop) CT-RT, which changed significantly the clinical practice and clinical research in gastric cancer.

This paper examines the current evidence from these various approaches and highlights the most recently reported clinical trials with focus on therapeutic options to further improve current treatment strategies for patients affected by this disease.

Combined Modality Treatment Options: First Generation of Randomized Clinical Trials

Adjuvant Chemoradiotherapy

Postop CT-RT has been the first strategy to provide a survival benefit in gastric cancer. The INT0116 trial demonstrated that postop CT-RT significantly improved relapse-free and overall survival, compared to surgery alone, in patients with locally advanced, stage Ib–IV M0, gastric or gastroesophageal (GEJ) cancer [15]. The CT-RT program consisted of one cycle of 5-fluorouracil (5-FU) and leucovorin for 5 days followed by CT-RT with 45 Gy and concurrent 5-FU/leucovorin on the first 4 and last 3 days of RT, followed by two further cycles of 5-FU/leucovorin. The survival at 3 years was 50% versus 40% ($p = 0.005$) in favor of the CT-RT group. The survival benefit was also maintained after a median follow-up of 10.3 years [16]. Despite these positive results, the study was criticized because of the low rate of D2 lymph node dissection, with 54% of patients having only a D1 lymphadenectomy, and because the survival rates in the Intergroup trial were not better than those observed in the negative European adjuvant trials. Moreover, grade 3–4 hematological and gastrointestinal toxicities occurred in 54% and 31% of patients, respectively, resulting in a limited compliance to treatment; only 64% of patients were able to complete postop RT-CT as planned.

As most patients had limited surgery and the impact on disease control and survival was mainly related to local control, it has been suggested that postop CT-RT compensated for inadequate surgery with the possible implications that such treatment could not be necessary in patients who have a more extensive D2 lymph node dissection and further investigations with this adjuvant approach were suggested.

Perioperative Chemotherapy

The MAGIC trial was the first trial to show an improvement in survival by periop CT in patients with gastric and GEJ cancers. The MAGIC trial consisted of three cycles of preop and three cycles of postop epirubicin, cisplatin, and infused 5-FU (ECF) that significantly increased the R0 resection rate compared to surgery alone (79% versus 69%, respectively) in operable gastric and GEJ cancers, stage II–IV M0. The CT arm showed a significant improvement in overall survival (36% vs 23% at 5 years, $p = 0.009$), downsizing (median tumor size 3 vs 5 cm, $p < 0.001$), and downstaging, both in the primary (T1–T2: 52% vs 37%, $p = 0.002$) and in nodal diseases (N1/N2: 84% vs 71%, $p = 0.01$). Notably, the few patients with EGJ cancer (11%) seemed to have more benefit from CT, suggesting a better tumor chemosensitivity. Rates of postop complications were similar in both groups of patients (46% and 45%, respectively) as well as the incidence of deaths within 30 days after surgery (5.6% and 5.9%, respectively), which demonstrates the feasibility and safety of preop CT. However, only 55% of patients in the arm with periop CT began the postop treatment, mainly due to early disease progression, postop complications, or patient refusal. Overall, only 42% of patients completed the planned six-cycle program, suggesting a problematic patient compliance to treatment mainly related to poor general conditions after preop CT and surgery [17].

These results were confirmed in a second periop trial reported by the French FNCLCC/FFCD 9703 phase III study [18]. Compared with the other adjuvant and periop trials, in this study most patients had GEJ (64%) and lower esophageal (11%) tumors; only 24% of patients had gastric cancer. Patients were randomized to receive either two or three preop cycles of continuous infusion 5-FU and cisplatin (FP regimen) followed by surgery or surgery alone. Four cycles of postop FP were planned in case of response to preop CT or stable disease with positive lymph nodes. Periop CT resulted in significantly improved 5-year overall survival (38% versus 24%) and 5-year DFS (34% versus 21%). Similarly to the MAGIC trial, the R0 resection rate was significantly improved, and the subgroup of EGJ tumors showed the greatest benefit from preop CT, but only a part of patients were able to complete the postop component of treatment.

The feasibility and tolerance of preop compared to postop approach was addressed by the Swiss Group for Clinical Cancer Research (SAKK); the group reported the data of a randomized trial demonstrating that docetaxel-based preop CT is better tolerated than postop CT, thus confirming the indications on patient compliance and further supporting the preop approach [19].

Adjuvant Chemotherapy

While adjuvant CT trials from Japan and Korea showed a clear benefit of adjuvant therapy for stage II and III gastric cancer using oral S1 for 1 year or intravenous oxaliplatin and capecitabine (XELOX) after surgery [20, 21], European trials have been disappointing so far. Three randomized trials evaluating adjuvant CT compared with surgery alone showed 5-year survival rates ranging between 40% and 50%, with no significant difference between arms [22–24]. Similarly, the most recently reported ITACA-S trial, evaluating an intensive adjuvant regimen with sequential FOLFIRI followed by docetaxel plus cisplatin, failed to show any benefit in disease-free and overall survival versus monotherapy with 5-FU/leucovorin alone. Based on these results, 5-FU/leucovorin has been considered as the standard treatment for patients radically operated with D2 dissection [25]. A recent meta-analysis based on individual patient data suggested a small but defined benefit with adjuvant CT, which remained constant after testing for heterogeneity according to the geographic region where the study was conducted (Europe, Asia, North America) and the CT regimen administered (monotherapy or combination CT), supporting the evidence of its indication [13, 14].

Preoperative Chemoradiotherapy

For operable gastric cancer, an increasing interest has emerged more recently in the preop CT-RT approach as a three-step strategy with induction CT followed by preop CT-RT and subsequent surgery delayed up to 18–20 weeks. Recent advances in clinical staging, including endoscopic ultrasound and laparoscopy, are now available to identify patients who are potentially candidates for this innovative treatment strategy [25]. The CT-RT approach appears to be better tolerated in the preop setting, and it may increase the likelihood of an R0 resection, as reported with preop CT alone. In addition, as the primary tumor is still in place, the radiation planning can be more accurate compared with the difficulties experienced with postop CT-RT [15]. Some phase II studies have shown the feasibility of this approach including two cycles of induction CT with 5-FU and cisplatin followed by preop concurrent CT-RT with 5-FU and cisplatin or Taxol combined with 45Gy of radiation followed by radical gastrectomy [26, 27]. Pathological complete response (pCR) ranged from 20% to 30% and R0 resection rate from 70% to 78%; pCR and

Table 8.1 Combined modality treatment: first generation of RCTs

Trial	N° Pts	Treatment	R0	pCR	5ys OS
INT0116 Stomach, 80% GEJ, 20%	559	Postop FU/LV + RT-FU/LV vs surgery alone	100%	–	35% vs 27%
MAGIC-B Stomach, 74% GEJ, 11% ES, 15%	503	Periop ECX 3 + 3 vs surgery alone	68% vs 66%	None	36% vs 23%
FFCD/ACCO Stomach, 25% GEJ, 64% ES, 11%	224	Periop CF 3 + 3 vs surgery alone	84% vs 74%	None	38% vs 24%
RTOG 9904 Stomach,100%	43	Preop FU/LV-DDP x2 + RT-FU	77%	26%	–

R0 resection were found to be independent prognostic factors for survival in a pooled analysis of these studies, and an excellent 5-year survival rate was reported. Grade 4 toxicity occurred in 21% of patients [28]. The major concern with this approach is the risk of tumor progression during neoadjuvant treatment, with unresectable or metastatic disease at the postponed planned surgery. Available data reported an incidence of 16–25% of disease progression at surgery in patients treated with neoadjuvant CT or CT-RT [28]. Whether patients who recur during preoperative treatment indicate a subset with more aggressive and rapidly progressive disease, in whom no benefit from surgery can be expected, or a disease progression in nonresponsive patients, remains a matter of debate. The identification of this high-risk group of patients could be better addressed by the biological characterization of the disease. Advances in molecular biology are in progress and could result in a more accurate determination of prognosis and individualized therapeutic strategies. The first generation of randomized clinical trials on combined modality treatment is reported in Table 8.1.

Beyond INT0116 and Magic: Highlights of the Second Generation of Randomized Trials and Novel Clinical Approaches

The INT0116 and MAGIC trials changed significantly the clinical practice and clinical research in gastric cancer in the last decade. To answer the several questions that emerged from these landmark trials, a new generation of adjuvant/neoadjuvant gastric RCTs and novel neoadjuvant approaches were planned and have been recently reported as follows.

Is Postoperative Chemoradiotherapy Beneficial Also After D2 Lymphadenectomy?

A first attempt to answer the question of whether postop CT-RT is beneficial after D2 lymphadenectomy was made by the Korean Adjuvant Chemoradiotherapy in Stomach Tumors (ARTIST) phase III trial, which compared adjuvant CT-RT with two cycles of capecitabine-cisplatin before and after capecitabine-based CT-RT versus six cycles of adjuvant capecitabine-cisplatin alone [29]. The study was negative, even if a trend toward an improved 3-year disease-free survival (78.2% vs 74.2%, $p = 0.09$) was noted in the CT-RT arm. In addition, in a subset analysis of patients with lymph node-positive disease, the 3-year DFS was significantly improved with CT-RT (77.5% vs 72.3%, $p = 0.04$). These results were confirmed at a longer follow-up of 7 years. The ARTIST trial differed from Intergroup trial in two important ways: firstly, all patients had D2 dissection with a median number of 40 examined lymph nodes, and, secondly, the control arm had adjuvant CT; thus, comparison of the two studies is somewhat difficult. One can speculate that postop CT-RT was beneficial also after D2 dissection, but this benefit was neutralized by postop

CT. It is also possible that postop CT-RT was better than postop CT in node-positive patients, but this is based only on a subset analysis with its relative limitations.

The ongoing ARTIST II 3-arm phase III trial is evaluating the efficacy of postop CT-RT (S1-oxaliplatin followed by radiation 45Gy and capecitabine) versus postop CT (S1 or S1-oxaliplatin) in patients with lymph node-positive gastric cancer receiving D2 lymph node dissection [30].

Does the Addition of a More Effective Chemotherapy Component Improve the Efficacy of Postoperative Chemoradiotherapy?

As the improvement in overall and disease-free survival for patients who underwent postop CT-RT in the INT0116 trial was mainly related to an increase of local control rather than to a decrease in the incidence of metastatic disease, the Cancer and Leukemia Group B (CALGB) promoted a new phase III trial testing a modern and more effective CT regimen with one cycle of epirubicin, cisplatin, and 5-FU (ECF) followed by radiation of 45Gy and concurrent continuous infusion 5-FU and by two more cycles of ECF versus the treatment arm of the INT0116 study (45 Gy and concurrent 5-FU/leucovorin). The results of this trial have been recently reported and demonstrated that the addition of epirubicin and cisplatin in postop CT-RT is not superior to standard 5-FU/leucovorin in terms of disease-free and overall survival (37% vs 39% and 44% vs 44%, respectively). Also, no significant differences were observed for either locoregional recurrences or distant metastasis rates between treatment arms and any patient subgroup, including the extended lymph node dissection group (55% of patients had >15 lymph nodes and 11% had <7 lymph node examined) [31].

Although surgical treatment was more standardized compared to the previous Intergroup study, these results are quite different from those reported in the abovementioned postop CT-RT ARTIST trial with the reported survival rates >70%. Again, comparison of these studies is difficult because of several implications in different patient populations, CT-RT and CT regimens, and some details in surgical approach.

Does the Addition of Targeted Agents or New Chemotherapy Combinations Improve the Efficacy of Perioperative Chemotherapy?

Following the MAGIC trial, there has been intensive clinical investigation to further improve the perioperative approach. The addition of bevacizumab to epirubicin, cisplatin, and capecitabine (ECX) in a phase III recently reported STO03 trial failed to demonstrate its superiority to periop ECX alone in patients with resectable gastric and EGJ adenocarcinoma [32]. Progression-free survival and overall survival were similar in the study arms, as were the rates of pathological response, with a pCR of 5% and 7% for ECX and ECX-bevacizumab, respectively.

More recently, results from the phase II part of the German FLOT4 phase III trial showed that preop docetaxel, oxaliplatin, and FU/leucovorin (FLOT) increased the pCR rate compared with ECF or ECX (16% vs 6%, $p = 0.015$) in resectable gastric (48%) or GEJ adenocarcinoma (52%). Interestingly, this favorable activity in terms of pCR was more evident in the intestinal-type histology (16%) compared with diffuse-type histology adenocarcinoma (3%, $p = 0.004$) [33]. This data of activity of docetaxel-based CT has been also reported in the phase I–II study with docetaxel, oxaliplatin, and capecitabine (DOC) currently ongoing in our Institute in advanced metastatic disease [34]. In the FLOT4 trial, postop morbidity was 40% with ECF-ECX and 25% with FLOT ($p = 0.02$), and postop mortality was 4% with ECF-ECX and 2% with FLOT (p = NS). The last update of the study confirmed also a significant impact of FLOT regimen for 5-year overall survival (39% vs 33%, $p = 0.001$) [35]. Importantly, also in this trial, only 50% of patients in the ECF-ECX group and 61% in the FLOT group started postop CT, thus confirming the problematic patient compliance for postoperative treatment after preop CT and surgery.

In summary, the use of periop CT for locally advanced gastric and EGJ adenocarcinoma is a well-established approach; periop CT has shown to improve survival in both the MAGIC and the FNCLCC-FFCD trials. Subsequent studies have confirmed these results. While the addition of bevacizumab to ECX of MAGIC failed to demonstrate superiority to ECX alone, docetaxel-based triplet regimen (FLOT) was superior to the standard anthracycline-based regimen ECF-ECX (FOLT4 trial). As result, the FLOT regimen expands the current available periop CT options for the treatment of resectable gastric and EGJ adenocarcinoma, and it could represent the preferred histology-driven option for patients with intestinal-type tumors. Patient compliance for postoperative treatment after preoperative chemotherapy and surgery still remains a problem.

Does the Addition of Postoperative Chemoradiotherapy Provide Additional Advantage to Perioperative Chemotherapy?

The results of phase III CRITICS trial, which evaluated three cycles of preop epirubicin, cisplatin, and capecitabine (ECX) followed by radical gastrectomy with D1+ lymphadenectomy and either three addictional cycles of postop ECX or CT-RT with 45Gy and capecitabine-cisplatin, have been recently reported [36]. This was the first trial that directly compared the two standard of care strategies for adjuvant treatment in resectable gastric cancer defined in the last decade: postop CT-RT, as investigated in the INT0116 trial, and periop CT, as investigated in MAGIC trial. The trial was designed with appropriate quality assurance criteria resulting in high standard of surgery as demonstrated by high D1+ resection rate of 86% and R0 resection rate of 81%. In addition, a detailed radiation therapy quality assurance was also included, consisting in a real-time pretreatment planning central review.

The trial did not show any superiority for postop CT-RT compared with postop CT alone in patients having preop CT and adequate surgery. There was no difference in overall or event-free survival or, surprisingly, in locoregional control. Tolerability was similar in the two treatment arms. Furthermore, it should be emphasized that also in this trial only half of the patients in both treatment groups were able to complete the postop component of treatment as planned. This difficulty in delivering postop treatment, in particular after preop CT-RT, confirms the poor postop patient compliance previously reported in both INT0116 and MAGIC trials and the necessity to better optimize the timing of combined modality treatment with surgery.

Does the Addition of Preoperative Chemoradiotherapy to Perioperative Chemotherapy and Postponed Surgery Provide Additional Advantage?

As benefits have been demonstrated in trials with periop CT, postop CT-RT, and preop CT-RT, questions about patient selection and the optimal sequence of treatments in a possible integrated approach still remain open.

The ongoing TOPGEAR trial (Trial of Preoperative therapy for Gastric and Esophagogastric Junction Adenocarcinoma), an international phase III study, is testing the addition of CT-RT to periop CT by administering it in the preop rather than in postop setting. The study design allows a comparison of the MAGIC regimen with the INT0116 regimen but with the specific intent to move CT-RT into the preop setting.

Patients in the periop-alone group receive three cycles of ECF CT, while patients in the CT-RT group receive two cycles of ECF followed by radiation with 45Gy and concurrent FU. Both groups of patients will receive three more cycles of ECF after surgery. This study is based on the potential advantages of preop therapy for tumor downstaging, with an increase R0 resection rate, and the better tolerability of preop compared to postop therapy. Indeed, the study represents also an evolving strategy of the several phase II studies of preop CT-RT in gastric cancer which have demonstrated safety, tolerability, and high rates of pathological response.

The recently reported interim analysis on the first 120 enrolled patients demonstrated that 93% of ECF group and 98% of CT-RT group patients received all cycles of preop CT and radiation as planned, while only 65% and 53%, respectively, received all cycles of postop CT. The proportion of patients proceeding to surgery was encouraging: 90% of patients in ECF group and 85% in CT-RT group underwent operation. Grade 3 or higher postop complications occurred in 22% of patients in both groups.

These results demonstrated that preop CT-RT can be safely delivered to the most part of patients after two cycles of induction ECF CT, without a significant increase in treatment toxicity or surgical morbidity. However, once again, also this study showed a limited patient compliance for postop CT after preop CT or CT-RT. The study is ongoing on the primary endpoint of overall survival, and results of the efficacy on adding preop CT-RT to periop CT are pending [37].

In order to further optimize preop CT-RT, a phase II study with a more effective systemic component including three cycles of induction CT (as MAGIC strategy) with new and potentially more active regimen including epirubicin, oxaliplatin, and capecitabine (EOX) [38], followed by preop CT-RT with modern drug-radiation combinations (3D-CRT or IMRT 45Gy and concurrent capecitabine and weekly oxaliplatin) and by standardized surgical procedure, postponed at the end of the overall neoadjuvant program (after 20–22 weeks), was activated at our Institute (Neoadjuvant Epirubicin, Oxaliplatin, Capecitabine, and Radiation Therapy, NEOX-RT study). Examples of structures and lymph node station delineation and IMRT plan are reported in Figs. 8.1 and 8.2 (NEOX-RT study). This was a multicentric phase II study aiming to assess the feasibility of a complete CT (three cycles) and CT-RT program both given preoperatively in order to improve patient compliance to the combined modality treatment and to further improve resectability, pCR, disease control, and overall survival in locally advanced, stage T3–T4 N0 or N+, gastric cancer. This approach had also the potential advantage that a greater proportion of patients could receive all components of the multimodality treatment. An accurate staging including laparoscopic examination and patient careful clinical monitoring with endoscopic ultrasound and FDG-PET during treatment to identify patients with early asymptomatic metastatic disease at diagnosis or rapidly progressive disease during treatment was planned.

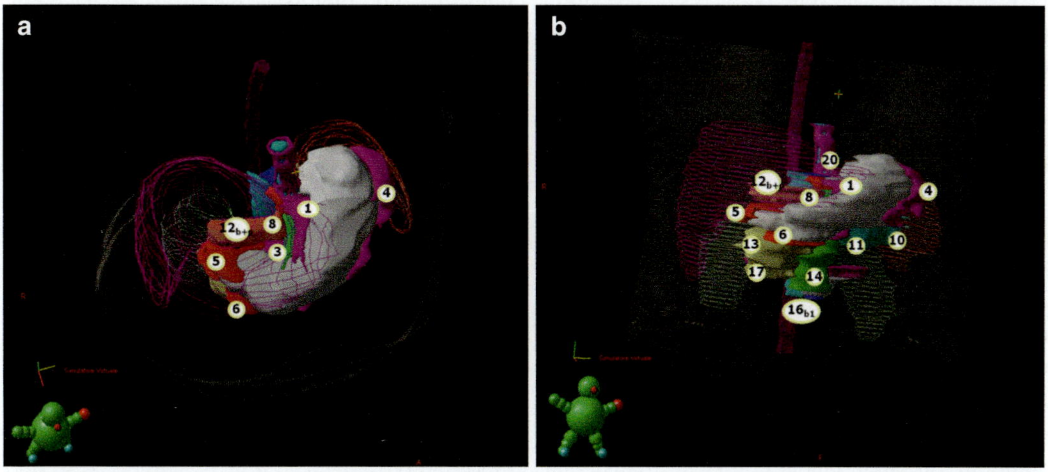

Fig. 8.1 Gastric cancer: structures and lymph node stations contouring in IMRT planning (NEOX-RT study). (**a**) Anterior 3D visualization. (**b**) Posterior 3D visualization (By courtesy of F.Cellini - GemelliArt, Roma)

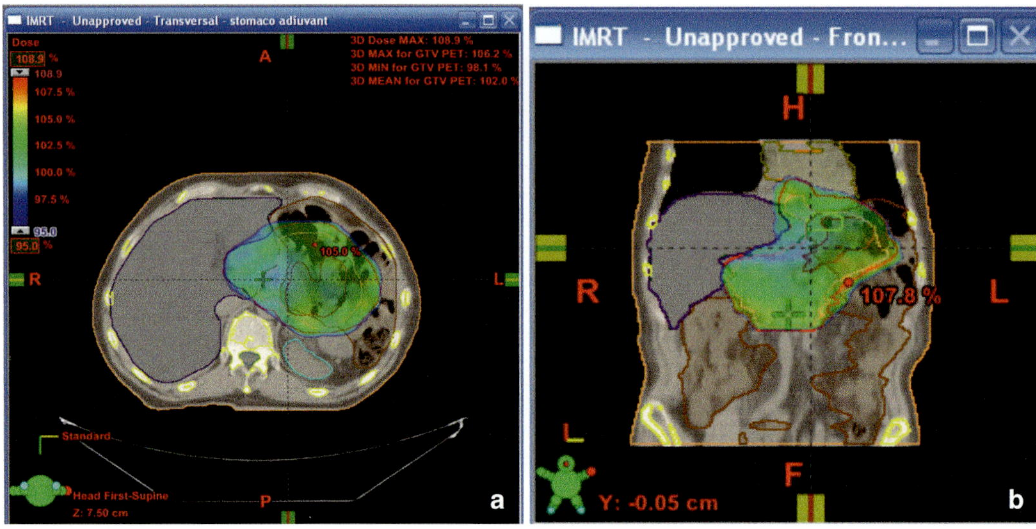

Fig. 8.2 Gastric cancer (antrum): IMRT plan for preop 45Gy/capecitabine-oxaliplatin (NEOX-RT study). (**a**) Target volume in transverse section. (**b**) Target volume in frontal section

In the reported interim analysis on the first 21 enrolled patients, tumor downstaging and nodal downstaging were 65% and 60%, respectively, with a pCR in 18% of patients. Compliance to treatment was good, and most patients completed the CT (87%) and CT-RT (86%) programs as planned. The most part of patients (90%) underwent R0 resection, and the median time to surgery was 23 weeks (planned 20–22 weeks). One patient had postop major complications. NEOX-RT appeared feasible and safe, and the pCR rate of 18% was remarkable [39]. The study has been recently concluded and final results will be reported.

Gastric and Gastroesophageal Junction Adenocarcinomas: Does Location and Histology Matter?

Because of different anatomic regions and lymph node compartments involved by the tumor, substantial differences between gastric and GEJ adenocarcinomas exist, with significant implications in the extension of surgical resection [40]. In addition, different epidemiological trends and histological characteristics between adenocarcinomas of these two anatomic regions have been also observed. GEJ cancer is a disease of smokers and drinkers. Gastric cancer is strongly associated with *Helicobacter pylori* infection, atrophic gastritis, and decreased acid production, while GEJ cancer is associated with a high acid production and Barrett's changes in the esophageal mucosa. Furthermore, tumors located in GEJ and cardia are predominantly of intestinal type (Lauren's classification) compared to distal stomach tumors, where diffuse types are more commonly located. While a decreased incidence of intestinal-type tumors in the distal stomach has been observed, the intestinal type, located in the proximal third, and the diffuse type at any location, have increased over time. Most importantly, tumor location and histology are associated to different clinical aggressiveness, treatment response, and prognosis. Proximal tumors, including GEJ, and diffuse histotype have usually a worse prognosis with a higher risk of lymph node and peritoneal spread [41]. However, GEJ tumors appear to be also the more responsive to preop CT(RT), and an unexpected high rate of pCR has been reported [33, 42, 43]. An important finding is that intestinal histotype tumors are more likely to achieve a pCR, compared to diffuse histotypes [33]. In addition, more rare histologic subgroups as signet-ring cell tumors, existing in any gastric and EGJ location, demonstrated to be inherently resistant to the current chemo(radio)therapy regimen, and implications on treatment programs should be considered [44]. Interestingly, both intestinal and diffuse tumor types showed different targetable biomarker expression profiles such as Her2 in the intestinal and EGFR in the non-intestinal pathway, indicating new therapy options [45].

Optimal management of patients with GEJ adenocarcinoma is still a controversial issue [46]. No randomized clinical trials have specifically selected this subset of patients, and clinical data are derived from studies addressing both esophageal and gastric cancers, including either squamous cell carcinoma or adenocarcinoma [47]. Most part of these trials evaluated the impact of neoadjuvant CT-RT [48–50] or neoadjuvant CT [33, 51, 52] as compared to surgery alone. A recently updated meta-analysis confirmed a strong evidence for a survival benefit of neoadjuvant CT-RT or CT over surgery alone [42, 43].

The most solid evidence in favor of neoadjuvant CT-RT was provided by the CROSS trial comparing surgery alone to preop RT with 41.4Gy with concurrent carboplatin and paclitaxel followed by surgical resection [48]. Up to 75% of enrolled patients had adenocarcinoma, and 22% had a GEJ tumor. Overall, a pCR of 29% was reported, and this was more frequent in patients with squamous cell carcinoma (49% vs 23%, $p = 0.008$). Overall 5-year survival was 47% versus 34% in favor of preoperative CT-RT [53]. To further optimize this CT-RT program, a phase II study is currently ongoing at our Institute to evaluate feasibility and efficacy of intensified IMRT of 52.5Gy with the same concurrent CT. The recently reported initial results demonstrated the feasibility and safety and encouraging activity of the treatment [54].

Few studies compared neoadjuvant CT-RT versus CT prior to surgery. A first randomized study enrolled 119 patients with adenocarcinoma of the lower esophagus or cardia to receive two cycles of DDP-5-FU/LV or the same preop CT followed by 30 Gy of RT with concurrent cisplatin and etoposide. Aimed for 354 patients, the study was concluded early due to poor accrual. The pCR rate was significantly superior in the CT-RT group (15% vs 2%); although the rate of postop mortality was somewhat higher with CT-RT (10.2% versus 3.8%, $p = 0.26$), a 5-year survival showed a trend in favor of preop CT-RT (48% vs 40%, $p = 0.055$). Another trial compared two cycles of FU and cisplatin with 35Gy of radiation to neoadjuvant FU and cisplatin alone. Also this study concluded early for the low accrual. A superior pCR rate for CT-RT was reported also in this study (13% vs 0%), but without significant difference in OS [49]. However, when these data were combined with the pooled results of other neoadjuvant CT or CT-RT trials in recent meta-analysis, a trend in favor of neoadjuvant CT-RT was reported ($p = 0.07$) [43]. Importantly, no difference in morbidity was reported between the two treatment approaches. The second generation of selected randomized clinical trials on combined modality treatment is reported in Table 8.2.

In summary, based on the available evidence, both neoadjuvant CT-RT and CT provide significant survival benefits over surgery alone in patients with GEJ carcinoma. A clear advantage of neoadjuvant CT-RT over neoadjuvant CT, in the few studies including patients with GEJ adenocarcinoma, has not yet been established, and further trials comparing these two strategies should be promoted on this emerging and well-defined tumor site.

Conclusions

After years of negative studies, two successful treatment strategies with postop CT-RT (INT0116 trial) or periop CT (MAGIC trial) became available as standard of care for adjuvant therapy of resectable gastric cancer in Western countries [15, 17]. Because of some limitation of these studies, a second generation of clinical trials was planned in the last decade to answer several questions that emerged from these two landmark trials.

The efficacy of postop CT-RT also after D2 lymph node dissection has not been clearly demonstrated in the ARTIST trial; even if a significant advantage in the subset of patients with

Table 8.2 Combined modality treatment: second generation of RCTs

Trial	N° Pts	Treatment	R0	pCR	5ys OS
CALGB 80101 Stomach, 78% GEJ, 22%	546	Postop ECF + RT-FU + ECF vs postop FU/ LV + RT-FU/LV	100%	–	44% vs 44%
ARTIST Stomach, 100%	458	D2 + postop X-P 2 + 2 + RT/Cape vs D2 + postop X-P x6	100%	–	77% vs 72% (3 years DFS)
STO03 Stomach, 36% GEJ, 50% ES, 14%	1063	ECX-bevacizumab vs ECX alone	61% vs 64%	7% vs 5%	48% vs 50% (3ys)
FLOT4 Stomach, 43% GEJ, 57%	265	Periop FLOT 4 + 4 vs periop ECF 3 + 3 or ECX	85% vs 74%	16% vs 6%	39% vs 33%
CRITICS Stomach, 83% GEJ, 17%	788	Periop ECX x3 vs periop ECX x3 + postop RT/X-P	80% vs 82%	6% vs 6%	42% vs 40%
TOPGEAR[a] Stomach, 73% GEJ, 27%	120	Periop ECF 2 + 3 + preop RT-FU vs periop ECF 3 + 3 alone	–	–	–
POET[b] GEJ, 100%	119	Preop FU/LV-DDP x14 weeks + preop RT/ DDP-VP16 vs preop FU/LV-DDP x14 weeks	96% vs 84%	16% vs 2%	39% vs 24%
CROSS[c] GEJ, 25% ES, 75%	366	Preop RT/Carbo-PTX vs surgery alone	82% vs 59%	23% vs na	47% vs 33%

[a]Interim data
[b]Stopped for poor accrual
[c]*SCC* 23%; Adenoca 75%

positive lymph nodes has been reported, the trial was negative [29]. In addition, both the CALGB and the CRITICS trials, in which a more standardized D2 dissection was provided, failed to demonstrate an advantage of postop CT-RT with an added more effective systemic CT component [31] or when compared to post-op CT only in a periop approach [36]. However, the 3–5-year survival rates of these two trials were well comparable or better than the treatment arms of the original INT0116 and MAGIC trials, confirming the superiority of postop CT-RT and periop CT to surgery alone (Tables 8.1 and 8.2).

While the addition of target therapy (bevacizumab) to periop ECF(ECX) failed to demonstrate superiority to standard ECF(ECX) [32], the docetaxel-based triplet FLOT was superior to triplet epirubicin-based CT in the periop FLOT4 trial in terms of pCR, postop morbidity, and survival [33, 35]. These results confirm the initial data of the DOC phase I–II study currently ongoing at our Institute, and docetaxel-based CT expands the current available periop options in locally advanced, resectable gastric cancer [34].

The more recent growing interest in preop CT-RT is further supported by the interim results of the TOPGEAR trial which demonstrated the feasibility and safety of delivering preop CT-RT after two cycles of ECF CT with high compliance rates to treatment (98%) and the high proportion of patients proceeding to surgery (85%) [37].

However, there are still open questions regarding the duration of the preop CT component, and whether the postop CT component is necessary. As in other recent periop trials, also in TOPGEAR trial, only about half of the patients were able to receive CT after surgery.

Considering the better patient tolerance of preop treatment, future studies should focus on the possibility to move a more complete CT component in the preop period. On this issue, the

NEOX-RT phase II study was activated at our Institute which included a more effective neoadjuvant component with three cycles of EOX (with no postop CT) followed by CT-RT, and surgery postponed at week 20–22 could be a useful contribution for a new preop treatment approach in locally advanced gastric cancer. Interim analysis demonstrated the feasibility and safety of this prolonged treatment time before surgery, and the final results of the study will be reported [39].

Future studies also need to give more focus on GEJ and stomach cancer as separate diseases to provide more solid data in these established tumor types. Furthermore, defined histologic subtypes (i.e., intestinal, diffuse, or mixed histotypes) are associated to different aggressiveness, treatment response, and prognosis. Therefore, future clinical studies should take into account these emerging evidences. New current insights into histological patterns [55–57] and molecular characterization of individual tumor subtypes [58–60] could address new and more individualized generation of combined modality treatment programs.

Acknowledgments The authors thank S. Flora and D. Michilin for manuscript editing assistance.

References

1. Siegel R, Naishadham D, Jemal A. Cancer statistics, 2012. CA Cancer J Clin. 2012;62(1):10–29.
2. Crew KD, Neugut AI. Epidemiology of gastric cancer. World J Gastroenterol. 2006;12(3):354–62.
3. Reim D, Loos M, Vogl F, Novotny A, Schuster T, Langer R, et al. Prognostic implications of the seventh edition of the international union against cancer classification for patients with gastric cancer: the Western experience of patients treated in a single-center European institution. J Clin Oncol Off J Am Soc Clin Oncol. 2013;31(2):263–71.
4. Lise M, Nitti D, Marchet A, Sahmoud T, Duez N, Fornasiero A, et al. Prognostic factors in resectable gastric cancer: results of EORTC study no. 40813 on FAM adjuvant chemotherapy. Ann Surg Oncol. 1995;2(6):495–501.
5. Yoo CH, Noh SH, Shin DW, Choi SH, Min JS. Recurrence following curative resection for gastric carcinoma. Br J Surg. 2000;87(2):236–42.
6. Wu C-W, Lo S-S, Shen K-H, Hsieh M-C, Chen J-H, Chiang J-H, et al. Incidence and factors associated with recurrence patterns after intended curative surgery for gastric cancer. World J Surg. 2003;27(2):153–8.
7. D'Angelica M, Gonen M, Brennan MF, Turnbull AD, Bains M, Karpeh MS. Patterns of initial recurrence in completely resected gastric adenocarcinoma. Ann Surg. 2004;240(5):808–16.
8. Songun I, Putter H, Kranenbarg EM-K, Sasako M, van de Velde CJH. Surgical treatment of gastric cancer: 15-year follow-up results of the randomised nationwide Dutch D1D2 trial. Lancet Oncol. 2010;11(5):439–49.
9. Sasako M, Sano T, Yamamoto S, Kurokawa Y, Nashimoto A, Kurita A, et al. D2 lymphadenectomy alone or with para-aortic nodal dissection for gastric cancer. N Engl J Med. 2008;359(5):453–62.
10. Verlato G, Roviello F, Marchet A, Giacopuzzi S, Marrelli D, Nitti D, et al. Indexes of surgical quality in gastric cancer surgery: experience of an Italian network. Ann Surg Oncol. 2009;16(3):594–602.
11. Sano T, Sasako M, Mizusawa J, Yamamoto S, Katai H, Yoshikawa T, et al. Randomized controlled trial to evaluate splenectomy in total gastrectomy for proximal gastric carcinoma. Ann Surg. 2017;265(2):277–83.
12. Mocellin S, McCulloch P, Kazi H, Gama-Rodrigues JJ, Yuan Y, Nitti D. Extent of lymph node dissection for adenocarcinoma of the stomach. Cochrane Database Syst Rev. 2015;8:CD001964.
13. GASTRIC (Global Advanced/Adjuvant Stomach Tumor Research International Collaboration) Group, Paoletti X, Oba K, Burzykowski T, Michiels S, Ohashi Y, et al. Benefit of adjuvant chemotherapy for resectable gastric cancer: a meta-analysis. JAMA. 2010;303(17):1729–37.
14. Sun P, Xiang J-B, Chen Z-Y. Meta-analysis of adjuvant chemotherapy after radical surgery for advanced gastric cancer. Br J Surg. 2009;96(1):26–33.
15. Macdonald JS, Smalley SR, Benedetti J, Hundahl SA, Estes NC, Stemmermann GN, et al. Chemoradiotherapy after surgery compared with surgery alone for adenocarcinoma of the stomach or gastroesophageal junction. N Engl J Med. 2001;345(10):725–30.
16. Smalley SR, Benedetti JK, Haller DG, Hundahl SA, Estes NC, Ajani JA, et al. Updated analysis of SWOG-directed intergroup study 0116: a phase III trial of adjuvant radiochemotherapy versus observation after curative gastric cancer resection. J Clin Oncol Off J Am Soc Clin Oncol. 2012;30(19):2327–33.
17. Cunningham D, Allum WH, Stenning SP, Thompson JN, Van de Velde CJH, Nicolson M, et al. Perioperative chemotherapy versus surgery alone for resectable gastroesophageal cancer. N Engl J Med. 2006;355(1):11–20.
18. Boige V, Pignon J, Saint-Aubert B, Lasser P, Conroy T, Bouché O, et al. Final results of a randomized trial comparing preoperative 5-fluorouracil (F)/cisplatin (P) to surgery alone in adenocarcinoma of stomach and lower esophagus (ASLE): FNCLCC ACCORD07-FFCD 9703 trial. J Clin Oncol. 2007;25(18_suppl):4510.

19. Fazio N, Biffi R, Maibach R, Hayoz S, Thierstein S, Brauchli P, et al. Preoperative versus postoperative docetaxel-cisplatin-fluorouracil (TCF) chemotherapy in locally advanced resectable gastric carcinoma: 10-year follow-up of the SAKK 43/99 phase III trial. Ann Oncol. 2016;27(4):668–73.
20. Sakuramoto S, Sasako M, Yamaguchi T, Kinoshita T, Fujii M, Nashimoto A, et al. Adjuvant chemotherapy for gastric cancer with S-1, an oral fluoropyrimidine. N Engl J Med. 2007;357(18):1810–20.
21. Bang Y-J, Kim Y-W, Yang H-K, Chung HC, Park Y-K, Lee KH, et al. Adjuvant capecitabine and oxaliplatin for gastric cancer after D2 gastrectomy (CLASSIC): a phase 3 open-label, randomised controlled trial. Lancet Lond Engl. 2012;379(9813):315–21.
22. De Vita F, Giuliani F, Orditura M, Maiello E, Galizia G, Di Martino N, et al. Adjuvant chemotherapy with epirubicin, leucovorin, 5-fluorouracil and etoposide regimen in resected gastric cancer patients: a randomized phase III trial by the Gruppo Oncologico Italia Meridionale (GOIM 9602 study). Ann Oncol. 2007;18(8):1354–8.
23. Cascinu S, Labianca R, Barone C, Santoro A, Carnaghi C, Cassano A, et al. Adjuvant treatment of high-risk, radically resected gastric cancer patients with 5-fluorouracil, leucovorin, cisplatin, and epidoxorubicin in a randomized controlled trial. J Natl Cancer Inst. 2007;99(8):601–7.
24. Nitti D, Wils J, Dos Santos JG, Fountzilas G, Conte PF, Sava C, et al. Randomized phase III trials of adjuvant FAMTX or FEMTX compared with surgery alone in resected gastric cancer. A combined analysis of the EORTC GI Group and the ICCG. Ann Oncol Off J Eur Soc Med Oncol. 2006;17(2):262–9.
25. Kwee RM, Kwee TC. Imaging in local staging of gastric cancer: a systematic review. J Clin Oncol Off J Am Soc Clin Oncol. 2007;25(15):2107–16.
26. Ajani JA, Mansfield PF, Janjan N, Morris J, Pisters PW, Lynch PM, et al. Multi-institutional trial of preoperative chemoradiotherapy in patients with potentially resectable gastric carcinoma. J Clin Oncol Off J Am Soc Clin Oncol. 2004;22(14):2774–80.
27. Ajani JA, Mansfield PF, Crane CH, Wu TT, Lunagomez S, Lynch PM, et al. Paclitaxel-based chemoradiotherapy in localized gastric carcinoma: degree of pathologic response and not clinical parameters dictated patient outcome. J Clin Oncol Off J Am Soc Clin Oncol. 2005;23(6):1237–44.
28. Ajani JA, Winter K, Okawara GS, Donohue JH, Pisters PWT, Crane CH, et al. Phase II trial of preoperative chemoradiation in patients with localized gastric adenocarcinoma (RTOG 9904): quality of combined modality therapy and pathologic response. J Clin Oncol Off J Am Soc Clin Oncol. 2006;24(24):3953–8.
29. Lee J, Lim DH, Kim S, Park SH, Park JO, Park YS, et al. Phase III trial comparing capecitabine plus cisplatin versus capecitabine plus cisplatin with concurrent capecitabine radiotherapy in completely resected gastric cancer with D2 lymph node dissection: the ARTIST trial. J Clin Oncol Off J Am Soc Clin Oncol. 2012;30(3):268–73.
30. National Institutes of Health. Phase III randomized trial of adjuvant chemotherapy with S-1 vs S-1/oxaliplatin ± radiotherapy for completely resected gastric adenocarcinoma: The ARTIST II Trial. [Internet]. 2014 [citato 3 maggio 2018]. Available at: https://clinicaltrials.gov/ct2/show/NCT01761461.
31. Fuchs CS, Niedzwiecki D, Mamon HJ, Tepper JE, Ye X, Swanson RS, et al. Adjuvant chemoradiotherapy with epirubicin, cisplatin, and fluorouracil compared with adjuvant chemoradiotherapy with fluorouracil and leucovorin after curative resection of gastric cancer: results from CALGB 80101 (Alliance). J Clin Oncol Off J Am Soc Clin Oncol. 2017;35(32):3671–7.
32. Cunningham D, Stenning SP, Smyth EC, Okines AF, Allum WH, Rowley S, et al. Peri-operative chemotherapy with or without bevacizumab in operable oesophagogastric adenocarcinoma (UK Medical Research Council ST03): primary analysis results of a multicentre, open-label, randomised phase 2-3 trial. Lancet Oncol. 2017;18(3):357–70.
33. Al-Batran S-E, Hofheinz RD, Pauligk C, Kopp H-G, Haag GM, Luley KB, et al. Histopathological regression after neoadjuvant docetaxel, oxaliplatin, fluorouracil, and leucovorin versus epirubicin, cisplatin, and fluorouracil or capecitabine in patients with resectable gastric or gastro-oesophageal junction adenocarcinoma (FLOT4-AIO): results from the phase 2 part of a multicentre, open-label, randomised phase 2/3 trial. Lancet Oncol. 2016;17(12):1697–708.
34. Frustaci S, Buonadonna A, Turchet E, Corona G, Tabaro G, Miolo G, et al. Phase I trial of docetaxel, oxaliplatin, and capecitabine (DOC) in untreated gastric cancer patients. Int J Clin Oncol. 2013;18(3):510–6.
35. Al-Batran SE, Homann N, Schmalenberg H. Perioperative chemotherapy with docetaxel, oxaliplatin, and fluorouracil/leucovorin (FLOT) versus epirubicin, cisplatin, and fluorouracil or capecitabine (ECF/ECX) for resectable gastric or gastroesophageal junction (GEJ) adenocarcinoma (FLOT4-AIO): a multicenter, randomized phase 3 trial. J Clin Oncol. 2017;35(15):4004.
36. Cats A, Jansen EPM, van Grieken NCT, Sikorska K, Lind P, Nordsmark M, et al. Chemotherapy versus chemoradiotherapy after surgery and preoperative chemotherapy for resectable gastric cancer (CRITICS): an international, open-label, randomised phase 3 trial. Lancet Oncol. 2018;19(5):616–28.
37. Leong T, Smithers BM, Haustermans K, Michael M, Gebski V, Miller D, et al. TOPGEAR: a randomized, phase III trial of perioperative ECF chemotherapy with or without Preoperative Chemoradiation for Resectable Gastric Cancer: interim results from an International, Intergroup Trial of the AGITG, TROG, EORTC and CCTG. Ann Surg Oncol. 2017;24(8):2252–8.
38. Cunningham D, Starling N, Rao S, Iveson T, Nicolson M, Coxon F, et al. Capecitabine and oxaliplatin for

advanced esophagogastric cancer. N Engl J Med. 2008;358(1):36–46.
39. De Paoli A, Buonadonna A, Turchet E, Cannizzaro R, Canzonieri V, Tumolo S, et al. Neoadjuvant epirubicin, oxaliplatin, capecitabine and radiation therapy (NEOX-RT) followed by surgery for locally advanced gastric cancer (LAGC): interim analysis of a phase II multicentric study. In. ECCO 2013 LBA43 49–3 S19.
40. Rüdiger Siewert J, Feith M, Werner M, Stein HJ. Adenocarcinoma of the esophagogastric junction: results of surgical therapy based on anatomical/topographic classification in 1,002 consecutive patients. Ann Surg. 2000;232(3):353–61.
41. Marrelli D, Pedrazzani C, Morgagni P, de Manzoni G, Pacelli F, Coniglio A, et al. Changing clinical and pathological features of gastric cancer over time. Br J Surg. 2011;98(9):1273–83.
42. Sjoquist KM, Burmeister BH, Smithers BM, Zalcberg JR, Simes RJ, Barbour A, et al. Survival after neoadjuvant chemotherapy or chemoradiotherapy for resectable oesophageal carcinoma: an updated meta-analysis. Lancet Oncol. 2011;12(7):681–92.
43. Ronellenfitsch U, Schwarzbach M, Hofheinz R, Kienle P, Kieser M, Slanger TE, et al. Preoperative chemo(radio)therapy versus primary surgery for gastroesophageal adenocarcinoma: systematic review with meta-analysis combining individual patient and aggregate data. Eur J Cancer. 2013;49(15):3149–58.
44. Messager M, Lefevre JH, Pichot-Delahaye V, Souadka A, Piessen G, Mariette C, et al. The impact of perioperative chemotherapy on survival in patients with gastric signet ring cell adenocarcinoma: a multicenter comparative study. Ann Surg. 2011;254(5):684–93. discussion 693
45. Rüschoff J. Adenocarcinoma of the GEJ: gastric or oesophageal cancer? In: Otto F, Lutz MP, editors. Early gastrointestinal cancers. Berlin, Heidelberg: Springer Berlin Heidelberg; 2012. p. 107–13.
46. Mariette C, Piessen G, Briez N, Gronnier C, Triboulet JP. Oesophagogastric junction adenocarcinoma: which therapeutic approach? Lancet Oncol. 2011;12(3):296–305.
47. De Paoli A, Di Bartolomeo M. Neoadjuvant therapy of gastroesophageal junction adenocarcinoma: chemoradiotherapy or chemotherapy. Eur J Oncol. 2014;19(1):21–3.
48. van Hagen P, Hulshof MCCM, van Lanschot JJB, Steyerberg EW, van Berge Henegouwen MI, Wijnhoven BPL, et al. Preoperative chemoradiotherapy for esophageal or junctional cancer. N Engl J Med. 2012;366(22):2074–84.
49. Burmeister BH, Thomas JM, Burmeister EA, Walpole ET, Harvey JA, Thomson DB, et al. Is concurrent radiation therapy required in patients receiving preoperative chemotherapy for adenocarcinoma of the oesophagus? A randomised phase II trial. Eur J Cancer. 2011;47(3):354–60.
50. Mariette C, Dahan L, Mornex F, Maillard E, Thomas P-A, Meunier B, et al. Surgery alone versus chemoradiotherapy followed by surgery for stage I and II esophageal cancer: final analysis of randomized controlled phase III trial FFCD 9901. J Clin Oncol Off J Am Soc Clin Oncol. 2014;32(23):2416–22.
51. Allum WH, Stenning SP, Bancewicz J, Clark PI, Langley RE. Long-term results of a randomized trial of surgery with or without preoperative chemotherapy in esophageal cancer. J Clin Oncol. 2009;27(30):5062–7.
52. Kelsen DP, Winter KA, Gunderson LL, Mortimer J, Estes NC, Haller DG, et al. Long-term results of RTOG trial 8911 (USA intergroup 113): a random assignment trial comparison of chemotherapy followed by surgery compared with surgery alone for esophageal cancer. J Clin Oncol. 2007;25(24):3719–25.
53. Shapiro J, van Lanschot JJB, Hulshof MCCM, van Hagen P, van Berge Henegouwen MI, Wijnhoven BPL, et al. Neoadjuvant chemoradiotherapy plus surgery versus surgery alone for oesophageal or junctional cancer (CROSS): long-term results of a randomised controlled trial. Lancet Oncol. 2015;16(9):1090–8.
54. Innocente R, Navarria F, Palazzari E, Matrone F, Boz G, Gigante M, et al. Intensified IMRT with concurrent chemotherapy for locally advanced esophageal carcinoma. In Proceeding ESTRO 2018 PO-0777.
55. Canzonieri V, Colarossi C, Del Col L, Perin T, Talamini R, Sigon R, et al. Exocrine and endocrine modulation in common gastric carcinoma. Am J Clin Pathol. 2012;137(5):712–21.
56. Takenaka Y, Tsukamoto T, Mizoshita T, Ogasawara N, Hirano N, Otsuka T, et al. Gastric and intestinal phenotypic correlation between exocrine and endocrine components in human stomach tumors. Histol Histopathol. 2007;22(3):273–84.
57. Jiang S-X, Mikami T, Umezawa A, Saegusa M, Kameya T, Okayasu I. Gastric large cell neuroendocrine carcinomas: a distinct clinicopathologic entity. Am J Surg Pathol. 2006;30(8):945–53.
58. Cancer Genome Atlas Research Network. Comprehensive molecular characterization of gastric adenocarcinoma. Nature. 2014;513(7517):202–9.
59. Shah MA, Khanin R, Tang L, Janjigian YY, Klimstra DS, Gerdes H, et al. Molecular classification of gastric cancer: a new paradigm. Clin Cancer Res. 2011;17(9):2693–701.
60. Caggiari L, Miolo G, Canzonieri V, De Zorzi M, Alessandrini L, Corona G, et al. A new mutation of the CDH1 gene in a patient with an aggressive signet-ring cell carcinoma of the stomach. Cancer Biol Ther. 2018;19(4):254–9.

Surgical Strategies in Gastric Cancer

9

Claudio Belluco, Matteo Olivieri, Andrea Lauretta, Danilo Antona, Antonino De Paoli, Federico Navarria, Angela Buonadonna, Michela Guardascione, Renato Cannizzaro, Vincenzo Canzonieri, and Giulio Bertola

Introduction

Surgical resection is the principal therapy for gastric cancer, as it offers the only potential for cure. Moreover, in the era of multimodality treatment, surgery plays a central role in the management of gastric cancer including staging evaluation, curative treatment, and when necessary palliation.

C. Belluco (✉) · M. Olivieri · A. Lauretta
D. Antona · G. Bertola
Surgical Oncology Department, IRCCS, CRO Aviano, National Cancer Institute, Aviano, PN, Italy
e-mail: cbelluco@cro.it

A. De Paoli · F. Navarria
Radiation Oncology Department, IRCCS, CRO Aviano, National Cancer Institute, Aviano, PN, Italy

A. Buonadonna · M. Guardascione
Medical Oncology Department, IRCCS, CRO Aviano, National Cancer Institute, Aviano, PN, Italy

R. Cannizzaro
Oncological Gastroenterology Department, IRCCS, CRO Aviano, National Cancer Institute, Aviano, PN, Italy

V. Canzonieri
Pathology Department, IRCCS, CRO Aviano, National Cancer Institute, Aviano, PN, Italy

Department of Medical, Surgical and Health Sciences, University of Trieste, Trieste, Italy

CRO Biobank, IRCCS, CRO Aviano, National Cancer Institute, Aviano, Italy

Department of Biology, Temple University, Philadelphia, PA, USA

Staging

In patients with gastric cancer, accurate staging is of main importance in order to plan optimal treatment strategies. Peritoneal carcinomatosis is one of the most frequently observed incurable factors in patients with gastric cancer. The prognosis of patients with peritoneal dissemination is dismal, and chemotherapy is indicated as first option. Peritoneal metastases are documented in up to one third of patients with previous negative staging abdominal CT scan. Staging laparoscopy allows for better definition of peritoneal spreading status by means of direct visualization, biopsy, and peritoneal washing cytology. Current indications for staging laparoscopy vary according to different societies' recommendations ranging from patients with cT3–cT4 tumors without evidence of lymph node or distant metastasis on CT scan to all patients with resectable gastric cancer [1–4]. Since chemotherapy and chemoradiotherapy regimens and indications depend on metastatic status, our indications for staging laparoscopy comprise all cases at risk of peritoneal spread including patients with doubtful cT2 tumors on endoscopic ultrasound and patients with cT3–cT4 N−/+ without evidence of peritoneal and distant metastasis on abdominal CT scan. In clear cT1–cT2 tumors on endoscopic ultrasound, we consider laparoscopy as initial procedure at the time of resective surgery in order to rule out peritoneal involvement, in which cases

© Springer Nature Switzerland AG 2019

V. Canzonieri, A. Giordano (eds.), *Gastric Cancer In The Precision Medicine Era*,
Current Clinical Pathology, https://doi.org/10.1007/978-3-030-04861-7_9

gastric resection is postponed to neoadjuvant treatment and restaging.

During staging laparoscopy peritoneal washing for cytology evaluation is also recommended. Since patients with positive peritoneal cytology are at high risk of peritoneal failure and oncologic outcome is poor when gastrectomy is performed as first step, neoadjuvant treatment and subsequent restaging are recommended in these patients [5].

Moreover, in patients with positive peritoneal cytology without the presence of peritoneal carcinomatosis, hyperthermic intraperitoneal chemotherapy (HIPEC) appears to increase overall survival rates. However, the efficacy of HIPEC as part of multimodality treatment approach in patients with gastric cancer should be tested in randomized clinical trials. HIPEC-related systemic drug toxicity should also be considered [6, 7].

Curative Treatment

The ultimate goal of gastric cancer treatment is radical surgical resection which offers the best chances for long-term survival. The extent of stomach resection and lymph node dissection are the two main issues to be considered when planning radical surgery for gastric cancer. Since macroscopically (R2) and microscopically (R1) positive resection margins are negative prognostic factors, the type of surgical procedure (total gastrectomy vs. partial gastrectomy) is determined by the site of the primary tumor in relation to the extent of free gross resection margins required to minimize the risk of positive microscopic resection margins. Depending on different guidelines, gross margin of resection is considered to be adequate which varies from 4 to 5 cm. Moreover, due to its more aggressive behavior, a wider free gross resection margin up to 8 cm has been suggested in cases with diffuse histologic tumor type. However, this implies a total gastrectomy for most of the patients with diffuse-type tumors [3, 8]. Intraoperative frozen section for resection margin evaluation is recommended; however conversion into a more extensive procedure (subtotal to total gastrectomy or from total gastrectomy to gastroesophagectomy) should be balanced with the stage of disease, the potential increased morbidity to the patient, and the potential oncologic benefit [9].

The extent and number of lymph node dissection during gastric resection procedures has both staging and curative implications. The *AJCC Cancer Staging Manual*, 8th edition, recommends that at least 16 regional nodes be assessed pathologically but that removal/evaluation of 30 or more nodes is desirable [10]. Adequate number of examined lymph nodes is important since it minimizes stage migration allowing for more precise staging and consequently better prognostic assessment [11]. The recommended extent of lymph node dissection is D2 lymphadenectomy (Fig. 9.1) which is an extended lymph node dissection, entailing removal of nodes along the hepatic, left gastric, celiac, and splenic arteries, as well as those in the splenic hilum (stations 1–12a). Moderate evidences based on a recent Cochrane meta-analysis including five randomized trials of D1 versus D2 dissection, comprising the 15-year follow-up data of the Dutch trial indicate that there is a significant difference favoring D2 lymphadenectomy in disease-specific survival, but not in overall survival or disease-free survival. Moreover, data suggested no significant difference in OS between more extended lymph node dissection (D3 lymphadenectomy) and D2 lymphadenectomy [12, 13].

Moreover, in spite of most studies reporting higher postoperative morbidity and mortality rate with D2 lymphadenectomy (especially if splenectomy is performed), it has been demonstrated that D2 dissection can be done with low operative mortality, similar to that of a D1 dissection [14].

Laparoscopic total and distal gastrectomy for gastric cancer has been demonstrated to be technically feasible and to result in lower complication rate compared to open surgery. Moreover, D2 lymphadenectomy can be equally obtained using laparoscopy. However, while in stage I gastric cancer oncologic outcome has been reported to be comparable between open and laparoscopic surgery, long-term oncologic data from prospective randomized trials in more advanced stages are not yet available [15–17].

At initial staging, unresectability criteria for gastric cancer are the presence of distant metastases, invasion of a major vascular structure, such

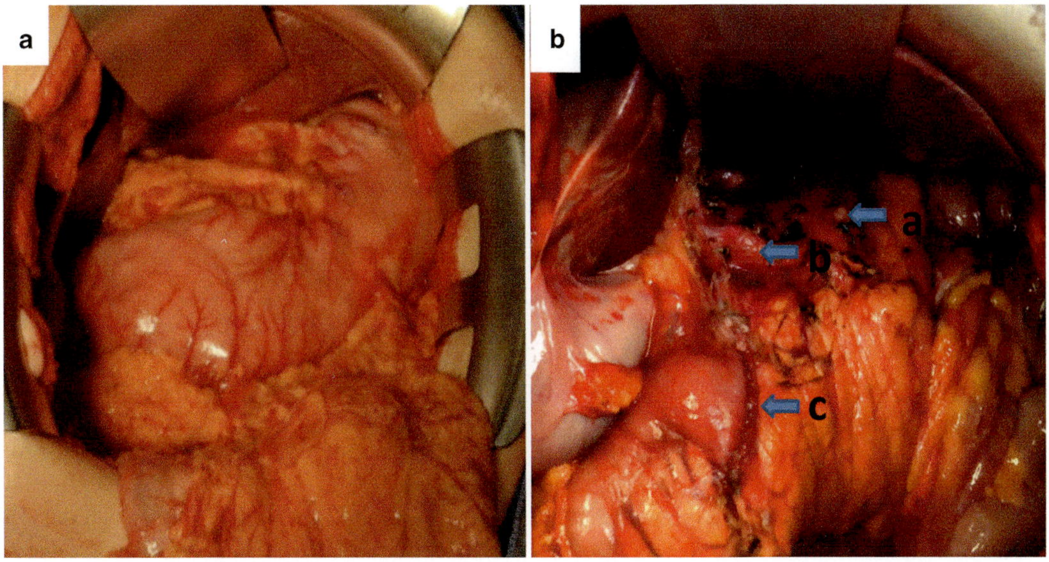

Fig. 9.1 (**a**, **b**) Adenocarcinoma of the greater curvature: (**a**) operative findings at laparotomy and (**b**) after total gastrectomy and lymphadenectomy (**a**) sectioned left gastric artery, (**b**) common hepatic artery, (**c**) duodenal stump

as the aorta, hepatic artery, or celiac axis. Conversion preoperative multimodality treatment including chemoradiotherapy with or without induction chemotherapy has been proposed for patients with locally advanced, initially unresectable, but nonmetastatic gastric cancer. Using this approach, potentially curative resectability rate as high as 70% has been reported with pathological complete response rates ranging from 5% to 30%. In these patients, one noncurative factor at initial diagnosis, complete pathological response, and R0 resection are all associated with favorable oncologic outcome. Therefore, initial staging, clinical evaluation after treatment, and extent of surgery aiming at curative resection are crucial for maximizing conversion treatment efficacy. In order to be adopted as a standard, this approach needs to be prospectively validated in clinical trials [18–21].

Gastric cancer presenting with a linitis plastica pattern (about 5% of all gastric cancer cases) is usually associated with diffuse histologic tumor type, peritoneal and distant metastasis, and a poor oncologic outcome. However, in the subset of nonmetastatic patients with linitis plastica amenable of radical resection, long-term survival rate similar to that of patients without linitis plastica has been reported. Therefore, optimal management of patients with linitis plastica should include accurate staging, neoadjuvant treatment, accurate restaging including laparoscopy, and intraoperative frozen section-guided radical surgery for achieving negative resection margins along with adequate lymphadenectomy [22, 23].

Liver Metastasis

Gastric cancer patients develop synchronous or metachronous liver metastasis in 5–14% of cases [24–28]. This disease has a dismal prognosis, and the median survival of patients with metastatic gastric cancer is approximately 6 months even with palliative chemotherapy [27, 29]. The role of surgical approach and hepatic metastases resection is controversial with some studies showing a doubtful effect on survival, while others reporting an improved outcome [30–39]. Rarely hepatic lesions are isolated, while in approximately 40% of cases, they are associated with peritoneal or extensive lymph node disease. The average survival following liver resection for metastasis from gastric cancer varies widely between 15% and 77% at 1 year and between 0% and 38% at 5 years with a median survival time of 5–31 months [25, 26, 28, 30, 35, 36, 38, 39]. Survival is significantly higher in case of single metastasis compared to multiple lesions and in metachronous compared to synchronous metastasis [25, 26, 39]. Therefore, in highly selected cases of single metachronous gastric cancer, liver metastasis, metastasectomy, or ablative procedures may be considered.

Palliative Treatment

Most patients with gastric cancer at the time of diagnosis are not amenable of surgical treatment with curative intent, and many of them will require a palliative treatment during the course of the disease. The role of palliative surgery resection is very questionable. Systemic chemotherapy is the treatment of choice for patients with not resectable gastric cancer, and it has been proven that it improves both quality of life and survival providing a median survival of approximately 10 months [40, 41]. Unfortunately, chemotherapy is not equally effective in palliation of symptoms and complications such as vomiting, pain, occlusion, bleeding, and perforation. Patients with unresectable locally advanced gastric cancer or metastatic gastric cancer require a multidisciplinary approach that includes radiotherapy and endoscopic and surgical techniques such as palliative resection and gastrojejunostomy. External beam radiotherapy (RT) has a clearly defined role in controlling pain, bleeding, and occlusion in patients affected by unresectable localized gastric neoplasia [42–44]. There are no controlled studies comparing the RT with endoscopy or surgery, but in case of gastric outlet obstruction, the response to radiotherapy is not immediate as in the case of endoscopic stenting or palliative surgery. Furthermore, the required dose for the treatment of occlusive status is greater than 40 Gy and is normally associated with more side effects [44]. Endoscopic stenting is an excellent alternative for the treatment of obstruction. A systematic review has shown that endoscopic stent has the same effectiveness of palliative gastrojejunostomy but is associated with reduced hospitalization and a faster relief of obstructive symptoms [45]. On the other hand, patients undergoing endoscopic treatment require more often reintervention than patients undergoing palliative bypass surgery. Finally, endoscopy with laser photocoagulation or with application of a hemostatic nanopowder (Hemospray) remains the established treatment of bleeding control in the first instance [46, 47].

In patients with locally advanced or metastatic gastric cancer, the role of palliative resection remains controversial. A French retrospective survey has identified four predictive factors of survival in these patients: the ASA score (I or II), incomplete resection without metastasis or carcinomatosis, single-site solid organ metastasis without peritoneal carcinomatosis, and localized carcinomatosis without signet ring cells without histology. Palliative surgery should not be supported in case of high-risk patients (ASA III or IV) or in case of diffuse carcinomatosis or solid organ metastasis associated with carcinomatosis or finally limited carcinomatosis but signet ring cell histology [48]. In the phase III REGATTA trial, 176 patients with locally advanced gastric cancer associated with hepatic lesion or peritoneal lesion or para-aortic lymphadenopathy were randomized to chemotherapy alone or gastrectomy followed by chemotherapy. The overall survival was not significantly improved by surgery, and the study was closed after an interim analysis. The 2-year survival with chemotherapy alone was 32% while with surgery followed by chemotherapy 25%. Moreover chemotherapy following gastrectomy was associated with a greater incidence of adverse events such as leukopenia and hyponatremia [49]. Palliative laparoscopic or open gastrojejunostomy is indicated in case of gastric cancer associated with obstruction; however it is indicated only in those cases where endoscopy or radiotherapy is not possible [50]. In conclusion, the impact of palliative surgery on symptomatic relief and survival should be balanced with morbidity and mortality. Patient and tumor characteristics should be considered in order to select the optimal candidate. However, both palliative gastrectomy and gastrojejunostomy are not recommended in most of the cases.

References

1. Board of Governors of the Society of American Gastrointestinal and Endoscopic Surgeons (SAGES), 2010. https://www.sages.org/publications/guidelines/guidelines-for-diagnostic-laparoscopy/.
2. Smyth EC, Verheij M, Allum W, Cunningham D, Cervantes A, Arnold D, ESMO Guidelines Committee. Gastric cancer: ESMO clinical practice

guidelines for diagnosis, treatment and follow-up. Ann Oncol. 2016;27:v38–49.
3. National Comprehensive Cancer Network (NCCN). *NCCN Clinical Practice Guidelines in Oncology*. Gastric Cancer (Version 1.2018). http://www.nccn.org/professionals/physician_gls/pdf/gastric.pdf. Accessed on May 2018.
4. De Manzoni G, Marrelli D, Baiocchi GL, et al. The Italian Research Group for Gastric Cancer (GIRCG) guidelines for gastric cancer staging and treatment: 2015. Gastric Cancer. 2017;20:20–30.
5. Japanese Gastric Cancer Association. Japanese gastric cancer treatment guidelines 2014 (ver. 4). Gastric Cancer. 2017;20(1):1–19. https://doi.org/10.1007/s10120-016-0622-4.
6. De Andrade JP, Mezhir JJ. The critical role of peritoneal cytology in the staging of gastric cancer: an evidence-based review. J Surg Oncol. 2014;110(3):291–7. https://doi.org/10.1002/jso.23632. Epub 2014 May 22. Review. PubMed PMID: 24850538.
7. Desiderio J, Chao J, Melstrom L, et al. The 30-year experience-a meta-analysis of randomised and high-quality non-randomised studies of hyperthermic intraperitoneal chemotherapy in the treatment of gastric cancer. Eur J Cancer. 2017;79:1–14. https://doi.org/10.1016/j.ejca.2017.03.030. Epub 2017 Apr 26. Review. PubMed PMID: 28456089; PubMed Central PMCID: PMC5568419.
8. Smyth EC, Verheij M, Allum W, Cunningham D, Cervantes A, Arnold D, ESMO Guidelines Committee. Gastric cancer: ESMO clinical practice guidelines for diagnosis, treatment and follow-up. Ann Oncol. 2016;27(suppl 5):v38–49. PubMed PMID: 27664260.
9. Postlewait LM, Maithel SK. The importance of surgical margins in gastric cancer. J Surg Oncol. 2016;113(3):277–82. https://doi.org/10.1002/jso.24110. Epub 2015 Dec 10. Review. PubMed PMID: 26662226.
10. Ajani JA, In H, Sano T, et al. Stomach. In: Amin MB, editor. AJCC cancer staging manual. 8th ed. Chicago: AJCC; 2017. p. 203.
11. de Manzoni G, Verlato G, Roviello F, et al. The new TNM classification of lymph node metastasis minimises stage migration problems in gastric cancer patients. Br J Cancer. 2002;87:171.
12. Songun I, Putter H, Kranenbarg EM, Sasako M, van de Velde CJ. Surgical treatment of gastric cancer: 15-year follow-up results of the randomized nationwide Dutch D1D2 trial. Lancet Oncol. 2010;11(5):439–49. https://doi.org/10.1016/S1470-2045(10)70070-X. Epub 2010 Apr 19. PubMed PMID: 20409751.
13. Mocellin S, McCulloch P, Kazi H, Gama-Rodrigues JJ, Yuan Y, Nitti D. Extent of lymph node dissection for adenocarcinoma of the stomach. Cochrane Database Syst Rev. 2015;8:CD001964. https://doi.org/10.1002/14651858.CD001964.pub4. Review. PubMed PMID: 26267122.
14. Hanna GB, Boshier PR, Knaggs A, Goldin R, Sasako M. Improving outcomes after gastroesophageal cancer resection: can Japanese results be reproduced in Western centers? Arch Surg. 2012;147(8):738–45. https://doi.org/10.1001/archsurg.2012.983. PubMed PMID: 22911070.
15. Kim W, Kim HH, Han SU, Kim MC, Hyung WJ, Ryu SW, Cho GS, Kim CY, Yang HK, Park DJ, Song KY, Lee SI, Ryu SY, Lee JH, Lee HJ, Korean Laparo-endoscopic Gastrointestinal Surgery Study (KLASS) Group. Decreased morbidity of laparoscopic distal gastrectomy compared with open distal gastrectomy for stage I gastric cancer: short-term outcomes from a multicenter randomized controlled trial (KLASS-01). Ann Surg. 2016;263(1):28–35. https://doi.org/10.1097/SLA.0000000000001346. PubMed PMID: 26352529.
16. Shi Y, Xu X, Zhao Y, Qian F, Tang B, Hao Y, Luo H, Chen J, Yu P. Short-term surgical outcomes of a randomized controlled trial comparing laparoscopic versus open gastrectomy with D2 lymph node dissection for advanced gastric cancer. Surg Endosc. 2018;32(5):2427–33. https://doi.org/10.1007/s00464-017-5942-x. Epub 2017 Dec 12. PubMed PMID: 29234941.
17. Hu Y, Huang C, Sun Y, Su X, Cao H, Hu J, Xue Y, Suo J, Tao K, He X, Wei H, Ying M, Hu W, Du X, Chen P, Liu H, Zheng C, Liu F, Yu J, Li Z, Zhao G, Chen X, Wang K, Li P, Xing J, Li G. Morbidity and mortality of laparoscopic versus open D2 distal gastrectomy for advanced gastric cancer: a randomized controlled trial. J Clin Oncol. 2016;34(12):1350–7. https://doi.org/10.1200/JCO.2015.63.7215. Epub 2016 Feb 22. PubMed PMID: 26903580.
18. Fukuchi M, Ishiguro T, Ogata K, Suzuki O, Kumagai Y, Ishibashi K, Ishida H, Kuwano H, Mochiki E. Prognostic role of conversion surgery for unresectable gastric cancer. Ann Surg Oncol. 2015;22(11):3618–24. https://doi.org/10.1245/s10434-015-4422-6. Epub 2015 Feb 7. PubMed PMID: 25663597.
19. Cho H, Nakamura J, Asaumi Y, Yabusaki H, Sakon M, Takasu N, Kobayashi T, Aoki T, Shiraishi O, Kishimoto H, Nunobe S, Yanagisawa S, Suda T, Ueshima S, Matono S, Maruyama H, Tatsumi M, Seya T, Tanizawa Y, Yoshikawa T. Long-term survival outcomes of advanced gastric cancer patients who achieved a pathological complete response with neoadjuvant chemotherapy: a systematic review of the literature. Ann Surg Oncol. 2015;22(3):787–92. https://doi.org/10.1245/s10434-014-4084-9. Epub 2014 Sep 16. Review. PubMed PMID: 25223927.
20. Tomasello G, Petrelli F, Ghidini M, Pezzica E, Passalacqua R, Steccanella F, Turati L, Sgroi G, Barni S. Tumor regression grade and survival after neoadjuvant treatment in gastro-esophageal cancer: a meta-analysis of 17 published studies. Eur J Surg Oncol. 2017;43(9):1607–16. https://doi.org/10.1016/j.ejso.2017.03.001. Epub 2017 Mar 18. Review. PubMed PMID: 28347525.
21. Li Z, Shan F, Wang Y, Zhang Y, Zhang L, Li S, Jia Y, Xue K, Miao R, Li Z, Ji J. Correlation of pathological complete response with survival after neoadjuvant chemotherapy in gastric or gastroesophageal junction cancer treated with radical surgery: a meta-analysis. PLoS One. 2018;13(1):e0189294. https://doi.org/10.1371/journal.pone.0189294. eCollection 2018. PubMed PMID: 29370182; PubMed Central PMCID: PMC5784899.

22. Blackham AU, Swords DS, Levine EA, Fino NF, Squires MH, Poultsides G, Fields RC, Bloomston M, Weber SM, Pawlik TM, Jin LX, Spolverato G, Schmidt C, Worhunsky D, Cho CS, Maithel SK, Votanopoulos KI. Is linitis plastica a contraindication for surgical resection: a multi-institution study of the U.S. gastric cancer collaborative. Ann Surg Oncol. 2016;23(4):1203–11. https://doi.org/10.1245/s10434-015-4947-8. Epub 2015 Nov 3. PubMed PMID: 26530447; PubMed Central PMCID: PMC4980579.
23. Chang JM, Lara KA, Gray RJ, Pockaj BA, Wasif N. Clinical outcomes after surgery for linitis plastica of the stomach: analysis of a population cancer registry. Am Surg. 2017;83(1):23–9. PubMed PMID: 28234115.
24. Marrelli D, Roviello F, De Stefano A, et al. Risk factors for liver metastases after curative surgical procedures for gastric cancer: a prospective study of 208 patients treated with surgical resection. J Am Coll Surg. 2004;198:51–8.
25. Okano K, Maeba T, Ishimura K, et al. Hepatic resection for metastatic tumors from gastric cancer. Ann Surg. 2002;235:86–91.
26. Sakamoto Y, Ohyama S, Yamamoto J, et al. Surgical resection of liver metastases of gastric cancer: an analysis of a 17-year experience with 22 patients. Surgery. 2003;133:507–11.
27. Zacherl J, Zacherl M, Scheuba C, et al. Analysis of hepatic resection of metastasis originating from gastric adenocarcinoma. J Gastrointest Surg. 2002;6:682–9.
28. Sakamoto Y, Sano T, Shimada K, et al. Favorable indications for hepatectomy in patients with liver metastasis from gastric cancer. J Surg Oncol. 2007;95:534–9.
29. Takahashi I, Kakeji Y, Emi Y, et al. S-1 in the treatment of advanced and recurrent gastric cancer: current state and future prospects. Gastric Cancer. 2003;6(Suppl 1):28–33.
30. Elias D, Cavalcanti de Albuquerque A, Eggenspieler P, et al. Resection of liver metastases from a non-colorectal primary: indications and results based on 147 monocentric patients. J Am Coll Surg. 1998;187:487–93.
31. Harrison LE, Brennan MF, Newman E, et al. Hepatic resection for non-colorectal, non-neuroendocrine metastases: a fifteen-year experience with ninety-six patients. Surgery. 1997;121:625–32.
32. Hirai I, Kimura W, Fuse A, et al. Surgical management for metastatic liver tumors. Hepatogastroenterology. 2006;53:757–63.
33. Ambiru S, Miyazaki M, Ito H, et al. Benefits and limits of hepatic resection for gastric metastases. Am J Surg. 2001;181:279–83.
34. Bines SD, England G, Deziel DJ, et al. Synchronous, metachronous, and multiple hepatic resections of liver tumors originating from primary gastric tumors. Surgery. 1993;114:799–805; discussion 804–795.
35. Miyazaki M, Itoh H, Nakagawa K, et al. Hepatic resection of liver metastases from gastric carcinoma. Am J Gastroenterol. 1997;92:490–3.
36. Ochiai T, Sasako M, Mizuno S, et al. Hepatic resection for metastatic tumours from gastric cancer: analysis of prognostic factors. Br J Surg. 1994;81:1175–8.
37. Saiura A, Umekita N, Inoue S, et al. Clinicopathological features and outcome of hepatic resection for liver metastasis from gastric cancer. Hepatogastroenterology. 2002;49:1062–5.
38. Shirabe K, Shimada M, Matsumata T, et al. Analysis of the prognostic factors for liver metastasis of gastric cancer after hepatic resection: a multi-institutional study of the indications for resection. Hepatogastroenterology. 2003;50:1560–3.
39. Cheon SH, Rha SY, Jeung HC, Im CK, Kim SH, Kim HR, Ahn JB, Roh JK, Noh SH, Chung HC. Survival benefit of combined curative resection of the stomach (D2 resection) and liver in gastric cancer patients with liver metastases. Ann Oncol. 2008;19(6):1146–53.
40. Catalano V, Labianca R, Beretta GD, Gatta G, de Braud F, Van Cutsem E. Gastric Cancer. Crit Rev Oncol Hematol. 2009;71:127–64.
41. Wagner AD, Unverzagt S, Grothe W, et al. Chemotherapy for advanced gastric cancer. Cochrane Database Syst Rev. 2010;3:CD004064.
42. Tey J, Back MF, Shakespeare TP, et al. The role of palliative radiation therapy in symptomatic locally advanced gastric cancer. Int J Radiat Oncol Biol Phys. 2007;67:385.
43. Harvey JA, Bessell JR, Beller E, et al. Chemoradiation therapy is effective for the palliative treatment of malignant dysphagia. Dis Esophagus. 2004;17:260.
44. Tey J, Choo BA, Leong CN, et al. Clinical outcome of palliative radiotherapy for locally advanced symptomatic gastric cancer in the modern era. Medicine (Baltimore). 2014;93:e118.
45. Jeurnink SM, van Eijck CH, Steyerberg EW, et al. Stent versus gastrojejunostomy for the palliation of gastric outlet obstruction: a systematic review. BMC Gastroenterol. 2007;7:18.
46. Barr H, Krasner N. Interstitial laser photocoagulation for treating bleeding gastric cancer. BMJ. 1989;299:659.
47. Pittayanon R, Rerknimitr R, Barkun A. Prognostic factors affecting outcomes in patients with malignant GI bleeding treated with a novel endoscopically delivered hemostatic powder. Gastrointest Endosc. 2018;87:994.
48. Mariette C, Bruyère E, Messager M, et al. Palliative resection for advanced gastric and junctional adenocarcinoma: which patients will benefit from surgery? Ann Surg Oncol. 2013;20:1240.
49. Fujitani K, Yang HK, Mizusawa J, et al. Gastrectomy plus chemotherapy versus chemotherapy alone for advanced gastric cancer with a single non-curable factor (REGATTA): a phase 3, randomised controlled trial. Lancet Oncol. 2016;17:309.
50. Takeno A, Takiguchi S, Fujita J, et al. Clinical outcome and indications for palliative gastrojejunostomy in unresectable advanced gastric cancer: multi-institutional retrospective analysis. Ann Surg Oncol. 2013;20:3527.

Part IV

Evolving Treatment Landscape in Gastric Cancer

From Molecular Classification to Targeted Therapy for Gastric Cancer in the Precision Medicine Era

10

Lara Alessandrini, Melissa Manchi, Fabrizio Italia, Tiziana Perin, and Vincenzo Canzonieri

Introduction

Gastric cancer (GC) is a common malignant neoplasm worldwide and one of the main causes of cancer-related deaths [1]. Despite some advances in therapies for GC, the long-term survival of patients with advanced disease remains poor. Historically, different types of classification have been used to stratify patients with GC for shaping the prognosis and treatment planning: anatomical classification (Borrmann classification and Siewert and Stein classification) [2, 3], histological classification (WHO classification and Lauren's classification) [4] and extent of disease (early gastric cancer vs advanced cancer) [5, 6]. More recently, the clinical impact of conceiving GC heterogeneity at diagnosis rather than a single disease has become evident. Therefore, based on new knowledge of molecular pathways associated with different aspects of GC, new pathogenetic classifications for GC have been and continue to be proposed. An improvement in the prognostic classification for GC is essential to develop a proper therapy for a selected patient population. The aim of this chapter is to discuss the state of the art on combining histological and molecular classifications of GC to provide an overview of the emerging therapeutic possibilities connected to the latest discoveries regarding GC.

L. Alessandrini
Pathology Department, IRCCS, CRO Aviano, National Cancer Institute, Aviano, PN, Italy

Department of Medicine (DIMED), Surgical Pathology & Cytopathology Unit, University Hospital of Padova, Padova, Italy

M. Manchi
Pathology Department, IRCCS, CRO Aviano, National Cancer Institute, Aviano, PN, Italy

F. Italia
Oncopath Lab, Floridia, SR, Italy

T. Perin
Pathology Department, IRCCS, CRO Aviano, National Cancer Institute, Aviano, PN, Italy

CRO Biobank, IRCCS, CRO Aviano, National Cancer Institute, Aviano, PN, Italy

V. Canzonieri (✉)
Pathology Department, IRCCS, CRO Aviano, National Cancer Institute, Aviano, PN, Italy

Department of Medical, Surgical and Health Sciences, University of Trieste, Trieste, Italy

CRO Biobank, IRCCS, CRO Aviano, National Cancer Institute, Aviano, PN, Italy

Department of Biology, Temple University, Philadelphia, PA, USA
e-mail: vcanzonieri@cro.it

Development of Histological and Molecular Classifications of GC

Tan et al. [7], based on the genomic signature found in GC cell lines and patient tissues, classified GC into two major subtypes that overlapped with the histological Lauren classification. The G-INT subtype is related with intestinal histology, and the G-DIF is related to diffuse histology.

© Springer Nature Switzerland AG 2019
V. Canzonieri, A. Giordano (eds.), *Gastric Cancer In The Precision Medicine Era*, Current Clinical Pathology, https://doi.org/10.1007/978-3-030-04861-7_10

G-INT is characterized by the deregulation of genes associated with carbohydrate metabolism. Accordingly, the FUT2 gene encoding the galactoside 2-alpha-L-fucosyltransferase 2 enzyme affects the Lewis blood group involved in *H. pylori* infection, the LGALS4 gene encoding galectin 4 is implicated in the interaction between cell-cell and cell-matrix and the peptide transporter cadherin-17 is encoded by the CDH17 gene.

G-DIF exhibits deregulation of genes related to high cell proliferation and a high energy requirement. The AURKB gene encoding Aurora B kinase, which functions in the attachment of the mitotic spindle to the centromere, and the ELOVL5 gene, encoding elongation of very long-chain fatty acid protein 5, are examples of alterations in G-DIF. Tumours of the G-DIF type show a poor prognosis and a reduced response to chemotherapy compared with those of the G-INT type. Moreover, in vitro cell lines from the G-INT tumour type are more sensitive to 5-FU and oxaliplatin, while G-DIF tumours are more sensitive to cisplatin [7, 8].

Subsequently, in 2013, Singapore researchers categorized GC into three main types based on their genomic profiles [9]:

1. A profile characterized by a high proliferating number of cells with high genomic instability and *TP53* gene mutation
2. A metabolic profile associated with higher anaerobic glycolysis instead of mitochondrial oxidative phosphorylation to generate the energy (a phenomenon known as the "Warburg effect") and resulting in tumour cells more sensitive to 5-FU therapy
3. A mesenchymal stem cell profile with a high capacity for self-renewal, immunomodulation and tissue regeneration showing a sensitivity to PIK3CA-mTOR pathway inhibitors

Thereafter, The Cancer Genome Atlas (TCGA) research group, comprising mainly of Western Europe and US members, introduced the new technologies of large-scale genome sequencing analyses (i.e. copy number variation (CNV), exome sequencing, DNA methylation profile, mRNA and micro-RNA sequencing) to further classify GC into four main groups [10] (Fig. 10.1):

I. Epstein-Barr virus (EBV)-positive cancers (9% of all GC) characterized by DNA hypermethylation, a high frequency of PIK3CA mutations and PDL1/PDL2 overexpression

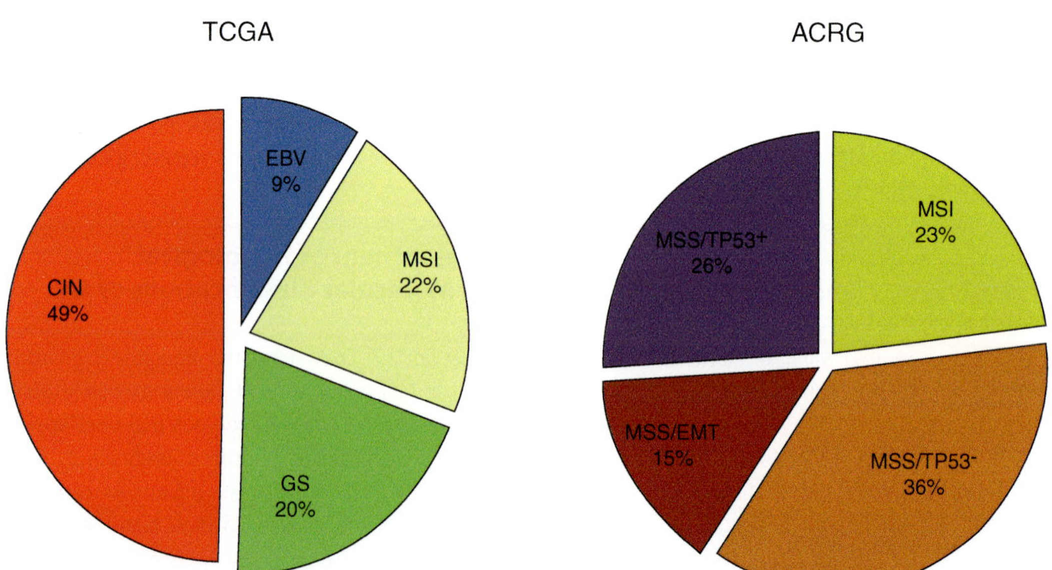

Fig. 10.1 Comparison of the different frequency rates of the molecular subtypes in TCGA and ACGR classifications

II. Microsatellite unstable tumours (MSI, 22%) showing a very high number of mutations and DNA methylation sites
III. Chromosome unstable tumours (CIN, 50%) mainly encoding alterations in tyrosine kinase receptors
IV. Genome stable tumours (GS, 20%)

In 2015, using similar approaches, the Asian Cancer Research Group (ACRG) also proposed a molecular classification for GC comprising four groups [11] (Fig. 10.1). They also proposed an MSI group (22.7%) but divided the remaining tumours based on the evidence of epithelial-mesenchymal transition (EMT) and p53 mutations (15.3% MSS/EMT microsatellite stable and EMT-associated tumours, 26.3% MSS/TP53+ active/intact and 35.7% MSS/TP53- inactive/altered tumours). Using these analyses, the MSI subtype had the best prognosis, while the MSS/EMT subtype had the worst. The former occurred predominantly at an early stage in the distal part of the stomach, showing mainly an intestinal histology (according to Lauren classification); the latter occurred at an advanced stage, at a younger age and with diffuse histology (>80%) and seeding in the peritonea with malignant ascites (64.1%) and had a frequency of 15–24% in the other subtypes. By contrast, liver metastasis was dominant in the MSI and MSS/TP53- types (approximately 20%). EBV infection was more frequent in the MSS/TP53 active group.

Similarities and Differences Between TCGA and ACRG Classification

ACRG validated their molecular sub-classification system using TCGA [10] and the Gastric Cancer Project '08 Singapore datasets [11]. The ACRG categories showed a significant overlap with TCGA subtypes: (i) regarding the tumours with an MSI profile, both classifications normally showed deregulation of the KRAS, NRAS and/or MLH1 gene; (ii) the enrichment of tumours with diffuse histology occurred more frequently in both the GS (TCGA) and MSS/EMT (ACRG) subtypes; (iii) both the EBV+ (TCGA) and MSS/P53+ (ACRG) subtypes showed PIK3CA and ARIDIA and rarely P53 mutations; and (iv) P53 mutations were often found in both CIN (TCGA) and MSS/P53- (ACRG) subtypes. However, ACRG did not classify tumours according to EBV status; CDH1 and RHOA mutations were rarely found in ACRG classification.

When the overall survival parameter was compared using TCGA and ACRG subtyping, only ACRG showed a significant association; TCGA classification only confirmed the association between better survival and the MSI subtype [12]. Nonetheless, presently, both TCGA and ACRG classifications raised sufficient potential to be used in clinical practice.

Limits of TCGA and ACRG Classifications

These novel classifications create a new paradigm in the definition of cancer biology and allow the identification of relevant genomic subsets using different techniques such as genomic screening, functional studies and molecular or epigenetic characterization. However, some limitations should also be openly recognized. First, these classifications are based on a highly complex methodology, and currently, they should not be replicated in standard laboratories lacking in the most recent technologies. Attempts towards simplification are ongoing, although the results may not fully capture the underpinning complexity of the disease. Second, these classifications lack prospective validation on a large scale, including patients of different ethnicities and age. Third, the two proposed classifications show more differences than similarities; in particular, they are different in terms of demographics, baseline molecular mechanisms, driver genes and association with prognosis. Moreover, there are notable dissimilarities in the distribution of Lauren's diffuse subtype among the different subgroups. Because different molecular subgroups may be identified across several independent gene expression profile studies, a collaborative international effort is warranted to aggregate a consensus classification. Fourth, the follow-up of included patients is limited, a factor that may decrease their prognostic power, and subgroups were evaluated on resected specimens, with a different prevalence of subgroups among localized, locally advanced and advanced settings. Fifth, both classifications require epithelial cells, but none considers active, non-malignant stromal cells. Not only gene expression profiles derived from stromal tissues may influence the assignment to a specific molecular category, thus creating interpretative challenges [13], but also novel stromal-based distinctive signatures have been proposed and are related to the predominant cancer phenotype [14].

Integrated Molecular Signatures to Discriminate Intestinal and Diffuse Histological GC Subtypes

Previous findings have indicated that diffuse GC and intestinal GC might be two distinct diseases with a different molecular basis, aetiology, epidemiology and response to therapies. Molecular profiling in a recent study based on 300 GC cases identified 40 genes specifically expressed in diffuse or intestinal GC [15]; among them, three genes were independently associated with the patient's prognosis (for diffuse GC, EFEMP1 encoding an extracellular matrix glycoprotein and FRZB encoding a secreted protein involved in the regulation of bone development, which could also influence Wnt/β-catenin signalling; for intestinal GC, KRT23, a member of the keratins, which is responsible for the structural integrity of epithelial cells).

Several gene expression profiles of GC were also analysed, but the prediction accuracy of these methods resulted in lower gene signatures [16]. In the last year, a 9-gene signature including two negative impact factors (NR1I2 and LGALSL) and seven positive ones (C1ORF198, CST2, LAMP5, FOXS1, CES1P1, MMP7 and COL8A1) was proposed as a potential useful classifier to predict the outcome of GC, and the model clustered patients well into high- and low-risk groups with significant differences in both survival time and reoccurrence [17].

Although molecular characterization studies have attempted to identify prognostic gene signatures in GC, they are inadequate and fail to accurately guide patient therapy. Identifying tumour markers or constructing featured gene models are still the focus of many studies.

TCGA Classification of GC and Related Signalling Pathways Targetable for Precision Therapy

The four molecular subtypes of GC identified by TCGA classification are detailed below (see also Fig. 10.2), along with potential targetable pathways for precision therapy (Fig. 10.3).

EBV-Related GC

The EBV subtype (9% tumours in TCGA) is characterized by a high EBV burden [10]. EBV-positive tumours are more frequently located in the gastric fundus or body, and 81% of cases occur in men. In addition, EBV-positive GC is more prevalent in younger patients than in older subjects (Fig. 10.2). The histology of EBV-related GC is poorly to moderately differentiated adenocarcinoma, often accompanied by dense lymphocytic infiltration [18–21]. Relevant targetable pathways identified in this subtype are related to the elevated expression of programmed death ligands 1 and 2 (PD-L1 and PD-L2), phosphatidylinositol-4,5-bisphosphate 3-kinase, catalytic subunit α (PIK3CA) mutation and Janus kinase 2 (JAK2) amplification.

PD-L1 is a ligand of programmed cell death protein 1 (PD-1), which is expressed on T cells. PD-L1, which is expressed on tumour cells or stromal immune cells, inhibits the activation of cytotoxic T cells through an interaction with PD-1 and helps cancer cells to evade antitumour immunity [22–24]. Because the expression of PD-L1 is observed in many malignant tumours and is associated with a poor prognosis, PD-L1 has been studied extensively as a therapeutic target. Several studies have demonstrated that PD-L1, expressed on cancer cells or tumour-

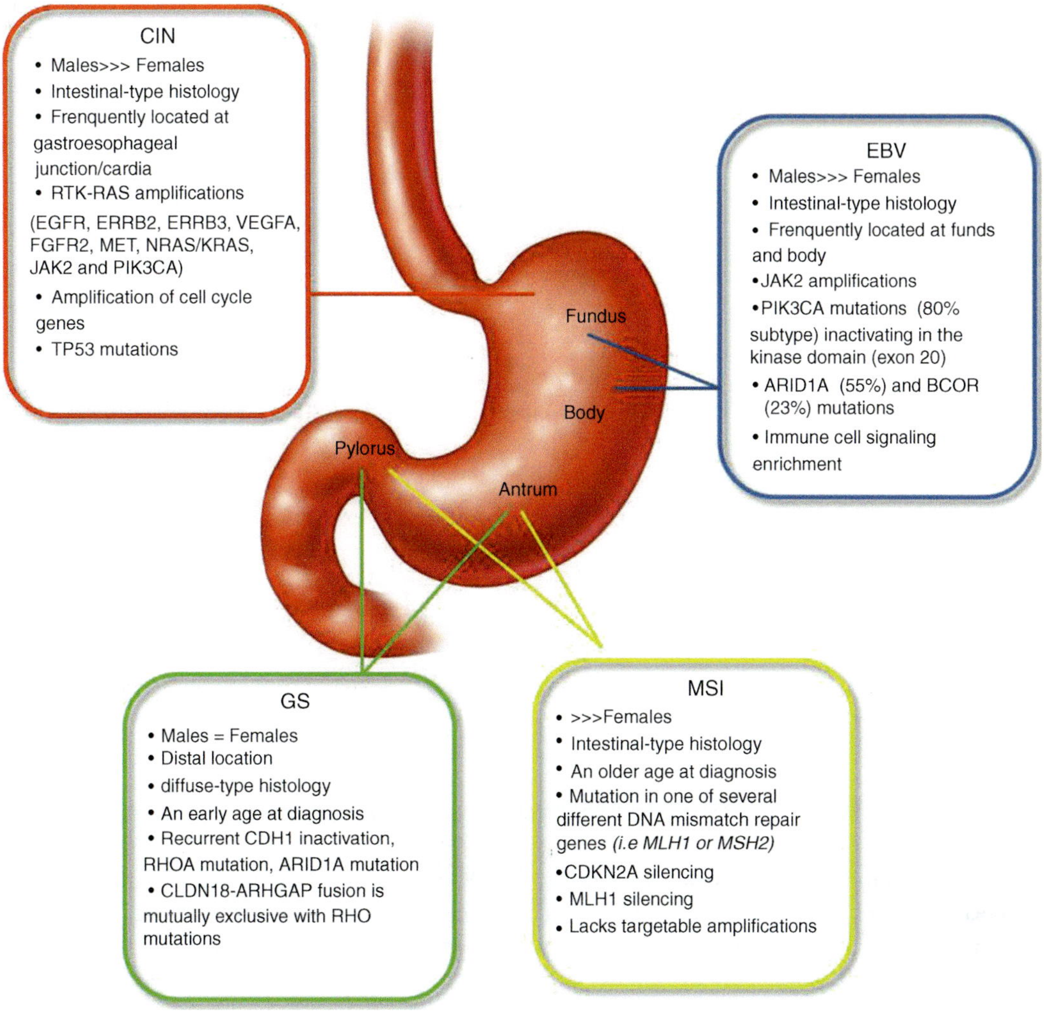

Fig. 10.2 The most relevant clinical-pathological and molecular features of TCGA subtypes

infiltrating immune cells, is a prognostic factor in GC, but the significance of PD-L1 in EBV-related GC has not yet been clarified [25–29]. In a recent study [30], both the expression of PD-L1 in cancer cells and PD-L1+ immune cell infiltration in EBV-related GC were significantly correlated with diffuse histology according to Lauren's classification and tumour invasion (pT1b or more). Therefore, this specific subtype of GC is potentially a good candidate for immunotherapy targeting of the PD-L1/PD-1 axis. Pembrolizumab, a highly selective immunoglobulin G4k humanized monoclonal antibody targeting the PD-1 receptor, demonstrated activity in the phase Ib KEYNOTE-012 trial in a cohort of heavily pretreated Asian and non-Asian patients with GC, with an acceptable toxicity profile [31]. On central review, the overall response rate was 22% [95% confidence interval (CI): 10–39%] with a median duration of response of 24 weeks (range: 8–33 weeks). Because most responses to chemotherapy in GC are short-lived, this is of significant interest. A correlation between PD-L1 expression (defined as PD-L1 ≥1% on archival tissue) and a response was subsequently demonstrated [32]. A double-checkpoint inhibition strategy targeting both the PD-1/PD-L1 and CTLA-4/B7 interactions, which has already

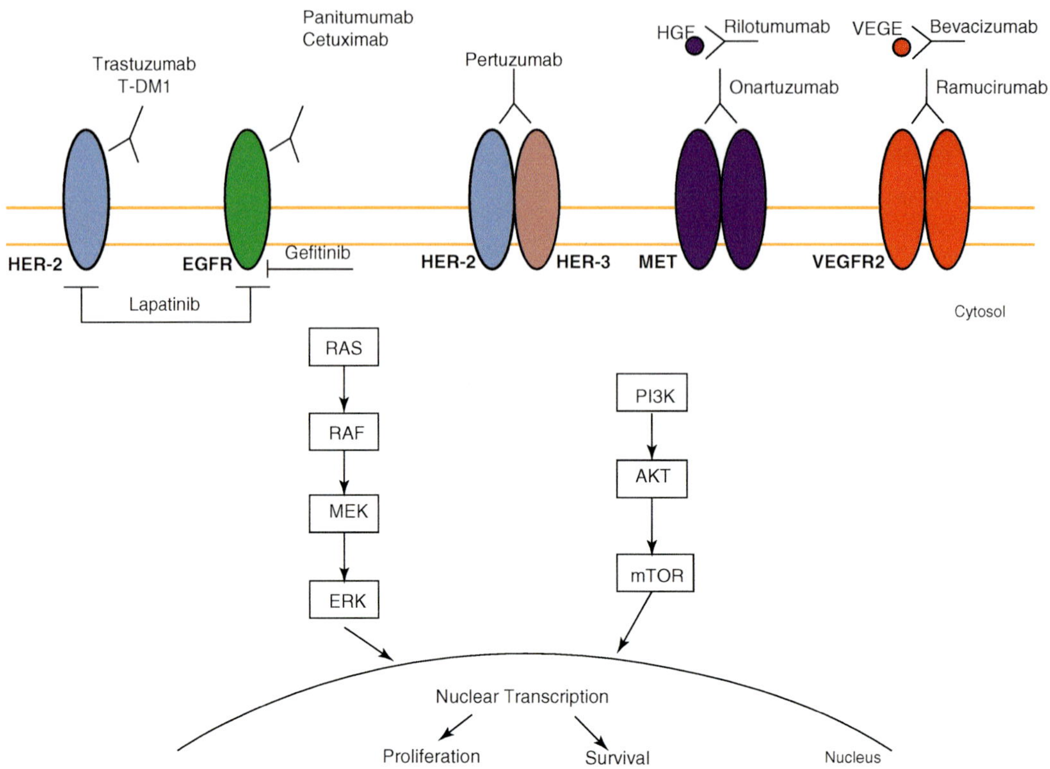

Fig. 10.3 Potential targetable pathways for precision therapy in GC addressed in the review

demonstrated efficacy in patients with melanoma, is under evaluation in several GC trials such as those using nivolumab + ipilimumab [ClinicalTrials.gov identifier: NCI01928394] and MEDI4734 and tremelimumab [ClinicalTrials.gov identifier: NCI02340975] [33].

The PI3K family of intracellular kinases mediates the regulation of cell survival, proliferation, differentiation, migration and metabolism [34]. The PI3K/AKT/mTOR pathway is frequently activated in GC, with the overexpression of *PI3KCA* described in 35–80% of GC cases [26–28] and phosphorylation of AKT described in 40–82% of GC cases [35, 37–39]. Expression of PI3KCA and phosphorylated AKT has also been associated with lymph node metastasis [35, 36, 38]. Furthermore, alterations in *PIK3CA* have been detected in 80% and 42% of the EBV and MSI molecular subtypes of GC, respectively [10]. The molecular mechanisms involved in the sensitivity to PI3K inhibitors are yet to be clarified to translate preclinical activity into a clinical benefit; to date, the development of PI3K inhibitors in advanced GC is still in the preclinical stage [40]. In gastric cancer, the PIK3CA mutation is an important biomarker for predicting the treatment response of everolimus and AKT inhibitors [41, 42]. It was hypothesized that AKT affects the BCL2 protein and NF-κB pathway, although PI3K may also induce upregulation of the chemoresistance proteins, MDR1/Pgp, BCL2 and XIAP, while downregulating the expression of BAX and caspase 3. In tumour tissues from GC patients, which were examined in vitro, AKT activation and *PTEN* loss were associated with increased resistance to multiple chemotherapeutic agents (5-FU, doxorubicin, mitomycin C and cisplatin) [43]. Similarly, a combination of PI3K and AKT inhibitors with chemotherapy agents successfully attenuated chemotherapeutic resistance in a synergistic manner in GC cell lines [44, 45].

JAK2 is overexpressed in a subset of EBV-subtype GCs, and the JAK/STAT signalling pathway has been detected in several types of tumours, including GC [46, 47]. Following the activation of JAK2 by phosphorylation, STAT phosphorylation is induced and gene expression involved in cell proliferation, and apoptosis arrest is stimulated [48]. Therefore, JAK2 inhibitors may also represent a potential therapeutic treatment for GC. To date, the JAK pathway has been primarily a targeted strategy for myeloproliferative and inflammatory disorders and has only recently extended to solid tumours [49]. Regarding gastrointestinal malignancies, ruxolitinib, a JAK1 and JAK2 inhibitor, has demonstrated preliminary efficacy in combination with capecitabine in pancreatic adenocarcinoma and is currently under evaluation in colorectal cancer in combination with regorafenib [ClinicalTrials.gov identifier: NCI02119676] [50]. To the authors' knowledge, there are no trials ongoing in GC.

GC with MSI

According to the TCGA molecular classification, enrichment for microsatellite instability (MSI) characterizes a distinct molecular subgroup of GC. MSI occurs in approximately 15–30% of GCs and more frequently correlates with intestinal histotype, location in the distal part of the stomach, female gender and older age at diagnosis [10, 51, 52] (Fig. 10.2). MSI is a genetic alteration consisting of the expansion or contraction of regions of repetitive nucleotide sequences, called microsatellites. The alteration is triggered by a dysfunction of DNA mismatch repair (MMR) enzymes, caused by mutations in one of several different DNA mismatch repair genes (i.e. *MLH1* or *MSH2*). In a single cell, biallelic inactivation of *MMR* genes causes an increased mutation rate (genomic instability) due to the failure of DNA mismatch repair that usually occurs during normal DNA synthesis [53]. Defective DNA mismatch repair is the hallmark of Lynch syndrome. Different *MMR* genes are probably involved in MSI-high (MSI-H) sporadic gastric cancer without *MLH1* hypermethylation, which represents the main mechanism leading to MMR deficiency in MSI GC [54, 55]. In gastric cancer, 5-FU is frequently used, and information about sensitivity to this agent may be very useful. A meta-analysis of Zhu et al. [56] showed a 37% mortality risk reduction and improved median OS in patients with MSI-H compared with MSI-L (low) or microsatellite-stable (MSS) GC patients. The relationship between MMRd, MSI and survival has been examined in patients with resectable GC randomized to surgery alone or perioperative chemotherapy within the MRC MAGIC trial. MSI and *MLH1* deficiency was associated with a better outcome in patients treated with surgery alone, while it had a negative prognostic effect in those treated with chemotherapy [54]. Although MSI cases generally lack targetable amplifications, mutations in *PIK3CA*, *ERBB3*, *ERB22* and *EGFR* are noted [10, 52]; *BRAF* V600E mutations, commonly seen in MSI colorectal cancer, are absent in MSI GC [10]. However, the predictive role of these mutations in MSI GC population is uncertain.

Major histocompatibility complex class I gene alterations are common in this subtype. This, together with the increased number of tumour-specific neoantigens derived from hypermutated genes, suggests a potential additional role of immunotherapy for this category of tumours. Evidence of the activity of pembrolizumab in a subset of patients with MSI-positive colorectal cancer has recently been presented; the immune-related objective response and progression-free survival rates were 40% and 78%, respectively [57]. One potential challenge in developing suitable candidate therapies for patients with MSI- and EBV-type tumours is that, paradoxically, these patients are likely to have improved survival following surgery compared with patients with other subtypes. Both MSI and EBV positivity have been validated as favourable prognostic factors in resected GC and, therefore, may be present in lower proportions in the metastatic setting, with subsequent difficulty in identifying cases hindering the trial design [58, 59].

GC with CIN

The largest group, the CIN subtype, accounts for approximately 50% of GCs, and its most frequent location is the oesophagogastric junction (EGJ)/cardia, as established by TCGA study [10]. CIN molecular features include alterations in both the DNA copy number and structural abnormalities in specific chromosomal regions. Those alterations could result in the gain or loss of entire chromosomes [60] (i.e. aneuploidy), nonreciprocal translocations, amplifications, deletion or the loss of one allele with the loss of heterozygosis. When CIN GC has an intestinal-type histology, it is associated with copy number gains of chromosomes 8q, 17q and 20q, whereas gains at 12q and 13q are more related to diffuse histology [61]. The final effect of the above-mentioned alterations is the loss or gain of function of oncogenes and tumour suppressor genes that may be efficaciously targeted by specific molecules [62]. Additionally, CIN subtype mutations in TP53 gene and receptor tyrosine kinases (RTKs) are frequently found as well as amplifications of cell cycle genes (Cyclin E1, Cyclin D1 and Cyclin-dependent kinase 6) and of the gene that encodes the ligand Vascular Endothelial Growth Factor A (VEGFA) [10, 63].

Furthermore, CIN displays amplification in oncogene pathways such as RTK/RAS/MAPK signalling, which includes HER2, BRAF, epidermal growth factor (EGFR), MET, FGFR2 and RAS [10, 64].

HER2

The proto-oncogene HER2 is a member of the EGF receptor tyrosine kinase family. The HER2 overexpression/amplification rate is different according to the site and histotype of GC: it is detected in more than 30% of tumours arising from the EGJ and in less than 20% of tumours in the gastric body; in addition, the intestinal and diffuse histotypes show rates of HER2 positivity of 34% and 6%, respectively [65]. Overexpression of HER2 has also been associated with HER2 amplification in 24% of CIN GC cases and subtypes other than CIN: in 12% of EBV cases and in 7% of MSI molecular subtypes [10]. Moreover, overexpression of HER2 has been associated with a poor prognosis and more aggressive disease. The established combination of chemotherapy and HER2-targeted therapy with trastuzumab had created a new standard of care for HER2-positive metastatic GC [33, 66, 67], as demonstrated in the trastuzumab for gastric cancer (ToGA) trial [66]. Following ToGA, several anti-HER2 agents were examined. The addition of pertuzumab (a monoclonal antibody blocking HER2/HER3 dimerization) to trastuzumab and docetaxel has already demonstrated a survival benefit in patients with breast cancer [68]. To evaluate this combination in GC, a phase III multicentre international clinical trial of pertuzumab or placebo in combination with trastuzumab and cisplatin-fluoropyrimidine regimen is ongoing. At this time, standard salvage treatment options for HER2-positive tumours are similar to those for HER2-negative disease; however, blockade of the HER2 pathway beyond trastuzumab progression is under investigation. The antibody-drug conjugate trastuzumab emtansine (T-DM1) has been evaluated in the second-line setting in a phase II clinical trial in previously treated patients with HER2-positive metastatic or advanced GC compared with docetaxel or paclitaxel. MM-111, a bispecific antibody fusion protein binding both HER2 and HER3 (the preferred dimerization partner of HER2), has been evaluated in a phase II clinical trial in combination with trastuzumab and paclitaxel [ClinicalTrials.gov identifier: NCT01774851]; however, this trial was terminated following inferior progression-free survival (PFS) results in the experimental arm. Lapatinib, a dual inhibitor of EGFR and HER2, has been examined as a first-line treatment in combination with capecitabine and oxaliplatin and second-line treatment in combination with paclitaxel [69, 70]. Both phase III studies failed to meet their primary endpoint (increased OS), and promising results were achieved. In the TRIO013/LOGiC trial, the primary endpoint of OS was not reached ($p = 0.35$), but patients of Asian ethnicity and patients younger than 60 years demonstrated a significant benefit in survival [69]. Similarly, in the TyTAN trial, patients with previously treated HER2 FISH-amplified GC were randomized to paclitaxel + lapatinib vs placebo, without having significantly longer OS ($p = 0.1044$). However, in patients with HER2 FISH amplification and 3+ score immunohistochemistry (IHC), a higher response rate was found [70]. Investment in dual inhibitors of the ERBB family continues; at a recent American Society of Medical Oncology (ASCO) Annual Meeting in 2015, an oral reversible tyrosine kinase inhibitor of EGFR and HER2 named S-222611 demonstrated a 15% response rate (including one complete response) in HER2-positive GC [71].

The acquired resistance to HER2 inhibitors has also been studied in GC, exploring various molecular mechanisms underlying this phenomenon. Lee et al. [72] discovered several patterns of synchronous molecular alterations in the group of HER2 GC. In the paper by Zuo et al. [73], trastuzumab-resistant NCI-N87/TR cells were derived from the human gastric carcinoma cell line NCI-N87 with high HER2 expression, by stepwise exposure to increasing doses of trastuzumab. Activation of the downstream PI3K-AKT signalling pathway was one of the major mechanisms of resistance of NCI-N87/TR gastric cancer cells to trastuzumab, likely associated with PTEN gene downregulation and mutation, as well as with overactivity of the IGF-1R signalling pathway [73]. The most relevant finding of the study by Piro and colleagues [74] was that the inhibition of FGFR3 could be a potential strategy to modulate this resistance. IQ-domain GTPase-activating protein 1 (IQGAP1) is a multifunctional scaffold protein that interacts with diverse proteins to regulate cell adhesion and cell migration [75]. It was demonstrated in breast cancer cell lines that IQGAP1 plays an important role in HER-2 expression, phosphorylation and signalling [76], and its overexpression is correlated with trastuzumab-induced resistance and aggressive forms of gastric cancer [77]. Recently, Arienti et al. [75] revealed that high IQGAP1 expression leads to resistance to trastuzumab in GC; in addition, they found two new mutations of the HER2 gene that may be correlated with acquired resistance to the drug. Moreover, functional crosstalk between the receptor tyrosine kinase MET and HER family members has been reported in the context of the acquisition of aggressive phenotypes [78]. Hepatocyte growth factor (HGF)-mediated activation of MET may also cause resistance to lapatinib in HER2-amplified GC cell lines by stimulating downstream signalling [79]. De Silva et al. [80] confirmed in vitro that MET is likely to be a significant mechanism of lapatinib resistance in vivo.

EGFR

EGFR gene amplification is the second most frequent RTK alteration reported in the GC TCGA study and is demonstrated in 10% of CIN subtype tumours. Unfortunately, disappointing results from two large randomized phase III trials have discouraged further investigation of anti-EGFR agents in molecularly unselected populations [81, 82]. Panitumumab added to epirubicin, capecitabine and oxaliplatin as first-line treatment for metastatic or locally advanced oesophagogastric adenocarcinomas resulted in detrimental outcomes compared with chemotherapy alone [82]. A possible explanation for this outcome was hypothesized to be a reduction in the chemotherapy dose intensity due to overlapping toxicity and potentially negative interactions between anti-EGFR agents and oxaliplatin-based regimens. In the EXPAND trial [81], cetuximab, another anti-EGFR agent, did not lead to a survival benefit when added to the cisplatin-capecitabine regimen in previously untreated advanced junctional or gastric adenocarcinoma. Additionally, two anti-EGFR tyrosine kinase inhibitors, erlotinib and gefitinib, were ineffective in phase II and phase III trials compared with best supportive care in oesophageal and junctional cancers [83, 84].

MET

In an unselected GC case series, MET protein expression by IHC was identified in wide ranges, from 22% to 90% [85, 86], whereas MET amplification ranged between 2% and 10% and was confirmed in 8% of CIN subtype tumours in the TCGA series [10]. Both MET overexpression and MET amplification have been validated as negative prognostic factors in GC, and this pathway was, therefore, considered a valid target for pharmacologically specific therapies [10]. Unfortunately, both monoclonal antibodies and RTK inhibitors targeting the MET pathway failed to realize their own potential [87, 88]. Rilotumumab, a fully human monoclonal antibody targeting hepatocyte growth factor (HGF), a ligand of the MET receptor, was associated with significantly longer PFS and OS when added to epirubicin, cisplatin and capecitabine chemotherapy in treatment-naïve molecularly unselected patients with advanced gastric or EGJ tumours in a multicentre phase II trial [89]. In patients selected for MET-positive expression/amplification, OS was longer in rilotumumab-treated patients compared with those on placebo (10.6 versus 5.7 months, respectively). However, the randomized phase III trial recently presented by Cunningham and colleagues in patients with MET-positive tumours by IHC was terminated prematurely due to an imbalanced number of deaths in the experimental arm [87]. Similarly, another anti-MET antibody, onartuzumab, showed no advantage in combination with mFOLFOX [88].

VEGFA Pathway

VEGFA is a member of the VEGF family, and it encodes a disulphide-linked homodimer that acts on endothelial cells and regulates vascular permeability, angiogenesis, vasculogenesis and endothelial cell growth, thereby promoting cell migration and inhibiting apoptosis.

VEGFA overexpression, reported in 54–90% of GC cases, is described as an early marker in the development of GC [90–92] and has been found to correlate with lymph node metastasis and poor prognosis. Other growth factors, VEGFC and VEGFD, are also overexpressed in 50–80% of GC cases, and high levels of expression correlate with lymphatic invasion [93, 94]. Interestingly, recurrent amplification of VEGFA has recently been reported to be a trait of the CIN subtype of GC, and this subgroup of cases may be a candidate for VEGF-targeting therapies [10].

Anti-angiogenesis therapies have been well-studied for cases of advanced-stage GC. For example, in the multinational, placebo-controlled phase III trial, Avastin in Gastric Cancer (AVAGAST), the efficacy of adding bevacizumab to an XP protocol for the first-line treatment of advanced-stage GC was examined. Unfortunately, AVAGAST did not accomplish its primary endpoint of extending the OS of patients with GC [95]. However, subgroup analyses demonstrated that significantly longer OS periods were achieved for patients from non-Asian regions [96]. Furthermore, in the RAINBOW trial, paclitaxel plus ramucirumab versus paclitaxel plus placebo were compared for the treatment of advanced, pretreated cases of GC. The results of this trial confirmed the survival advantage of ramucirumab plus paclitaxel for the treatment of GC in the non-Asian population [97]. The absence of a survival benefit in the RAINBOW and AVAGAST trials in the Asian subset population could be explained by various reasons: (i) the OS in Asian patients is always longer than that in the non-Asian population; (ii) patients from Asia had a better performance status; and (iii) the molecular differences between Asian and Western patients (i.e. different rates of the TCGA subgroups in the two ethnicities) could have affected the results.

FGFR

FGFR2 amplification is associated with tumour cell proliferation and survival of GC cell lines and is related to a poor prognosis. In TCGA classification, approximately 9% of CIN GC patients had FGFR2 gene amplification. Several drugs and studies targeting this mutation are ongoing [10]. A phase II randomized trial is evaluating the activity of AZD4547 (a FGFR 1–2 and 3 inhibitor) compared with paclitaxel in second-line treatment. Other ongoing trials are testing dovitinib in FGFR2-amplified GC patients or in combination with docetaxel [33].

KRAS and BRAF

KRAS mutation occurs in less than 5% of GC and is considered to have a negative prognostic impact in GC patients. KRAS activates critical pathways involved in carcinogenesis and tumour progression, including PI3K-Akt, RAF, MEK-extracellular signal-regulated kinase and NF-κB. However, no target therapies are currently approved for this alteration [98].

Genomically Stable (GS) GC

The GS subgroup includes all tumours that did not meet the criteria for the previously discussed three subtypes [10]. This subtype represents 20% of the TCGA samples and has been associated with diffuse histology, earlier age at presentation (median: 59 years) and distal localization, and it occurs equally in males and females (Fig. 10.2). Several unique subtype-specific molecular changes have been described for GS tumours. The principal somatic genomic alterations observed in GS gastric tumours involve *CDH1*, *ARID1A* and *RHOA*. In addition, recurrent interchromosomal translocation (between *CLDN18* and *ARHGAP26*) implicated in cell motility was found in GS GC [10].

CDH1

The *CDH1* gene is located on chromosome 16q22.1 and encodes E-cadherin, which belongs to the cadherin superfamily of calcium-dependent cell adhesion molecules. Inactivating mutations in the *CDH1* gene are frequently found in gastric cancer, especially in hereditary diffuse gastric cancer [99], whereas CDH1 epigenetic promoter methylation is also frequently found in sporadic gastric cancer [100]. In the analysis of TCGA Research Network [10], *CDH1* somatic mutations were more frequent in the GS subtype (37% of cases). Li et al. [101] discovered that, in diffuse-type GC, *CDH1* mutation is associated with shortened OS, independent of disease stage.

ARID1A

Inactivating mutations of *ARID1A* were found in both GS and EBV-related GC [10]. The *ARID1A* gene, located in chromosome 1p35.3, encodes for adenine-thymine-rich interactive domain-containing protein 1A, which is involved in chromatin remodelling and regulating cellular processes, including DNA repair, differentiation and development [102]. As shown by Wang et al. [103], the loss of *ARID1A* expression was significantly correlated with tumour stage, grade and poor survival in GC patients.

RHOA

Rho GTPases are important intracellular signalling molecules that regulate cytoskeleton organization, cell cycle and cell motility. In cancer, Rho activity promotes metastasis by disrupting the epithelial layer, increasing motility and inducing degradation of the extracellular matrix [104]. *RHOA* mutations have been found to be strongly related to GC with a diffuse histotype [10].

Ripasudil, a selective inhibitor of Rho-associated coiled coil-containing protein kinase (ROCK), was approved in Japan in September 2014 for the treatment of glaucoma and ocular hypertension [105]. Accordingly, it is expected that newly developed drugs inhibiting the RhoA pathway will be evaluated in clinical trials for GC.

TCGA network analysis discovered a recurrent interchromosomal translocation between claudin 18 (*CLDN18*), a component of the tight junction adhesion structures [106], and Rho GTPase-activating protein 6 (*ARHGAP26*), resulting in the *CLDN18-ARHGAP26* fusion gene, which primarily occurs in GS GC [10]. ARHGAP26 is a GTPase-activating protein that facilitates the conversion of RHO GTPases to the GDP state and has been implicated in enhancing cellular motility. Yao et al. [107] showed that the expression of the *CLDN18-ARHGAP26* fusion gene resulted in the epithelial-mesenchymal transition of gastric epithelial cells and, therefore, in cell transformation and cancer development. A recent trial tested IMAB362, a chimeric IgG1 antibody against CLDN18.2 showing clinical activity in patients with 2+/3+ immunostaining [108]. The *CLDN18-ARHGAP* fusions were mutually exclusive with *RHOA* mutations; within the GS subtype, 30% of cases had either *RHOA* or *CLDN18-ARHGAP* alterations [10].

Patient-Derived Preclinical Models of GC

The lack of effective preclinical models of human tumours, reflecting the complexity and heterogeneity of cancer, has consistently limited the development of targeted drugs. Available models include cancer cell line in vitro and cell line xenograft mouse in vivo models, as well as organoids (Table 10.1). However, cell lines cannot replicate the heterogeneity of tumour cells or the relationship between the tumour and microenvironment.

Table 10.1 Patient-derived preclinical models of GC: advantages and disadvantages

	Cons	Pros
Cell line xenografts	Monodimensional No tumour microenvironment interaction Loss of architecture Genetic modifications	Rapid analysis of drug response Immortal cell lines allow an unlimited source of material Low cost, low complexity
PDX models	Limited source of material High failure rate of engraftment Long time for establishment Expensive Tissue must be rapidly processed	Reliable representation of tumour heterogeneity Includes microenvironment Can predict response to drugs
Organoids	No tumour microenvironment interaction	High level of architectural and physiological similarity to native tissue Intermediate cost, easy to handle Large-scale drug screening

Moreover, cell lines are usually established from aggressive tumours and are derived from a specific cell population; irreversible genomic alterations in the process of generating cancer cell lines have been observed [109–111]. For these reasons, this model failed to meet expectations in clinical trials, necessitating an alternative preclinical model to bypass these issues.

PDX models are xenograft mouse tumour models that are established by transplanting human tumour fragments into immunodeficient mice. The neoplastic tissue contains not only cancer cells but also the stroma, and this model can represent cancer heterogeneity. However, there are some inconveniences in the PDX models: the source of original material is limited, transplantation must be conducted rapidly and it is expensive and labour-intensive to establish and maintain the models [109]. A clearly important aspect is that PDX models of human GC constructed using subcutaneous or orthotopic implantation of surgical tissues or gastroscopic biopsies can reliably replicate the morphology and genetic alterations of native tumours [112–115]. Moreover, orthotopic implantation of GC tissue can lead to primary and metastatic tumour growth mimicking the progression of tumour stage, as seen in patients [112]. In one study using PDX models generated by subcutaneous implantation, CD44v8-10 was verified as a GC stem cell marker [116]. In another study, in vivo high-throughput screening using a 1 × 1 × 1 experimental design (a "one animal per model per treatment" approach) with PDX models assessed population responses to 62 treatments across 6 indications, including GC112; these latter data demonstrated the reproducibility and clinical translatability of PDX clinical trials by identifying associations between a genotype and a drug response and established mechanisms of resistance [117]. Similarly, based on the genomically defined GC PDX models, combination therapy of irinotecan with a BCL2L1-targeted drug was confirmed to effectively reduce the tumour size [118].

Organoids are miniature replicas of tissues cultured three-dimensionally in a semi-solid extracellular matrix and growth factor-enriched medium. Organoids sustain high levels of architectural and physiological similarity to native organ systems, superior to traditional two-dimensional homogeneous cell lines [119]. Additional advantages of organoids are that they are self-organizing, easy to handle, acceptable in cost, accessible to genetic engineering and amenable to large-scale drug screening with shorter turnaround times [120]. In a study using pluripotent stem cell-derived gastric organoids, *H. pylori* induced robust activation of c-Met by tyrosine phosphorylation and a twofold increase in epithelial cell proliferation. Cytotoxin-associated gene A played a pivotal role in this process, forming a complex with the c-Met receptor [121]. In another related study, gastric organoids exhibited dysplasia and readily generated adenocarcinomas in mice characterized by activating mutations in KRAS or loss of TP53 [122]. The potential metastatic role of TGFBR2 loss-of-function mutations was shown in CDH1−/−; TP53−/− murine epithelial-mesenchymal organoids used to model hereditary GC, with short hairpin RNA knockdown of TGFBR2 [123]. A critical role of RHOA function in mediating anoikis in diffuse-type gastric carcinogenesis was confirmed in mouse intestinal organoids containing stably expressed RHOA mutations [124]. Thus, organoids constitute a robust model system that may facilitate personalized therapy development by enabling high-throughput drug screening to identify gene-drug associations and by testing specific individual responses to different therapeutic agents [116, 125].

Conclusions

The recent molecular research on GC has generated plentiful data that are currently not integrated into clinical practice.

However, they may be of help in the design of future clinical trials to personalize treatment in several ways: (i) by helping to identify the driving pathways of tumour growth, (ii) by discovering potential drugs targeting such pathways and (iii) by finding predictable mechanisms of resistance and strategies to overcome them.

It must be emphasized that each targetable molecular alteration/pathway is not specific to a distinct subtype of GC; therefore, molecular subgroups alone are not sufficient to assign a patient to a clinical trial. By contrast, molecular characterization of patients is useful to select a small population to be screened for protocol-eligible molecular aberrations. To select the most appropriate therapies for patients with advanced-stage GC, the implementation of GC research and clinical trials in which patients can be classified based on molecular characteristics or molecular subtypes is required.

References

1. Siegel RL, Miller KD, Jemal A. Cancer statistics, 2016. CA Cancer J Clin. 2016;66:7–30.
2. Borrmann R. Geschwulste des margens. In: Henke F, Lubarsch O, editors. Handbuch spez pathol anat und histo. Berlim: Springer; 1926. p. 864–71.
3. Siewert JR, Stein HJ. Classification of adenocarcinoma of the oesophagogastric junction. Br J Surg. 1998;85:1457.
4. Lauren P. The two histological main types of gastric carcinoma: diffuse and so called intestinal-type carcinoma: an attempt at a histo-clinical classification. Acta Pathol Microbiol Scand. 1965;64:31–49.
5. Lauwers GY, Carneiro F, Graham DY. Gastric carcinoma. In: Bowman FT, Carneiro F, Hruban RH, editors. Classification of tumours of the digestive system. 4th ed. Lyon: IARC; 2010.
6. Japanese Research Society for Gastric Cancer. The general rules for the gastric cancer study in surgery and pathology I: clinical classification. Jpn J Surg. 1981;11:127.
7. Tan IB, Ivanova T, Lim KH, et al. Intrinsic subtypes of gastric cancer, based on gene expression pattern, predict survival and respond differently to chemotherapy. Gastroenterology. 2011;141(2):476–85, 85 e1e11.
8. Choi YY, Cheong JH. Beyond precision surgery: molecularly motivated precision care for gastric cancer. Eur J Surg Oncol. 2017;43(5):856–64. https://doi.org/10.1016/j.ejso.2017.02.013. Epub 2017 Mar 1.
9. Lei Z, Tan IB, Das K, Deng N, Zouridis H, Pattison S, Chua C, Feng Z, Guan YK, Ooi CH, Ivanova T, Zhang S, Lee M, Wu J, Ngo A, Manesh S, Tan E, Teh BT, So JB, Goh LK, Boussioutas A, Lim TK, Flotow H, Tan P, Rozen SG. Identification of molecular subtypes of gastric cancer with different responses to PI3-kinase inhibitors and 5-fluorouracil. Gastroenterology. 2013;145:554–65.
10. Cancer Genome Atlas Research Network. Comprehensive molecular characterization of gastric adenocarcinoma. Nature. 2014;513:202–9.
11. Ooi CH, Ivanova T, Wu J, Lee M, Tan IB, Tao J, Ward L, Koo JH, Gopalakrishnan V, Zhu Y, Cheng LL, Lee J, Rha SY, Chung HC, Ganesan K, So J, Soo KC, Lim D, Chan WH, Wong WK, Bowtell D, Yeoh KG, Grabsch H, Boussioutas A, Tan P. Oncogenic pathway combinations predict clinical prognosis in gastric cancer. PLoS Genet. 2009;5:e1000676.
12. Cristescu R, Lee J, Nebozhyn M, Kim KM, Ting JC, Wong SS, Liu J, Yue YG, Wang J, Yu K, Ye XS, Do IG, Liu S, Gong L, Fu J, Jin JG, Choi MG, Sohn TS, Lee JH, Bae JM, Kim ST, Park SH, Sohn I, Jung SH, Tan P, Chen R, Hardwick J, Kang WK, Ayers M, Hongyue D, Reinhard C, Loboda A, Kim S, Aggarwal A. Molecular analysis of gastric cancer identifies subtypes associated with distinct clinical outcomes. Nat Med. 2015;21:449–56.
13. Dunne PD, McArt DG, Bradley CA, O'Reilly PG, Barrett HL, Cummins R, O'Grady T, Arthur K, Loughrey MB, Allen WL, McDade SS, Waugh DJ, Hamilton PW, Longley DB, Kay EW, Johnston PG, Lawler M, Salto-Tellez M, Van Schaeybroeck S. Challenging the cancer molecular stratification dogma: intratumoral heterogeneity undermines consensus molecular subtypes and potential diagnostic value in colorectal cancer. Clin Cancer Res. 2016;22:4095–104.
14. Uhlik MT, Liu J, Falcon BL, Iyer S, Stewart J, Celikkaya H, O'Mahony M, Sevinsky C, Lowes C, Douglass L, Jeffries C, Bodenmiller D,

Chintharlapalli S, Fischl A, Gerald D, Xue Q, Lee JY, Santamaria-Pang A, Al-Kofahi Y, Sui Y, Desai K, Doman T, Aggarwal A, Carter JH, Pytowski B, Jaminet SC, Ginty F, Nasir A, Nagy JA, Dvorak HF, Benjamin LE. Stromal-based signatures for the classification of gastric cancer. Cancer Res. 2016;76:2573–86.
15. Min L, Zhao Y, Zhu S, Qiu X, Cheng R, Xing J, Shao L, Guo S, Zhang S. Integrated analysis identifies molecular signatures and specific prognostic factors for different gastric cancer subtypes. Transl Oncol. 2017;10:99–107.
16. Brettingham-Moore KH, Duong CP, Heriot AG, Thomas RJ, Phillips WA. Using gene expression profiling to predict response and prognosis in gastrointestinal cancers-the promise and the perils. Ann Surg Oncol. 2011;18:1484–91.
17. Wang Z, Chen G, Wang Q, Lu W, Xu M. Identification and validation of a prognostic 9-genes expression signature for gastric cancer. Oncotarget. 2017;8:73826–36.
18. Shinozaki-Ushiku A, Kunita A, Fukayama M. Update on Epstein–Barr virus and gastric cancer [review]. Int J Oncol. 2015;46:1421–34.
19. Abe H, Kaneda A, Fukayama M. Epstein–Barr virus associated gastric carcinoma: use of host cell machineries and somatic gene mutations. Pathobiology. 2015;82:212–23.
20. Fukayama M, Hino R, Uozaki H. Epstein–Barr virus and gastric carcinoma: virus–host interactions leading to carcinoma. Cancer Sci. 2008;99:1726–33.
21. Song HJ, Srivastava A, Lee J, et al. Host inflammatory response predicts survival of patients with Epstein–Barr virus-associated gastric carcinoma. Gastroenterology. 2010;139:84–92.
22. Iwai Y, Ishida M, Tanaka Y, et al. Involvement of PD-L1 on tumor cells in the escape from host immune system and tumor immuno- therapy by PD-L1 blockade. Proc Natl Acad Sci U S A. 2002;99:12293–7.
23. Blank C, Gajewski TF, Mackensen A. Interaction of PD-L1 on tumor cells with PD-1 on tumor-specific T cells as a mechanism of immune evasion:implications for tumor immunotherapy. Cancer Immunol Immunother. 2005;54:307–14.
24. Francisco LM, Sage PT, Sharpe AH. The PD-1 pathway in tolerance and autoimmunity. Immunol Rev. 2010;236:219–42.
25. Zhang L, Qiu M, Jin Y, et al. Programmed cell death ligand 1 (PD-L1) expression on gastric cancer and its relationship with clinicopathologic factors. Int J Clin Exp Pathol. 2015;8:11084–91.
26. Qing Y, Li Q, Ren T, et al. Upregulation of PD-L1 and APE1 is associated with tumorigenesis and poor prognosis of gastric cancer. Drug Des Devel Ther. 2015;9:901–9.
27. Kim JW, Nam KH, Ahn SH, et al. Prognostic implications of immunosuppressive protein expression in tumors as well as immune cell infiltration within the tumor microenvironment in gastric cancer. Gastric Cancer. 2016;19:42–52.
28. Thompson ED, Zahurak M, Murphy A, et al. Patterns of PD-L1 expression and CD8 T cell infiltration in gastric adenocarcinomas and associated immune stroma. Gut; Available from: URL: http://gut.bmj.com/content/early/2016/01/22/gutjnl-2015-310839.long.
29. Liu YX, Wang XS, Wang YF, et al. Prognostic significance of PD-L1 expression in patients with gastric cancer in East Asia: a meta-analysis. Onco Targets Ther. 2016;9:2649–54.
30. Saito R, Abe H, Kunita A, Yamashita H, Seto Y, Fukayama M. Overexpression and gene amplification of PD-L1 in cancer cells and PD-L1+ immune cells in Epstein-Barr virus-associated gastric cancer: the prognostic implications. Mod Pathol. 2017;30(3):427–39. https://doi.org/10.1038/modpathol.2016.202. Epub 2016 Dec 9.
31. Shankaran V, Muro K, Bang Y, Geva R, Catenacci D, Gupta S, et al. Correlation of gene expression signatures and clinical outcomes in patients with advanced gastric cancer treated with pembrolizumab (MK-3475). J Clin Oncol. 2015;33:3026.
32. Bang Y, Im S, Lee K, Cho J, Song E, Lee K, et al. Randomized, double-blind phase II trial with prospective classification by ATM protein level to evaluate the efficacy and tolerability of olaparib plus paclitaxel in patients with recurrent or metastatic gastric cancer. J Clin Oncol. Epub ahead of print 17 August 2015. 2015b;33:3858. https://doi.org/10.1200/JCO.2014.60.0320.
33. Fontana E, Smyth EC. Novel targets in the treatment of advanced gastric cancer: a perspective review. Ther Adv Med Oncol. 2016;8(2):113–25. https://doi.org/10.1177/1758834015616935.
34. Liu JF, Zhou XK, Chen JH, Yi G, Chen HG, Ba MC, Lin SQ, Qi YC. Up-regulation of PIK3CA promotes metastasis in gastric carcinoma. World J Gastroenterol. 2010;16(39):4986–91.
35. Ye B, Jiang L, Xu H, Zhou D, Li Z. Expression of PI3K/AKT pathway in gastric cancer and its blockade suppresses tumor growth and metastasis. Int J Immunopathol Pharmacol. 2012;25(3):627–36.
36. Tapia O, Riquelme I, Leal P, Sandoval A, Aedo S, Weber H, Letelier P, Bellolio E, Villaseca M, Garcia P, Roa J. The PI3K/AKT/mTOR pathway is activated in gastric cancer with potential prognostic and predictive significance. Virchows Arch. 2014;465(1):25–33.
37. Cinti C, Vindigni C, Zamparelli A, Sala D, Epistolato M, Marrelli D, Cevenini G, Tosi P. Activated Akt as an indicator of prognosis in gastric cancer. Virchows Arch. 2008;453(5):449–55.
38. Sangawa A, Shintani M, Yamao N, Kamoshida S. Phosphorylation status of Akt and caspase-9 in gastric and colorectal carcinomas. Int J Clin Exp Pathol. 2014;7(6):3312–7.
39. Welker ME, Kulik G. Recent syntheses of PI3K/Akt/mTOR signaling pathway inhibitors. Bioorg Med Chem. 2013;21(14):4063–91.

40. Janku F, Tsimberidou AM, Garrido-Laguna I, Wang X, Luthra R, Hong DS, Naing A, Falchook GS, Moroney JW, Piha-Paul SA, Wheler JJ, Moulder SL, Fu S, Kurzrock R. PIK3CA mutations in patients with advanced cancers treated with PI3K/AKT/mTOR axis inhibitors. Mol Cancer Ther. 2011;10(3):558–65.
41. Davies B, Greenwood H, Dudley P. Preclinical pharmacology of AZD5363, an inhibitor of AKT: pharmacodynamics, antitumor activity, and correlation of monotherapy activity with genetic background. Mol Canc Ther. 2012;11:873–87.
42. Li V, Wong C, Chan T. Mutations of PIK3CA in gastric adenocarcinoma. BMC Cancer. 2005;5:29.
43. Yu H-G, Ai Y-W, Yu L-L, Zhou X-D, Liu J, Li J-H, Xu X-M, Liu S, Chen J, Liu F, Qi Y-L, Deng Q, Cao J, Liu S-Q, Luo H-S, Yu J-P. Phosphoinositide 3-kinase/Akt pathway plays an important role in chemoresistance of gastric cancer cells against etoposide and doxorubicin induced cell death. Int J Cancer. 2008;122(2):433–43.
44. Oki E, Kakeji Y, Tokunaga E. Impact of PTEN/AKT/PI3K signal pathway on the chemotherapy for gastric cancer. J Clin Oncol. 2006;24(18):4034.
45. Im S, Lee K, Nam E. Tumori. 2005;91:513–21.
46. Wu H, Huang M, Cao P, Wang T, Shu Y, Liu P. MiR-135a targets JAK2 and inhibits gastric cancer cell proliferation. Cancer Biol Ther. 2012;13(5):281–8.
47. Brooks AJ, Dai W, O'Mara ML, Abankwa D, Chhabra Y, Pelekanos RA, Gardon O, Tunny KA, Blucher KM, Morton CJ, Parker MW, Sierecki E, Gambin Y, et al. Mechanism of activation of protein kinase JAK2 by the growth hormone receptor. Science. 2014;344(6185):1249783.
48. Levine RL, Wadleigh M, Cools J, Ebert BL, Wernig G, Huntly BJ, Boggon TJ, Wlodarska I, Clark JJ, Moore S, Adelsperger J, Koo S, Lee JC, et al. Activating mutation in the tyrosine kinase JAK2 in polycythemia vera, essential thrombocythemia, and myeloid metaplasia with myelofibrosis. Cancer Cell. 2005;7(4):387–97.
49. Buchert M, Burns C, Ernst M. Targeting JAK kinase in solid tumors: emerging opportunities and challenges. Oncogene. Epub ahead of print 18 May 2015. 2015;35:939. https://doi.org/10.1038/onc.2015.150.
50. Hurwitz H, Uppal N, Wagner S, Bendell J, Beck J, Wade S, et al. A randomized doubleblind phase 2 study of ruxolitinib (RUX) or placebo (PBO) with capecitabine (CAPE) as second-line therapy in patients (pts) with metastatic pancreatic cancer (mPC). J Clin Oncol. 2014;32:4000.
51. Pedrazzani C, Corso G, Velho S, Leite M, Pascale V, Bettarini F, Marrelli D, Seruca R, Roviello F. Evidence of tumor micro satellite instability in gastric cancer with familial aggregation. Fam Cancer. 2009;8:215–20. https://doi.org/10.1007/s10689-008-9231-7. PMID: 19152022.
52. Velho S, Fernandes MS, Leite M, Figueiredo C, Seruca R. Causes and consequences of microsatellite instability in gastric carcinogenesis. World J Gastroenterol. 2014;20:16433–42. https://doi.org/10.3748/wjg.v20.i44.16433. PMID: 25469011.
53. Chung DC, Rustgi AK. DNA mismatch repair and cancer. Gastroenterology. 1995;109:1685–99. [PMID: 7557155].
54. Correlation between mismatch repair deficiency (MMRd), microsatellite instability (MSI) and survival in MAGIC. J Clin Oncol [Internet]. Accessed 28 Jul 2016.
55. Pinto M, Wu Y, Mensink RG, Cirnes L, Seruca R, Hofstra RM. Somatic mutations in mismatch repair genes in sporadic gastric carcinomas are not a cause but a consequence of the mutator phenotype. Cancer Genet Cytogenet. 2008;180:110–4. https://doi.org/10.1016/j.cancergencyto.2007.09.022. PMID:18206535.
56. Zhu L, Li Z, Wang Y, Zhang C, Liu Y, Qu X. Microsatellite instability and survival in gastric cancer: a systematic review and meta-analysis. Mol Clin Oncol. 2015;3:699–705. https://doi.org/10.3892/mco.2015.506. PMID: 26137290.
57. Le D, Uram J, Wang H, Bartlett B, Kemberling H, Eyring A, et al. PD-1 blockade in tumors with mismatch-repair deficiency. N Engl J Med. 2015;372:2509–20.
58. Camargo M, Kim W, Chiaravalli A, Kim K, Corvalan A, Matsuo K, et al. Improved survival of gastric cancer with tumour Epstein-Barr virus positivity: an international pooled analysis. Gut. 2014;63:236–43.
59. Choi Y, Bae J, An J, Kwon I, Cho I, Shin H, et al. Is microsatellite instability a prognostic marker in gastric cancer? a systematic review with meta-analysis. J Surg Oncol. 2014;110:129–35.
60. Giam M, Rancati G. Aneuploidy and chromosomal instability in cancer: a jackpot to chaos. Cell Div. 2015;10:3.
61. Chia NY, Tan P. Molecular classification of gastric cancer. Ann Oncol. 2016;27:763–9. https://doi.org/10.1093/annonc/mdw040. PMID: 26861606.
62. Aprile G, Giampieri R, Bonotto M, Bittoni A, Ongaro E, Cardellino GG, Graziano F, Giuliani F, Fasola G, Cascinu S, Scartozzi M. The challenge of targeted therapies for gastric cancer patients: the beginning of a long journey. Expert Opin Investig Drugs. 2014;23:925–42.
63. Chen T, Xu XY, Zhou PH. Emerging molecular classifications and therapeutic implications for gastric cancer. Chin J Cancer. 2016;35:49.
64. Tan P, Yeoh KG. Genetics and molecular pathogenesis of gastric adenocarcinoma. Gastroenterology. 2015;149:1153–1162.e3.
65. Gravalos C, Jimeno A. HER2 in gastric cancer: a new prognostic factor and a novel therapeutic target. Ann Oncol. 2008;19:1523–9.
66. Bang YJ, Van Cutsem E, Feyereislova A, Chung HC, Shen L, Sawaki A, Lordick F, Ohtsu A, Omuro Y, Satoh T, Aprile G, Kulikov E, Hill J, Lehle M, Rüschoff J, Kang YK. Trastuzumab in combination

with chemotherapy versus chemotherapy alone for treatment of HER2-positive advanced gastric or gastro-oesophageal junction cancer (ToGA): a phase 3, open-label, randomised controlled trial. Lancet. 2010;376:687–97.
67. Hecht JR, Bang YJ, Qin SK, Chung HC, Xu JM, Park JO, Jeziorski K, Shparyk Y, Hoff PM, Sobrero A, Salman P, Li J, Protsenko SA, Wainberg ZA, Buyse M, Afenjar K, Houé V, Garcia A, Kaneko T, Huang Y, Khan-Wasti S, Santillana S, Press MF, Slamon D. Lapatinib in combination with capecitabine plus oxaliplatin in human epidermal growth factor receptor 2-positive advanced or metastatic gastric, esophageal, or gastroesophageal adenocarcinoma: TRIO-013/LOGiC–A randomized phase III trial. J Clin Oncol. 2016;34:443–51.
68. Baselga J, Cortés J, Kim S, Im S, Hegg R, Im Y, et al. Pertuzumab plus trastuzumab plus docetaxel for metastatic breast cancer. N Engl J Med. 2012;366:109–19.
69. Hecht J, Bang Y, Qin S, Chung H, Xu J, Park J, et al. Lapatinib in combination with capecitabine plus oxaliplatin (CapeOx) in HER2 positive advanced or metastatic gastric (A/MGC), esophageal (EAC), or astroesophageal (GEJ) adenocarcinoma: the logic trial. J Clin Oncol. 2013;31:LBA4001.
70. Satoh T, Xu R, Chung H, Sun G, Doi T, Xu J, et al. Lapatinib plus paclitaxel versus paclitaxel alone in the second-line treatment of HER2-amplified advanced gastric cancer in Asian populations: TyTAN-a randomized, phase III study. J Clin Oncol. 2014b;32:2039–49.
71. Deva S, Baird R, Cresti N, Garcia-Corbacho J, Hogarth L, Frenkel E, et al. Phase I expansion of S-222611, a reversible inhibitor of EGFR and HER2, in advanced solid tumors, including patients with brain metastases. J Clin Oncol. 2015;33(15_suppl):2511.
72. Lee JY, Hong M, Kim ST, Park SH, Kang WK, Kim KM, Lee J. The impact of concomitant genomic alterations on treatment outcome for trastuzumab therapy in HER2-positive gastric cancer. Sci Rep. 2015;5:9289. https://doi.org/10.1038/srep09289. PMID: 25786580.
73. Zuo Q, Liu J, Zhang J, Wu M, Guo L, Liao W. Development of trastuzumab-resistant human gastric carcinoma cell lines and mechanisms of drug resistance. Sci Rep. 2015;5:11634.
74. Piro G, Carbone C, Cataldo I, Di Nicolantonio F, Giacopuzzi S, Aprile G, Simionato F, Boschi F, Zanotto M, Mina MM, Santoro R, Merz V, Sbarbati A, de Manzoni G, Scarpa A, Tortora G, Melisi D. An FGFR3 autocrine loop sustains acquired resistance to trastuzumab in gastric cancer patients. Clin Cancer Res. 2016;22:6164–75.
75. Arienti C, Zanoni M, Pignatta S, Del Rio A, Carloni S, Tebaldi M, Tedaldi G, Tesei A. Preclinical evidence of multiple mechanisms underlying trastuzumab resistance in gastric cancer. Oncotarget. 2016;7:18424–39.
76. White CD, Brown MD, Sacks DB. IQGAPs in cancer: a family of scaffold proteins underlying tumorigenesis. FEBS Lett. 2009;583:1817–24.
77. Walch A, Seidl S, Hermannstädter C, Rauser S, Deplazes J, Langer R, von Weyhern CH, Sarbia M, Busch R, Feith M, Gillen S, Höfler H, Luber B. Combined analysis of Rac1, IQGAP1, Tiam1 and E-cadherin expression in gastric cancer. Mod Pathol. 2008;21:544–52.
78. Khoury H, Naujokas MA, Zuo D, Sangwan V, Frigault MM, Petkiewicz S, Dankort DL, Muller WJ, Park M. HGF converts ErbB2/Neu epithelial morphogenesis to cell invasion. Mol Biol Cell. 2005;16:550–61.
79. Chen CT, Kim H, Liska D, Gao S, Christensen JG, Weiser MR. MET activation mediates resistance to lapatinib inhibition of HER2- amplified gastric cancer cells. Mol Cancer Ther. 2012;11:660–9.
80. De Silva N, Schulz L, Paterson A, Qain W, Secrier M, Godfrey E, Cheow H, O'Donovan M, Lao-Sirieix P, Jobanputra M, Hochhauser D, Fitzgerald R, Ford H. Molecular effects of Lapatinib in the treatment of HER2 overexpressing oesophago-gastric adenocarcinoma. Br J Cancer. 2015;113:1305–12.
81. Lordick F, Kang Y, Chung H, Salman P, Oh S, Bodoky G, et al. Capecitabine and cisplatin with or without cetuximab for patients with previously untreated advanced gastric cancer (EXPAND): a randomised, open-label phase 3 trial. Lancet Oncol. 2013;14:490–9.
82. Waddell T, Chau I, Cunningham D, Gonzalez D, Okines A, Okines C, et al. Epirubicin, oxaliplatin, and capecitabine with or without panitumumab for patients with previously untreated advanced oesophagogastric cancer (REAL3): a randomised, open-label phase 3 trial. Lancet Oncol. 2013;14:481–9.
83. Dragovich T, Mccoy S, Fenoglio-Preiser C, Wang J, Benedetti J, Baker A, et al. Phase II trial of erlotinib in gastroesophageal junction and gastric adenocarcinomas: SWOG 0127. J Clin Oncol. 2006;24:4922–7.
84. Dutton S, Ferry D, Blazeby J, Abbas H, Dahle-Smith A, Mansoor W, et al. Gefitinib for oesophageal cancer progressing after chemotherapy (COG): a phase 3, multicentre, double-blind, placebocontrolled randomised trial. Lancet Oncol. 2014;15:894–904.
85. Ha S, Lee J, Kang S, Do I, Ahn S, Park J, et al. MET overexpression assessed by new interpretation method predicts gene amplification and poor survival in advanced gastric carcinomas. Mod Pathol. 2013;26:1632–41.
86. Scagliotti G, Novello S, Von Pawel J. The emerging role of MET/HGF inhibitors in oncology. Cancer Treat Rev. 2013;39:793–801.
87. Cunningham D, Tebbutt N, Davidenko I, Murad A, Al-Batran S, Ilson D, et al. Phase III, randomized, double-blind, multicenter, placebo (P)-controlled trial of rilotumumab (R) plus epirubicin, cisplatin and capecitabine (ECX) as first-line therapy in patients (pts) with advanced MET-positive (pos) gas-

tric or gastroesophageal junction (G/GEJ) cancer: RILOMET-1 study. J Clin Oncol. 2015;33:4000.
88. Shah M, Bang Y, Lordick F, Tabernero J, Chen M, Hack S, et al. Metgastric: a phase III study of onartuzumab plus mFOLFOX6 in patients with metastatic HER2-negative (HER2-) and METpositive (MET+) adenocarcinoma of the stomach or gastroesophageal junction (GEC). J Clin Oncol. 2015;33:4012.
89. Iveson T, Donehower R, Davidenko I, Tjulandin S, Deptala A, Harrison M, et al. Rilotumumab in combination with epirubicin, cisplatin, and capecitabine as first-line treatment for gastric or oesophagogastric junction adenocarcinoma: an open-label, dose de-escalation phase 1b study and a double-blind, randomised phase 2 study. Lancet Oncol. 2014;15:1007–18.
90. Chen J, Zhou SJ, Zhang Y, Zhang GQ, Zha TZ, Feng YZ, Zhang K. Clinicopathological and prognostic significance of galectin-1 and vascular endothelial growth factor expression in gastric cancer. World J Gastroenterol. 2013;19(13):2073–9.
91. Lee SJ, Kim JG, Sohn SK, Chae YS, Moon JH, Kim SN, Bae HI, Chung HY, Yu W. No association of vascular endothelial growth factor-A (VEGF-A) and VEGF-C expression with survival in patients with gastric cancer. Cancer Res Treat. 2009;41(4):218–23.
92. Deguchi K, Ichikawa D, Soga K, Watanabe K, Kosuga T, Takeshita H, Konishi H, Morimura R, Tsujiura M, Komatsu S, Shiozaki A, Okamoto K, Fujiwara H, Otsuji E. Clinical significance of vascular endothelial growth factors C and D and chemokine receptor CCR7 in gastric cancer. Anticancer Res. 2010;30(6):2361–6.
93. Gou HF, Chen XC, Zhu J, Jiang M, Yang Y, Cao D, Hou M. Expressions of COX-2 and VEGF-C in gastric cancer: correlations with lymphangiogenesis and prognostic implications. J Exp Clin Canc Res. 2011;30:14.
94. Ohtsu A, Shah MA, Van Cutsem E, Rha SY, Sawaki A, Park SR, Lim HY, Yamada Y, Wu J, Langer B, Starnawski M, Kang YK. Bevacizumab in combination with chemotherapy as first-line therapy in advanced gastric cancer: a randomized, double-blind, placebo-controlled phase III study. J Clin Oncol. 2011;29(30):3968–76.
95. Van Cutsem E, de Haas S, Kang YK, Ohtsu A, Tebbutt NC, Ming Xu J, Peng Yong W, Langer B, Delmar P, Scherer SJ, Shah MA. Bevacizumab in combination with chemotherapy as first-line therapy in advanced gastric cancer: a biomarker evaluation from the AVAGAST randomized phase III trial. J Clin Oncol. 2012;30(17):2119–27.
96. Fuchs CS, Tomasek J, Yong CJ, Dumitru F, Passalacqua R, Goswami C, Safran H, dos Santos LV, Aprile G, Ferry DR, Melichar B, Tehfe M, Topuzov E, et al. Ramucirumab monotherapy for previously treated advanced gastric or gastro-oesophageal junction adenocarcinoma (REGARD): an international, randomised, multicentre, placebocontrolled,phase 3 trial. Lancet. 2014;383(9911):31–9.
97. Li J, Qin S, Xu J, Guo W, Xiong J, Bai Y, Sun G, Yang Y, Wang L, Xu N, Cheng Y, Wang Z, Zheng L, et al. Apatinib for chemotherapy-refractory advanced metastatic gastric cancer: results from a randomized, placebocontrolled,parallel-arm, phase II trial. J Clin Oncol. 2013;31(26):3219–25.
98. Choi YY, Noh SH, Cheong JH. Molecular dimensions of gastric cancer: translational and clinical perspectives. J Pathol Transl Med. 2016;50:1–9.
99. Corso G, Marrelli D, Pascale V, Vindigni C, Roviello F. Frequency of CDH1 germline mutations in gastric carcinoma coming from high- and low-risk areas: metanalysis and systematic review of the literature. BMC Cancer. 2012;12:8.
100. Liu YC, Shen CY, Wu HS, Hsieh TY, Chan DC, Chen CJ, Yu JC, Yu CP, Harn HJ, Chen PJ, Hsieh CB, Chen TW, Hsu HM. Mechanisms inactivating the gene for E-cadherin in sporadic gastric carcinomas. World J Gastroenterol. 2006;12:2168–73.
101. Li X, Wu WK, Xing R, Wong SH, Liu Y, Fang X, Zhang Y, Wang M, Wang J, Li L, Zhou Y, Tang S, Peng S, Qiu K, Chen L, Chen K, Yang H, Zhang W, Chan MT, Lu Y, Sung JJ, Yu J. Distinct subtypes of gastric cancer defined by molecular characterization include novel mutational signatures with prognostic capability. Cancer Res. 2016;76:1724–32.
102. Weissman B, Knudsen KE. Hijacking the chromatin remodeling machinery: impact of SWI/SNF perturbations in cancer. Cancer Res. 2009;69:8223–30.
103. Wang DD, Chen YB, Pan K, Wang W, Chen SP, Chen JG, Zhao JJ, Lv L, Pan QZ, Li YQ, Wang QJ, Huang LX, Ke ML, He J, Xia JC. Decreased expression of the ARID1A gene is associated with poor prognosis in primary gastric cancer. PLoS One. 2012;7:e40364.
104. Shang X, Marchioni F, Evelyn CR, Sipes N, Zhou X, Seibel W, Wortman M, Zheng Y. Small-molecule inhibitors targeting G-protein-coupled Rho guanine nucleotide exchange factors. Proc Natl Acad Sci U S A. 2013;110(8):3155–60.
105. Shang X, Marchioni F, Sipes N, Evelyn CR, Jerabek-Willemsen M, Duhr S, Seibel W, Wortman M, Zheng Y. Rational design of small molecule inhibitors targeting RhoA subfamily Rho GTPases. Chem Biol. 2012;19(6):699–710.
106. Türeci O, Koslowski M, Helftenbein G, Castle J, Rohde C, Dhaene K, Seitz G, Sahin U. Claudin-18 gene structure, regulation, and expression is evolutionary conserved in mammals. Gene. 2011;481:83–92.
107. Yao F, Kausalya JP, Sia YY, Teo AS, Lee WH, Ong AG, Zhang Z, Tan JH, Li G, Bertrand D, Liu X, Poh HM, Guan P, Zhu F, Pathiraja TN, Ariyaratne PN, Rao J, Woo XY, Cai S, Mulawadi FH, Poh WT, Veeravalli L, Chan CS, Lim SS, Leong ST, Neo SC, Choi PS, Chew EG, Nagarajan N, Jacques PÉ, So JB, Ruan X, Yeoh KG, Tan P, Sung WK, Hunziker W, Ruan Y, Hillmer AM. Recurrent fusion genes in gastric cancer: CLDN18-ARHGAP26 induces loss of epithelial integrity. Cell Rep. 2015;12:272–85.

108. FAST: An international, multicenter, randomized, phase II trial of epirubicin, oxaliplatin, and capecitabine (EOX) with or without IMAB362, a first-in-class anti-CLDN18.2 antibody, as firstline therapy in patients with advanced CLDN18.2 gastric and gastroesophageal junction (GEJ) adenocarcinoma. J Clin Oncol [Internet]. Accessed 31 Jul 2016. Available from: URL: http://meetinglibrary.asco.org/content/164788-176.
109. Hidalgo M, Amant F, Biankin AV, et al. Patient-derived xenograft models: an emerging platform for translational cancer research. Cancer Discov. 2014;4(9):998–1013.
110. Hausser HJ, Brenner RE. Phenotypic instability of Saos-2 cells in long-term culture. Biochem Biophys Res Commun. 2005;333(1):216–22.
111. Gillet JP, Calcagno AM, Varma S, et al. Redefining the relevance of established cancer cell lines to the study of mechanisms of clinical anti-cancer drug resistance. Proc Natl Acad Sci U S A. 2011;108(46):18708.
112. Furukawa T, Kubota T, Watanabe M, et al. Orthotopic transplantation of histologically intact clinical specimens of stomach cancer to nude mice: correlation of metastatic sites in mouse and individual patient donors. Int J Cancer. 1993;53:608–12.
113. Furukawa T, Fu X, Kubota T, et al. Nude mouse metastatic models of human stomach cancer constructed using orthotopic implantation of histologically intact tissue. Cancer Res. 1993;53:1204–8.
114. Zhang L, Yang J, Cai J, et al. A subset of gastric cancers with EGFR amplification and overexpression respond to cetuximab therapy. Sci Rep. 2013;3:2992.
115. Zhu Y, Tian T, Li Z, et al. Establishment and characterization of patient-derived tumor xenograft using gastroscopic biopsies in gastric cancer. Sci Rep. 2015;5:8542.
116. Lau WM, Teng E, Chong HS, et al. CD44v8-10 is a cancer-specific marker for gastric cancer stem cells. Cancer Res. 2014;74:2630–41.
117. Gao H, Korn JM, Ferretti S, et al. High-throughput screening using patient-derived tumor xenografts to predict clinical trial drug response. Nat Med. 2015;21:1318–25.
118. Park H, Cho S-Y, Kim H, et al. Genomic alterations in BCL2L1 and DLC1 contribute to drug sensitivity in gastric cancer. Proc Natl Acad Sci U S A. 2015;112:12492–7.
119. Dedhia PH, Bertaux-Skeirik N, Zavros Y, et al. Organoid models of human gastrointestinal development and disease. Gastroenterology. 2016;150:1098–112.
120. Hill DR, Spence JR. Gastrointestinal organoids: understanding the molecular basis of the host-microbe interface. Cell Mol Gastroenterol Hepatol. 2017;3:138–49.
121. McCracken KW, Catá EM, Crawford CM, et al. Modelling human development and disease in pluripotent stemcell- derived gastric organoids. Nature. 2014;516:400–4.
122. Li X, Nadauld L, Ootani A, et al. Oncogenic transformation of diverse gastrointestinal tissues in primary organoid culture. Nat Med. 2014;20:769–77.
123. Nadauld LD, Garcia S, Natsoulis G, et al. Metastatic tumor evolution and organoid modeling implicate TGFBR2 as a cancer driver in diffuse gastric cancer. Genome Biol. 2014;15:428.
124. Wang K, Yuen ST, Xu J, et al. Whole-genome sequencing and comprehensive molecular profiling identify new driver mutations in gastric cancer. Nat Genet. 2014;46:573–82.
125. van de Wetering M, Francies HE, Francis JM, et al. Prospective derivation of a living organoid biobank of colorectal cancer patients. Cell. 2015;161:933–45.

Part V

Future Medicine in Gastric Cancer

Noncoding RNA in Gastric Cancer with Potential Prognostic and Predictive Role

11

Federica Rao, Flavio Rizzolio, Clara Rizzardi, Tiziana Perin, and Vincenzo Canzonieri

Introduction

GC is one of the most frequent malignant tumors; every year in the world, there are 723,000 cancer-related deaths caused by GC according to the World Health Organization (WHO). It is the fifth most common cancer in the world and the third cause of death among cancer pathologies [1]. Due to the lack of specific diagnostic markers, most patients with GC do not receive an appropriate diagnosis and treatment; this leads to a progression of the pathological state with development of metastases [2]. Previous studies have hypothesized that GC is a genetic disease involving multi-step changes in the genome [3]. However, the human genome contains nearly 20,000 protein-coding genes, but they represent less than 2% of the whole genome [4]. In contrast, according to the Encyclopedia of DNA Elements (ENCODE) project, more than 80% of functional DNA elements in the human genome do not code for proteins [5]. A large part of these functional DNA elements is represented by ncRNAs [6].

In the last years, several studies have shown that ncRNAs play a significant role in different cellular and physiological processes including gene regulation, genomic imprinting, chromatin packaging, dosage compensation, cell differentiation, and embryonic development [6, 7]. Accordingly, the dysregulation of ncRNAs, as pivotal modulators of gene expression, has been documented in different human complex diseases including cancer [8]. In fact, they are able to influence different mechanisms in cancer cells,

F. Rao
Pathology Department, IRCCS, CRO Aviano, National Cancer Institute, Aviano, PN, Italy

F. Rizzolio (✉)
Pathology Department, IRCCS, CRO Aviano, National Cancer Institute, Aviano, PN, Italy

Department of Molecular Sciences and Nanosystems, Ca' Foscari University, Venice-Mestre, VE, Italy

Department of Biology, Temple University, Philadelphia, PA, USA
e-mail: flavio.rizzolio@unive.it

C. Rizzardi
Department of Medical, Surgical and Health Sciences, University of Trieste, Trieste, TS, Italy

T. Perin
Pathology Department, IRCCS, CRO Aviano, National Cancer Institute, Aviano, PN, Italy

CRO Biobank, IRCCS, CRO Aviano, National Cancer Institute, Aviano, PN, Italy

V. Canzonieri (✉)
Pathology Department, IRCCS, CRO Aviano, National Cancer Institute, Aviano, PN, Italy

Department of Medical, Surgical and Health Sciences, University of Trieste, Trieste, TS, Italy

CRO Biobank, IRCCS, CRO Aviano, National Cancer Institute, Aviano, PN, Italy

Department of Biology, Temple University, Philadelphia, PA, USA
e-mail: vcanzonieri@cro.it

© Springer Nature Switzerland AG 2019
V. Canzonieri, A. Giordano (eds.), *Gastric Cancer In The Precision Medicine Era*, Current Clinical Pathology, https://doi.org/10.1007/978-3-030-04861-7_11

such as proliferation, apoptosis, invasion, and metastasis as well as neoangiogenesis [9]. Expression profiling studies on ncRNAs in a variety of cancer types have revealed a broad range of lncRNAs with aberrant expression [10]. Moreover, it has been shown that ncRNAs are promising candidate prognostic biomarkers for GC detection and potential therapeutic targets. Several ncRNAs could be secreted into body fluids, suggesting that tumor cells may change their extracellular environments through RNA-based, hormone-like mechanisms [11].

In this chapter, we discussed the different roles of ncRNAs in GC and the possible diagnostic, prognostic, and therapeutic applications.

ncRNAs

ncRNAs refer to a class of RNAs with no protein-coding function that are widely expressed in organisms [12]. ncRNAs can be divided into two groups: housekeeping ncRNAs and regulatory ncRNAs. The latter can further be divided into three types, according to their length: (1) short ncRNAs, including miRNAs, small interfering RNAs (siRNAs), and Piwi-interacting RNAs (piRNAs), (2) mid-size ncRNAs, and (3) lncRNAs [13–15].

Short ncRNAs are shorter than 50 nucleotides (nt), mid-size ncRNAs have a length between 50 and 200 nt, and lncRNAs are longer than 200 nt [16].

Currently, numerous studies have found that miRNAs and lncRNAs play important roles in GC progression.

Table 11.1 summarizes the characteristics of different groups of ncRNAs.

miRNAs in GC

miRNAs are a class of small ncRNAs of approximately 18–24 nt. Genes encoding miRNAs could be single copy, multiple copies, or clusters; other forms exist in the region of protein-coding genes, including introns. They are highly conserved sequences and have temporal and tissue specificity [17].

Although miRNAs do not code for proteins, they have an important role in the regulation of gene expression at the posttranscriptional level. Through complete or incomplete complementary binding to the 3′-untranslated regions (3′-UTRs) of target mRNAs, miRNAs promote the degradation of targeted-mRNA or their translational suppression. As a consequence of this process, which involves the recruitment of a number of other proteins, miRNAs are able to regulate negatively the expression of target genes [18, 19].

One miRNA interacts with several different mRNAs in different regions. A mRNA could also combine with several miRNAs on the basis of complete or incomplete sequence complementarity.

The synthesis of miRNA involves the production of a primary transcript (pri-miRNA) from genomic DNA by polymerase II within the nucleus. Then, the pri-miRNA is cut by the Drosha enzyme of RNase 3 endonuclease enzyme family into hairpin precursors of miRNA (pre-miRNA), which are approximately 70 nt [20]. Finally, the synergistic effect of Ran-GTP and transporter protein Exportin 5 transports pre-miRNA out of the nucleus, and the enzyme Dicer cuts it to produce the approximately 22 nt mature miRNA [21]. At this point, the synthesized miRNA is ready to exert its function.

Through the latest approaches of microarray technology, bioinformatics, and other genetics methods, the ectopic expression of miRNAs in GC has been found to be closely related to different steps of cancer initiation and progression including metastasis. By upregulation of the expression of oncogenes or downregulation of the expression of tumor suppressor genes, miRNAs play an important role in the regulation of cancer-related genes. A first example can be given by miRNA-106b-25. Petrocca et al. reported that an abnormal regulation of the transcription factor E2F1 and transforming growth factor-β (TGF-β) plays a critical role in gastric carcinogenesis. E2F1 activates its own promoter and miR-106b-25 cluster expression simultaneously with its host gene, Mcm7. Furthermore, the TGF-β tumor suppressor pathway was impaired by overexpression of the miR-106b-25 cluster, but also the expres-

Table 11.1 Classification of human genomic ncRNAs

RNA type	Symbol	Length (nt)	Function	References
Housekeeping ncRNAs				
Transfer RNAs	tRNA	70–80	Connect amino acids with mRNA [1]	(1) Lodish H, Berk A, Zipursky SL, et al. Molecular cell biology. 4th ed. New York: W. H. Freeman; 2000
Ribosomal RNAs	rRNA	121–5070	Component of ribosomes [1]	
Small nuclear RNAs	snRNA	≈ 150	Assemble with proteins into spliceosomes to remove introns during mRNA processing [2]	(2) Valadkhan S, Gunawardane LS. Role of small nuclear RNAs in eukaryotic gene expression. Essays in Biochemistry. May 03, 2013, 5479–90. https://doi.org/10.1042/bse0540079
Small nucleolar RNAs	snoRNA	70–200	Guide modifications of other ncRNAs, alternative splicing; or function as miRNA [3]	(3) Scott MS, Ono M. From snoRNA to miRNA: dual function regulatory non-coding RNAs. Biochimie. 2011;93(11):1987–92. https://doi.org/10.1016/j.biochi.2011.05.026
Telomerase RNAs	TERC	451	Provide template for de novo synthesis of telomeric DNA [4]	(4) Theimer CA, Feigon J. Structure and function of telomerase RNA. Curr Opin Struct Biol. 2006;16(3):307–18. https://doi.org/10.1016/j.sbi.2006.05.005
Ribonuclease P	RPPH1	341	RNA component of ribonuclease P [5]	(5) Altman S, Ribonuclease P. Philos Trans R Soc Lond B Biol Sci. 2011;366(1580):2936–41. https://doi.org/10.1098/rstb.2011.0142
Regulatory ncRNA				
Small interfering RNAs	siRNA	21–22	Silencing genes in a sequence-specific manner [6]	(6) Dana H, Chalbatani GM, Gharagouzlo E. Molecular mechanisms and biological functions of siRNA. Int J Biomed Sci. 2017;13(2):48–57. Available on: https://www.ncbi.nlm.nih.gov/pmc/articles/PMC5542916/#__ffn_sectitle
MicroRNAs	miRNA	20–23	Regulating gene expression [7]	(7) MacFarlane L-A, Murphy PR. MicroRNA: Biogenesis, function and role in cancer. Curr Genomics. 2010;11(7):537–61. https://doi.org/10.2174/138920210793175895
Piwi-interacting RNAs	piRNA	25–33	Repress transposons and maintain germline genome integrity [8]	(8) Iwasaki YW, Siomi MC, Siomi H. PIWI-Interacting RNA: its biogenesis and functions. Ann Rev Biochem. 2015;84:405–33. d https://doi.org/10.1146/annurev-biochem-060614-034258
Promoter-associated RNAs	paRNA	<200	Regulating gene expression [9]	(9) Yan BX, Ma JX. Promoter-associated RNAs and promoter-targeted RNAs. Cell Mol Life Sci. 2012;69(17):2833–42. https://doi.org/10.1007/s00018-012-0953-1
Long noncoding RNAs	lncRNA	>200	Various [10]	(10) Ahmad Bhat S, Mudasir Ahmad S, et al. Long non-coding RNAs: mechanism of action and functional utility, Non-coding RNA Res. 2016;1(1):43–50. https://doi.org/10.1016/j.ncrna.2016.11.002

sion of the factors CDKN1A (p21Waf1/Cip1) and BCL2L11 (Bim) is altered. Finally, CDKN1A and BCL2L11 disrupted the G1/S checkpoint and conferred resistance to TGF-β-dependent apoptosis, respectively (Fig. 11.1) [22].

A different example can be given by miRNA-9, which is downregulated in GC. A direct target of the miRNA-9 molecule is the nuclear factor of kappa light polypeptide gene enhancer in B-cells 1 (NF-κB1). A study conducted by Wan et al. has

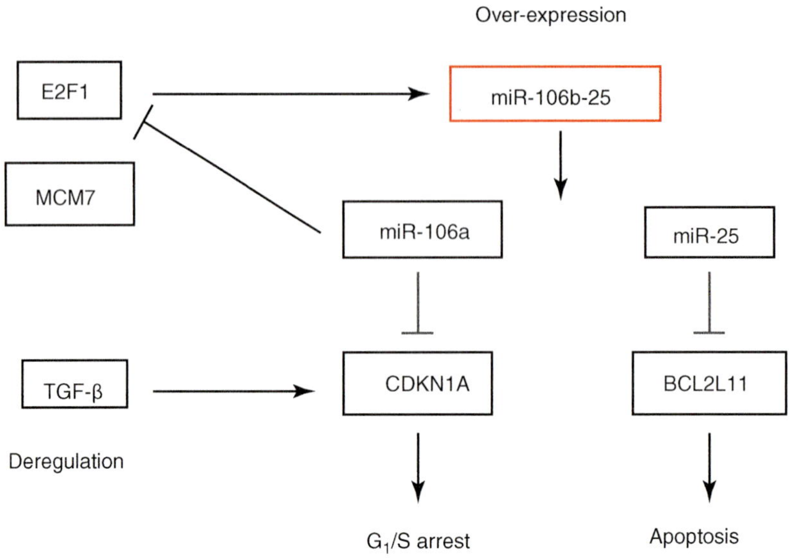

Fig. 11.1 Functions of microRNA-106b-25. miRNA-106b-25 interferes with the expression of CDKN1 and BCL2L11. The interaction of miRNA-106b-25 with E2F1 and transforming growth factor-β (TGF-β) affects the cell cycle and apoptosis

shown that cell growth and proliferation were significantly inhibited by overexpression of miR-9 that not only inversely regulates endogenous NF-κB1 protein expression but also reduces endogenous NF-κB1 mRNA levels [23].

In a more recent study by Tae-Su Han and his colleagues, several GC-specific miRNAs have been identified through comprehensive miRNA profiling using a next-generation sequencing (NGS) platform. It was discovered that miR-29c expression was downregulated in GC tissues. Moreover, a tumor suppressor role was identified for miR-29c, which regulates its downstream target gene, ITGB1, in GC. The suppression of miR-29c is an early event in gastric carcinogenesis [24].

Chemotherapeutic resistance is a big problem that has not yet been solved in GC treatment. Multiple reports have suggested that miRNAs are associated with the sensitivity of GC cell lines to chemotherapy. For example, miR-375 was conspicuously downregulated in cisplatin (DDP)-resistant cells compared with the DDP-sensitive human GC cell line. Western blot analyses showed that upregulation of miR-375 increased GC cell sensitivity to DDP treatment by targeting ERBB2 and phosphorylated Akt. The antiproliferative and apoptosis-inducing effects of DDP could be reversed by reducing the level of miR-375 [25].

Many other miRNAs, like miR-448, miR-15a, and miR-485-5p, were found to suppress proliferation, invasion, or migration in GC cell lines via their target genes such as IGF1R, Bmi1, and Flot1, respectively [26–28].

Other miRNAs, such as miR-1290 and miR-543, could promote gastric tumor cell proliferation or metastasis by targeting their downstream genes FOXA1 and SIRT1 [29, 30].

lncRNA in GC

lncRNAs are the largest class of ncRNAs ranging from 200 nt to several kilobases in length. It is possible to classify them into different groups based on their genomic localization, mode of action, and function. On the base of their genomic location, five main types can be distinguished: antisense, intronic, intergenic, bidirectional, and sense-overlapping lncRNAs. Based on their mode of action on DNA sequences, there are two classes of lncRNAs: cis-acting lncRNAs and trans-acting lncRNAs. Functionally, lncRNAs may be grouped into four types: signaling, decoy, guide, and scaffold (Fig. 11.2) [6, 31]. lncRNAs take part in various cellular and physiological processes such as gene regulation, genomic imprinting, chromatin packaging, dosage compensation, cell differentia-

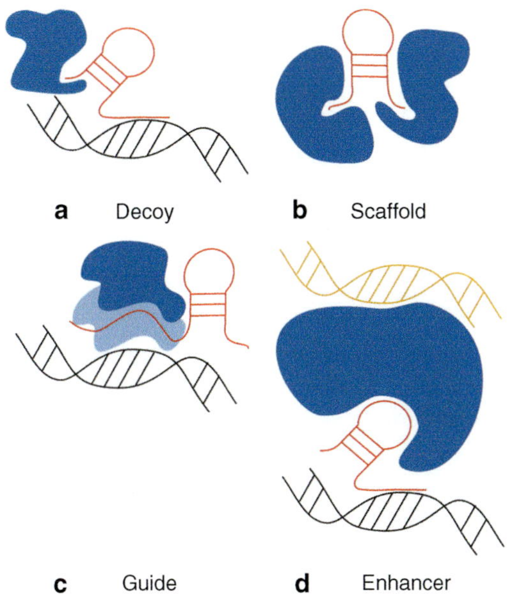

Fig. 11.2 Four types of lncRNA mechanisms: (**a**) The lncRNAs can act as decoys, titrating away DNA-binding proteins (e.g., transcription factors); (**b**) lncRNAs may act as scaffolds to bring two or more proteins to spatial proximity or into a complex; (**c**) lncRNAs may act as guides to recruit proteins to DNA (e.g., chromatin modification enzymes); and (**d**) lncRNA guidance can also be exerted through chromosome looping in an enhancer-like model in cis. lncRNA (red), DNA (black), section of DNA loop (yellow), DNA-binding proteins (blue). (Source: Luka Bolha et al. [31], Article ID 7243968, 14 pages, Fig. 1, https://doi.org/10.1155/2017/7243968, an open access article distributed under the Creative Commons Attribution License)

tion, and embryonic development [6]. Being pivotal regulators of gene expression, alterations of lncRNA can be found in different diseases including cancer. In fact, they influence the main mechanisms related to cancer including proliferation, apoptosis, invasion, and metastasis as well as neoangiogenesis [9].

lncRNAs expression profiling in a variety of cancer types has revealed a broad range of lncRNAs with aberrant expression.

lncRNA Upregulated in GC

Ak058003 is transcribed from its locus at chromosome 10q22, and it has a length of 1197 base pairs (bp). Wang et al. have discovered that the expression of Ak058003 increased during hypoxia. Moreover, this lncRNA is upregulated in GC, and its elevated level is accompanied by an increase in cell migration in vivo and in vitro. Furthermore, this lncRNA targets the γ-synuclein (SNCG), a prometastatic oncogene. Increased AK058003 expression decreases SNCG promoter methylation and consequently upregulates the expression of this oncogene, which promotes hypoxia-induced GC cell metastasis [32].

ANRIL is transcribed in an antisense direction by a locus located on 9p21.3 [33]. It has been shown that ANRIL can act as a scaffold or guide to chromatin [34]. According to recent studies, ANRIL binds to PRC2 and epigenetically represses the expression of miR-99a and miR-449a. In GC, the levels of ANRIL and miR-99a/miR-449a are inversely related so that the expression of these two miRNAs is decreased and the level of ANRIL expression is high in GC samples. This leads to a high tumor-node-metastasis (TNM) stage and tumor size [35].

BANCR The BRAF-activated noncoding RNA (BANCR) gene is located on 9q21.1 and contains four exons. It encodes a lncRNA with a length of 693 bp. BANCR expression is elevated in many GC tissues and cell lines. It has been assessed that this lncRNA influences GC cell growth and apoptosis through regulating NF-κB1 expression via miR-9. Upregulation of BANCR contributes to a decline in NF-κB1 expression that leads to an increase in cell numbers and a decrease in apoptosis in GC cells [36]. Several studies have shown that overexpression of BANCR in GC tissues is correlated with clinical stage, lymph node, and distant metastases [37].

CCAT1 Colon cancer-associated transcript 1 (CCAT1) is 2628 nt long, and its gene is located at 8q24 [38]. CCAT1 is overexpressed in some GC tissues with a significant correlation with primary tumor growth, lymph node, and distant metastases. c-Myc oncogene physically interacts with E-box element in the CCAT1 promoter and increases its expression. In vitro, CCAT1 regulates cell proliferation and migration [39]. Other studies have demonstrated that CCAT1 activates the ERK/MAPK pathway and suppresses cell cycle arrest and apoptosis.

GACAT3 Located at 2p24, GACAT3 encodes a lncRNA of 1096 nt in length. It was observed that it is upregulated in GC tissues and this upregulation is positively correlated with TNM stages, tumor size, and distant metastasis [40].

H19 As a maternally imprinted gene, H19 is located on 11p15.5. H19 plays an important role during embryogenesis, and its expression is low in most adult tissues except for cardiac and skeletal muscles [41, 42]. It is associated with p53 protein, and reciprocally, p53 protein has repressing effects on H19 levels [43, 44]. H19 gene contains a 23 nt RNA, miR-675 [45]. It has been shown that H19 works via its miR-675 product to silence the transcription factor RUNX1, a tumor suppressor in GC, in turn inducing cell proliferation [41]. The amount of H19 and miR-675 is increased in GC tissues with a significant correlation with lymph node metastases and clinical stage [46]. H19 and miR-675 have different targets, but they both function as oncogenes to increase proliferation, migration, invasion, and metastases in human GC [47].

HOTAIR HOX transcript antisense RNA (HOTAIR) is transcribed from 12q13.13 and plays an important role in GC progression [48]; for this reason it is one of the most studied lncRNAs. HOTAIR is expressed from the HOXC locus, and its length is of 2158 nt [49]. Functioning as a scaffold, HOTAIR is involved in epigenetic silencing. It directs polycomb repression complex 2 (PRC2) to trimethylate histone H3 lysine-27 of specific HOXD genes and thus repressing their expression.

It is believed that HOTAIR can promote metastasis through this pathway by inhibiting certain metastasis suppressor genes [50]. It has been demonstrated that HOTAIR expression is markedly raised in GC tissues, which is associated with poor prognosis, higher TNM stage, perineural invasion, larger tumor size, and lymph node and distant metastases [49, 51].

MALAT1 Encoded at chromosome 11q13 with 8000 nt in length, metastasis-associated lung adenocarcinoma transcript 1 (MALAT1) is a lncRNA [52, 53]. It was observed that MALAT1 is overexpressed in GC tissues, which correlates with peritoneal metastasis in patients [54]. Furthermore, MALAT1 increases cellular proliferation by regulating alternative splicing factor 1 (ASF1) and pre-mRNA-splicing factor (SF2) (SF2/ASF1) [55]. These proteins are pivotal players in inflammatory disorders and also in cancer [56].

PVT1 Plasmacytoma variant translocation 1 gene (PVT1) is located on human 8q24, 57 kb downstream of c-Myc [57]. The 8q24 region with both genes is involved in a variety of cancer types.

It has been reported that this lncRNA has a role in the suppression of apoptotic genes in different types of cancer. Upregulation of PVT1 is essential for the increased level of c-Myc in cancer cells [58]. PVT1 expression is elevated in GC tissues as well. Furthermore, PVT1 may be involved in the silencing process of *CDKN2B/p15* and *CDKN2A/p16* genes through its association with EZH2 during the progression of GC [59]. Its overexpression is linked to lymph node metastases [57].

UCA1 Urothelial carcinoma associated 1 (UCA1) is located on 19p13.12, and it contains three exons [60]. UCA1 presents higher expression in GC tissues and cell lines. The expression was associated with tumor size, worse differentiation, invasion depth, and TNM stages. Analyses conducted in GC have reported that excessive amount of UCA1 correlates with poor overall survival and disease-free survival in patients [61].

lncRNA Downregulated in GC

AA174084 is a lncRNA downregulated in GC tissues compared with adjacent normal tissues. Studies conducted on samples of gastric juice in patients with gastric ulcer, chronic atrophic gastritis, or GC have shown that levels of this lncRNA were highest in GC patients, suggesting its potential value as a GC biomarker. AA174084 expression levels in GC tissues were associated with age, Borrmann type, and perineural invasion. Expression in gastric juice was associated with tumor size, tumor stage, Lauren type, and CEA levels. Overall, the current data show that the AA174084 level in gastric juice may be used as a screening biomarker for detecting GC at early stages [62].

FENDRR FOXF1 adjacent noncoding developmental regulatory RNA (FENDRR) is located on 16q24.1 and contains seven exons. Through binding to PRC2 and/or TrxG/MLL complexes, FENDRR lncRNA regulates histone methylation and chromatin structure [63]. Furthermore, FENDRR is diminished in GC tissues and cell lines, which correlate with depth of invasion, advanced tumor stage, and lymphatic metastasis.

FER1L4 Fer-1-like protein 4 (FER1L4) is located at 20q11. Its expression is reduced in GC tissues, and it is correlated with histological grade, tumor size, severity of invasion, vessel or nerve invasion, and lymph node and distant metastases [64]. FER1L4 is one of the targets of miR-106a-5p. Low quantity of this lncRNA increases the amount of free miR-106a-5p, making it more available for its targets such as the retinoblastoma gene, *RB1* [65].

GACAT2 Gastric cancer-associated transcript 2 (GACAT2) is encoded at 18p11, and it has a length of 818 nt. GACAT2 is markedly decreased in GC tissues and cell lines, which is associated with distal metastasis and neural and blood vessel invasion in GC tissues [66].

MEG3 Maternally expressed gene 3 (MEG3) is a tumor suppressor lncRNA transcribed from an imprinted gene cluster at 14q32, with a length of 1700 nt [67]. It has been demonstrated a significant decrease of MEG3 levels in GC tissues, and this was linked with TNM stage, tumor size, depth of invasion, and shorter overall survival time in GC patients [68].

MT1JP Metallothionein 1 J gene is located on 16q13. It has considerably lower expression in GC tissue samples than in matched normal tissues. Zhongchuan et al. have demonstrated that MT1JP is necessary for maintaining the normal life activities of cells and played a critical function as a tumor suppressor. lncRNA MT1JP is involved in many steps of tumor progression, including cell proliferation, migration, and invasion. For this reason, it may be a potential diagnostic marker and could have a potential therapeutic value in the prevention of GC [2].

ncRuPAR Noncoding RNA upstream of the PAR-1 (ncRuPAR) [69] increases the expression of protease activator-1 (PAR1) during embryonic growth. The study conducted by Liu et al. reports that it works as a tumor suppressor in cancer.

Its gene is located on human 5q13. Decreased expression of this lncRNA in GC samples was inversely correlated with the amount of PAR-1. Its level was negatively associated with tumor size, tumor invasion depth, lymph node, and distant metastases [70].

TUSC7 Tumor suppressor candidate 7 (TUSC7) is located on 3q13.31 and contains four exons. Some studies have reported that TUSC7 is downregulated in GC tissues contributing to an augmentation in cell growth. In addition, p53 is a regulator of TUSC7 in GC, and *TP53* mutations or deletions are the likely cause of TUSC7 downregulation. Furthermore, TUSC7 negatively regulates the level of miR-23b, which promotes cell growth in GC samples [71].

miRNA as Biomarker in GC

Numerous miRNAs are aberrantly expressed in the plasma and serum of GC patients [72–74]. For example, miR223, miR-233, miR-378, miR-421, miR-451, miR-4865p, and miR-199-3p are overexpressed in sera of GC patients [75–78]. Wang et al. found that miR-233 was overexpressed in GC patient sera, and its level was positively associated with tumor differentiation grade, TNM stage, tumor size, and metastasis status [75].

Wu et al. found that miR-421 was overexpressed in 90 cases of GC patient sera compared to 90 controls. The high expression of miR-421 in cancer cells acts as a biomarker for GC circulating tumor cells, which may be used for early diagnosis for gastric metastasis [76]. Furthermore, in vivo and in vitro experiments demonstrated that the onco-miR-421 promotes tumor proliferation, invasion, and metastasis but had no significant association with the clinic-pathological features [79, 80].

In contrast, the expression of miRNAs such as let-7a, miR-375, miR-20a-5p, and miR-320 was relatively reduced in GC patient sera [81, 82]. A study demonstrated that let-7a exhibited relatively low expression in plasma of GC patients compared with healthy controls, whereas the expression of miR-17-5p, miR-106a, miR-106b, and miR-21 was significantly elevated in GC plasma [83]. Other studies demonstrated that miR375 was suppressed in GC. Overexpression of miR-375 suppresses GC progression by targeting p53, JAK2, ERBB2, and STAT3 [84, 85]. These studies indicate that miRNA could be useful diagnostic biomarkers. However, large-scale clinical research is needed to demonstrate that miRNA can serve as a diagnostic biomarker for GC.

Several studies have demonstrated that miRNAs could be used not only as biomarkers but also as potential therapeutic targets for cancer. miRNA-based drugs that act by suppressing miRNAs or inhibit the onco-miRNAs can inhibit tumor progression by suppressing the relative signal pathway [86, 87]. For example, miR-34 is one of the most characterized tumor suppressor miRNAs in a variety of tumors including GC. In literature, it is reported that it is lost or expressed at minimum levels in numerous tumor tissues, and the reintroduction of miR-34 mimics was found to inhibit cancer cell growth both in vitro and in vivo. Therefore, miR-34a has proved to be a tumor suppressor in cancer cells and an ideal therapeutic tool to reduce metastasis, chemoresistance, and tumor recurrence [88–90].

However, some problems should be considered; as one miRNA can target multiple genes and signaling, the off-target effect is not easily predictable. Thus, miRNA therapy needs more detailed studies [91].

lncRNA as Biomarkers in GC

In recent years, detection of cancer-associated lncRNAs in body fluids of cancer patients has proven itself as a valuable method to effectively diagnose cancer. Cancer diagnosis and prognosis through the use of circulating lncRNAs are preferred when compared to classical biopsies of tumor tissues, because of their noninvasiveness and great potential for routine applications in clinical practice.

Among main advantages of lncRNAs, which make them suitable as cancer diagnostic and prognostic biomarkers, is their high stability while circulating in body fluids, especially when included in exosomes or apoptotic bodies [92]. It has been shown that lncRNAs are able to resist the multiple ribonucleases in body fluids [93]. In addition, lncRNA deregulation in primary tumor tissues is clearly mirrored in various bodily fluids, including whole blood, plasma, urine, saliva, and gastric juice [94, 95]. These characteristics make the lncRNAs of potential prognostic and predictive biomarkers for GC, easy to take and evaluate, bringing great benefits to patients compared to a classic tissue biopsy [96].

The detection of circulating lncRNAs could represent an excellent method in the evaluation of cancer to distinguish tumor patients from healthy people at early stages with both high sensitivity and specificity. In addition, the prognosis of tumor patients and the risk of tumor metastasis and recurrence after surgery could be assessed [93]. Good results have been obtained from the diagnostic performances of lncRNAs BANCR, H19, CCAT, and AA174084 evaluated in body fluid samples (e.g., plasma and gastric juice) of GC patients. These lncRNAs had the ability to differentiate GC patients from healthy individuals and to effectively detect different stages of GC (from early to metastatic cancer forms). However, despite their overall positive diagnostic performances, similar to those obtained by several conventional cancer biomarkers, false-positive and false-negative detections were observed [95, 97, 98].

Stability of lncRNAs in body fluids of tumor patients has not been thoroughly explored. Studies revealed that some lncRNAs remained stable in plasma under extreme conditions, such as several freeze-thawed cycles and prolonged incubation at elevated temperatures [99]. So far, three mechanisms have been identified by which lncRNAs are released into body fluids. First, extracellular RNAs may package themselves into specific membrane vesicles, such as exosomes and microvesicles, in order to be secreted and resist to RNase activity. Different studies revealed that exosomes most frequently protect plasma lncRNAs [100–103]. Second, extracellular RNAs can be actively released by tumor tissues and cells [104]. Third, extracellular RNAs may encapsulate themselves into high-density lipoprotein (HDL) or apoptotic bodies or be associated with protein complexes, for example, Argonaute (Ago)-miRNA complex and nucleophosmin 1 (NPM1)-miRNA complex [105, 106]. However, despite many performed studies, secretion and transport mechanisms of lncRNAs to the circulation system remain yet poorly understood.

In order to introduce circulating lncRNAs into clinical practice, further studies and improvements should be performed regarding the standardization of sample preparation protocols and the extraction methods [93].

Conclusion

In recent years, the role of ncRNAs in GC has been clarified. Multiple studies have already demonstrated the potential clinical applications of several ncRNAs in GC diagnosis and prognosis. Circulating ncRNAs are regarded as an emerging biomarker for GC, but the applications of circulating ncRNAs need to be further investigated because of the interactions between ncRNAs and GC that are very complex.

Among these, several ncRNAs are promising neoplastic biomarkers to be detected in the patient's body fluids, including miR-34, H19, HOTAIR, MALAT1, UCA1, and AA174084. For many of these ncRNAs, it has been proven that they could be used in clinical practice as diagnostic and prognostic GC biomarkers. ncRNA research will likely take a big step forward with the identification of more molecules in the next years.

References

1. Anvara MS, Minuchehra Z, Shahlaeib M, Kheitana S. Gastric cancer biomarkers; A systems biology approach; 2405–5808/ © 2018 Published by Elsevier B.V. https://doi.org/10.1016/j.bbrep.2018.01.001.
2. Lv Z, Zhang Y, Yu X, Lin Y, Ge Y. The function of long non-coding RNA MT1JP in the development and progression of gastric cancer. Pathol Res Pract. 2018;214(8):1218–23. https://doi.org/10.1016/j.prp.2018.07.001.
3. Yan X, Hu Z, Feng Y, Hu X, Yuan J, Zhao SD, Zhang Y, Yang L, Shan W, He Q, Fan L, Kandalaft LE, Tanyi JL, Li C, Yuan CX, Zhang D, Yuan H, Hua K, Lu Y, Katsaros D, Huang Q, Montone K, Fan Y, Coukos G, Boyd J, Sood AK, Rebbeck T, Mills GB, Dang CV, Zhang L. Comprehensive genomic characterization of long non-coding RNAs across human cancers. Cancer Cell. 2015;28:529–40. https://doi.org/10.1016/j.ccell.2015.09.006.
4. Ezkurdia I, Juan D, Rodriguez JM, Frankish A, Diekhans M, Harrow J, Vazquez J, Valencia A, Tress ML. Multiple evidence strands suggest that there may be as few as 19,000 human protein-coding genes. Hum Mol Genet. 2014;23:5866–78. https://doi.org/10.1093/hmg/ddu309.
5. Consortium EP. An integrated encyclopedia of DNA elements in the human genome. Nature. 2012;489(7414):57–74. Available on: https://www.nature.com/articles/nature11247
6. Bhan A, Mandal SS. Long noncoding RNAs: emerging stars in gene regulation, epigenetics and human disease. ChemMedChem. 2014;9(9):1932–56. https://doi.org/10.1002/cmdc.201300534. Epub 2014 Mar 26.
7. Amaral PP, Dinger ME, Mercer TR, Mattick JS. The eukaryotic genome as an RNA machine. Science. 2008;319:1787–9. https://doi.org/10.1126/science.1155472.
8. Taft RJ, Pang KC, Mercer TR, Dinger M, Mattick JS. Non-coding RNAs: regulators of disease. J Pathol. 2010;220:126–39. https://doi.org/10.1002/path.2638.
9. Zhao J, Liu Y, Huang G, et al. Long non-coding RNAs in gastric cancer: versatile mechanisms and potential for clinical translation. Am J Cancer Res. 2015;5(3):907–27. Available on: https://www.ncbi.nlm.nih.gov/pmc/articles/PMC4449426/#__ffn_sectitle
10. Yang G, Lu X, Yuan L. LncRNA: a link between RNA and cancer. Biochim Biophys Acta. 2014;1839(11):1097–109. https://doi.org/10.1016/j.bbagrm.2014.08.012. Epub 2014 Aug 23
11. Kahlert C, Kalluri R. Exosomes in tumor microenvironment influence cancer progression and metastasis. J Mol Med (Berl). 2013;91:431–7. https://doi.org/10.1007/s00109-013-1020-6.
12. Li PF, Chen SC, Xia T, Jiang XM, Shao YF, Xiao BX, Guo JM. Non-coding RNAs and gastric cancer. World J Gastroenterol. 2014;20:5411–9. https://doi.org/10.3748/wjg.v20.i18.5411.
13. Place RF, Noonan EJ. Non-coding RNAs turn up the heat: an emerging layer of novel regulators in the mammalian heat shock response. Cell Stress Chaperones. 2014;19:159–72. https://doi.org/10.1007/s12192-013-0456-5.
14. Gomes AQ, Nolasco S, Soares H. Non-coding RNAs: multi-tasking molecules in the cell. Int J Mol

Sci. 2013;14:16010–39. https://doi.org/10.3390/ijms140816010.
15. Zhang XM, Ma ZW, Wang Q, Wang JN, Yang JW, Li XD, Li H, Men TY. A new RNA-seq method to detect the transcription and non-coding RNA in prostate cancer. Pathol Oncol Res. 2014;20:43–50. https://doi.org/10.1007/s12253-013-9618-0.
16. Lv J, Liu H, Huang Z, Su J, He H, Xiu Y, Zhang Y, Wu Q. Long non-coding RNA identification over mouse brain development by integrative modeling of chromatin and genomic features. Nucleic Acids Res. 2013;41:10044–61. https://doi.org/10.1093/nar/gkt818.
17. Kim VN, Nam JW. Genomics of microRNA. Trends Genet. 2006;22:165–73. https://doi.org/10.1016/j.tig.2006.01.003.
18. Singh TR, Gupta A, Suravajhala P. Challenges in the miRNA research. Int J Bioinforma Res Appl. 2013;9:576–83. https://doi.org/10.1504/IJBRA.2013.056620.
19. Zhang Y, Wang Z, Gemeinhart RA. Progress in microRNA delivery. J Control Release. 2013;172:962–74. https://doi.org/10.1016/j.jconrel.2013.09.015.
20. Lee Y, Ahn C, Han J, Choi H, Kim J, Yim J, Lee J, Provost P, Rådmark O, Kim S, et al. The nuclear RNase III Drosha initiates microRNA processing. Nature. 2003;425:415–9. https://doi.org/10.1038/nature01957.
21. Lund E, Güttinger S, Calado A, Dahlberg JE, Kutay U. Nuclear export of microRNA precursors. Science. 2004;303:95–8. https://doi.org/10.1126/science.1090599.
22. Petrocca F, Visone R, Onelli MR, Shah MH, Nicoloso MS, de Martino I, Iliopoulos D, Pilozzi E, Liu CG, Negrini M, et al. E2F1-regulated microRNAs impair TGFbeta-dependent cell-cycle arrest and apoptosis in gastric cancer. Cancer Cell. 2008;13:272–86. https://doi.org/10.1016/j.ccr.2008.02.013.
23. Wan HY, Guo LM, Liu T, Liu M, Li X, Tang H. Regulation of the transcription factor NF-kappaB1 by microRNA-9 in human gastric adenocarcinoma. Mol Cancer. 2010;9:16. https://doi.org/10.1186/1476-4598-9-16.
24. Han TS, Hur K, Xu G, Choi B, Okugawa Y, Toiyama Y, Oshima H, Oshima M, Lee HJ, Kim VN, et al. MicroRNA-29c mediates initiation of gastric carcinogenesis by directly targeting ITGB1. Gut. 2015;64:203–14. https://doi.org/10.1136/gutjnl-2013-306640.
25. Zhou N, Qu Y, Xu C, Tang Y. Upregulation of microRNA-375 increases the cisplatin-sensitivity of human gastric cancer cells by regulating ERBB2. Exp Ther Med. 2016;11:625–30. https://doi.org/10.3892/etm.2015.2920.
26. Wu X, Tang H, Liu G, Wang H, Shu J, Sun F. miR-448 suppressed gastric cancer proliferation and invasion by regulating ADAM10. Tumour Biol. 2016. Epub ahead of print; https://doi.org/10.1007/s13277-016-4942-0.
27. Wu C, Zheng X, Li X, Fesler A, Hu W, Chen L, Xu B, Wang Q, Tong A, Burke S, et al. Reduction of gastric cancer proliferation and invasion by miR-15a mediated suppression of Bmi-1 translation. Oncotarget. 2016;7:14522–36. https://doi.org/10.18632/oncotarget.7392.
28. Kang M, Ren MP, Zhao L, Li CP, Deng MM. miR-485-5p acts as a negative regulator in gastric cancer progression by targeting flotillin-1. Am J Transl Res. 2015;7:2212–22. Available on: https://www.ncbi.nlm.nih.gov/pmc/articles/PMC4697701/
29. Lin M, Shi C, Lin X, Pan J, Shen S, Xu Z, Chen Q. sMicroRNA-1290 inhibits cells proliferation and migration by targeting FOXA1 in gastric cancer cells. Gene. 2016;582:137–42. https://doi.org/10.1016/j.gene.2016.02.001.
30. Li J, Dong G, Wang B, Gao W, Yang Q. miR-543 promotes gastric cancer cell proliferation by targeting SIRT1. Biochem Biophys Res Commun. 2016;469:15–21. https://doi.org/10.1016/j.bbrc.2015.11.062.
31. Bolha L, Ravnik-Glavač M, Glavač D. Long Noncoding RNAs as Biomarkers in Cancer. Dis Markers. 2017;2017, 7243968:14. https://doi.org/10.1155/2017/7243968
32. Wang Y, Liu X, Zhang H, et al. Hypoxia-inducible lncRNA-AK058003 promotes gastric cancer metastasis by targeting gamma-synuclein. Neoplasia. 2014;16(12):1094–106. https://doi.org/10.1016/j.neo.2014.10.008.
33. Kotake Y, Nakagawa T, Kitagawa K, Suzuki S, Liu N, Kitagawa M, Xiong Y. Long non-coding RNA ANRIL is required for the PRC2 recruitment to and silencing of p15(INK4B) tumor suppressor gene. Oncogene. 2011 Apr 21;30(16):1956–62. https://doi.org/10.1038/onc.2010.568.
34. Holdt LM, Hoffmann S, Sass K, Langenberger D, Scholz M, Krohn K, Finstermeier K, Stahringer A, Wilfert W, Beutner F, Gielen S, Schuler G, Gäbel G, Bergert H, Bechmann I, Stadler PF, Thiery J, Teupser D. Alu elements in ANRIL non-coding RNA at chromosome 9p21 modulate atherogenic cell functions through trans-regulation of gene networks. PLoS Genet. 2013;9(7):e1003588. https://doi.org/10.1371/journal.pgen.1003588.
35. Zhang EB, Kong R, Yin DD, et al. Long noncoding RNA ANRIL indicates a poor prognosis of gastric cancer and promotes tumor growth by epigenetically silencing of miR-99a/miR-449a. Oncotarget. 2014;5(8):2276–92. https://doi.org/10.18632/oncotarget.1902.
36. Zhang ZX, Liu ZQ, Jiang B, et al. BRAF activated non-coding RNA (BANCR) promoting gastric cancer cells proliferation via regulation of NF-kappaB1. Biochem Biophys Res Commun. 2015;465(2):225–31. https://doi.org/10.1016/j.bbrc.2015.07.158.
37. Li L, Zhang L, Zhang Y, et al. Increased expression of LncRNA BANCR is associated with clinical progression and poor prognosis in gastric cancer. Biomed Pharmacother. 2015;72:109–12. https://doi.org/10.1016/j.biopha.2015.04.007.

38. Nissan A, Stojadinovic A, Mitrani-Rosenbaum S, et al. Colon cancer associated transcript-1: a novel RNA expressed in malignant and pre-malignant human tissues. Int J Cancer. 2012;130(7):1598–606. https://doi.org/10.1002/ijc.26170.
39. Yang F, Xue X, Bi J, et al. Long noncoding RNA CCAT1, which could be activated by c-Myc, promotes the progression of gastric carcinoma. J Cancer Res Clin Oncol. 2013;139(3):437–45. https://doi.org/10.1007/s00432-012-1324-x.
40. Shen W, Yuan Y, Zhao M, Li J, Xu J, Lou G, Zheng J, Bu S, Guo J, Xi Y. Novel long non-coding RNA GACAT3 promotes gastric cancer cell proliferation through the IL-6/STAT3 signaling pathway. Tumour Biol. 2016;37(11):14895–902. https://doi.org/10.1007/s13277-016-5372-8.
41. Zhuang M, Gao W, Xu J, et al. The long non-coding RNA H19-derived miR-675 modulates human gastric cancer cell proliferation by targeting tumor suppressor RUNX1. Biochem Biophys Res Commun. 2014;448(3):315–22. https://doi.org/10.1016/j.bbrc.2013.12.126.
42. Zhang EB, Han L, Yin DD, et al. c-Myc-induced, long, noncoding H19 affects cell proliferation and predicts a poor prognosis in patients with gastric cancer. Med Oncol. 2014;31(5):914. https://doi.org/10.1007/s12032-014-0914-7.
43. Yang F, Bi J, Xue X, et al. Up-regulated long non-coding RNA H19 contributes to proliferation of gastric cancer cells. FEBS J. 2012;279(17):3159–65. https://doi.org/10.1111/j.1742-4658.2012.08694.x.
44. Dugimont T, Montpellier C, Adriaenssens E, et al. The H19 TATA-less promoter is efficiently repressed by wild-type tumor suppressor gene product p53. Oncogene. 1998;16(18):2395–401. https://doi.org/10.1038/sj.onc.1201742.
45. Zhang Y, Ma M, Liu W, et al. Enhanced expression of long noncoding RNA CARLo-5 is associated with the development of gastric cancer. Int J Clin Exp Pathol. 2014;7(12):8471–9. Available on: https://www.ncbi.nlm.nih.gov/pmc/articles/PMC4314006/#__ffn_sectitle
46. Cai X, Cullen BR. The imprinted H19 noncoding RNA is a primary microRNA precursor. RNA. 2007;13(3):313–6. https://doi.org/10.1261/rna.351707.
47. Luo J, Tang L, Zhang J, et al. Long non-coding RNA CARLo-5 is a negative prognostic factor and exhibits tumor pro-oncogenic activity in non-small cell lung cancer. Tumour Biol. 2014;35(11):11541–9. https://doi.org/10.1007/s13277-014-2442-7.
48. Pan W, Liu L, Wei J, et al. A functional lncRNA HOTAIR genetic variant contributes to gastric cancer susceptibility. Mol Carcinog. 2016;55:90–6. https://doi.org/10.1002/mc.22261.
49. Emadi-Andani E, Nikpour P, Emadi-Baygi M, et al. Association of HOTAIR expression in gastric carcinoma with invasion and distant metastasis. Adv Biomed Res. 2014;3:135. https://doi.org/10.4103/2277-9175.133278.
50. Endo H, Shiroki T, Nakagawa T, et al. Enhanced expression of long non-coding RNA HOTAIR is associated with the development of gastric cancer. PLoS One. 2013;8(10):e77070. https://doi.org/10.1371/journal.pone.0077070.
51. Liu XH, Sun M, Nie FQ, et al. Lnc RNA HOTAIR functions as a competing endogenous RNA to regulate HER2 expression by sponging miR-331-3p in gastric cancer. Mol Cancer. 2014;13:92. https://doi.org/10.1186/1476-4598-13-92.
52. Gutschner T, Hammerle M, Diederichs S. MALAT1 – a paradigm for long noncoding RNA function in cancer. J Mol Med (Berl). 2013;91(7):791–801. https://doi.org/10.1007/s00109-013-1028-y.
53. Ji P, Diederichs S, Wang W, et al. MALAT-1, a novel noncoding RNA, and thymosin beta4 predict metastasis and survival in early-stage non-small cell lung cancer. Oncogene. 2003;22(39):8031–41. https://doi.org/10.1038/sj.onc.1206928.
54. Okugawa Y, Toiyama Y, Hur K, et al. Metastasis-associated long non-coding RNA drives gastric cancer development and promotes peritoneal metastasis. Carcinogenesis. 2014;35(12):2731–9. https://doi.org/10.1093/carcin/bgu200.
55. Wang J, Su L, Chen X, et al. MALAT1 promotes cell proliferation in gastric cancer by recruiting SF2/ASF. Biomed Pharmacother. 2014;68(5):557–64. https://doi.org/10.1016/j.biopha.2014.04.007.
56. Chalaris A, Garbers C, Rabe B, et al. The soluble Interleukin 6 receptor: generation and role in inflammation and cancer. Eur J Cell Biol. 2011;90(6–7):484–94. https://doi.org/10.1016/j.ejcb.2010.10.007.
57. Ding J, Li D, Gong M, et al. Expression and clinical significance of the long non-coding RNA PVT1 in human gastric cancer. Onco Targets Ther. 2014;7:1625–30. https://doi.org/10.2147/OTT.S68854.
58. Tseng YY, Moriarity BS, Gong W, et al. PVT1 dependence in cancer with MYC copy-number increase. Nature. 2014;512(7512):82–6. https://doi.org/10.1038/nature13311.
59. Kong R, Zhang EB, Yin DD, et al. Long noncoding RNA PVT1 indicates a poor prognosis of gastric cancer and promotes cell proliferation through epigenetically regulating p15 and p16. Mol Cancer. 2015;14:82. https://doi.org/10.1186/s12943-015-0355-8.
60. Wang XS, Zhang Z, Wang HC, et al. Rapid identification of UCA1 as a very sensitive and specific unique marker for human bladder carcinoma. Clin Cancer Res. 2006;12(16):4851–8. https://doi.org/10.1158/1078-0432.
61. Zheng Q, Wu F, Dai WY, et al. Aberrant expression of UCA1 in gastric cancer and its clinical significance. Clin Transl Oncol. 2015;17(8):640–6. https://doi.org/10.1007/s12094-015-1290-2.
62. ShaoY YM, Jiang X, et al. Gastric juice long noncoding RNA used as a tumor marker for screening gastric cancer. Cancer. 2014;120(21):3320–8. https://doi.org/10.1002/cncr.28882.

63. Khalil AM, Guttman M, Huarte M, et al. Many human large intergenic noncoding RNAs associate with chromatin modifying complexes and affect gene expression. Proc Natl Acad Sci U S A. 2009;106(28):11667–72. https://doi.org/10.1073/pnas.0904715106.
64. Liu Z, Shao Y, Tan L, et al. Clinical significance of the low expression of FER1L4 in gastric cancer patients. Tumour Biol. 2014;35(10):9613–7. https://doi.org/10.1007/s13277-014-2259-4.
65. Xia T, Liao Q, Jiang X, et al. Long noncoding RNA associated-competing endogenous RNAs in gastric cancer. Sci Rep. 2014;4:6088. https://doi.org/10.1038/srep06088.
66. Shao Y, Chen H, Jiang X, et al. Low expression of lncRNAHMlincRNA717 in human gastric cancer and its clinical significances. Tumour Biol. 2014;35(10):9591–5. https://doi.org/10.1007/s13277-014-2243-z.
67. Zhang X, Rice K, Wang Y, et al. Maternally expressed gene 3 (MEG3) noncoding ribonucleic acid: isoform structure, expression and functions. Endocrinology. 2010;151(3):939–47. https://doi.org/10.1210/en.2009-0657.
68. Sun M, Xia R, Jin F, et al. Downregulated long noncoding RNA MEG3 is associated with poor prognosis and promotes cell proliferation in gastric cancer. Tumour Biol. 2014;35:1065–73. https://doi.org/10.1007/s13277-013-1142-z.
69. Madamanchi NR, Hu ZY, Li F, et al. A noncoding RNA regulates human protease-activated receptor-1 gene during embryogenesis. Biochim Biophys Acta. 2002;1576(3):237–45. https://doi.org/10.1016/S0167-4781(02)00308-1.
70. Liu L, Yan B, Yang Z, et al. ncRuPAR inhibits gastric cancer progression by down-regulating protease-activated receptor-1. Tumour Biol. 2014;35(8):7821–9. https://doi.org/10.1007/s13277-014-2042-6.
71. Qi P, Xu MD, Shen XH, et al. Reciprocal repression between TUSC7 and miR-23b in gastric cancer. Int J Cancer. 2015;137(6):1269–78. https://doi.org/10.1002/ijc.29516.
72. Liu HS, Xiao HS. MicroRNAs as potential biomarkers for gastric cancer. World J Gastroenterol. 2014;20:12007–17. https://doi.org/10.3748/wjg.v20.i34.12007.
73. Ishiguro H, Kimura M, Takeyama H. Role of microRNAs in gastric cancer. World J Gastroenterol. 2014;20:5694–9. https://doi.org/10.3748/wjg.v20.i19.5694.
74. He Y, Lin J, Kong D, Huang M, Xu C, Kim TK, Etheridge A, Luo Y, Ding Y, Wang K. Current state of circulating microRNAs as cancer biomarkers. Clin Chem. 2015 Sep;61(9):1138–55. https://doi.org/10.1373/clinchem.2015.241190.
75. Wang H, Wang L, Wu Z, Sun R, Jin H, Ma J, Liu L, Ling R, Yi J, Wang L, Bian J, Chen J, Li N, et al. Three dysregulated microRNAs in serum as novel biomarkers for gastric cancer screening. Med Oncol. 2014;31:298. https://doi.org/10.1007/s12032-014-0298-8.
76. Wu J, Li G, Yao Y, Wang Z, Sun W, Wang J. MicroRNA-421 is a new potential diagnosis biomarker with higher sensitivity and specificity than carcinoembryonic antigen and cancer antigen 125 in gastric cancer. Biomarkers. 2015;20:58–63. https://doi.org/10.3109/1354750X.2014.992812
77. Liu H, Zhu L, Liu B, Yang L, Meng X, Zhang W, Ma Y, Xiao H. Genome-wide microRNA profiles identify miR-378 as a serum biomarker for early detection of gastric cancer. Cancer Lett. 2012;316:196–203. https://doi.org/10.1016/j.canlet.2011.10.034.
78. Li BS, Zhao YL, Guo G, Li W, Zhu ED, Luo X, Mao XH, Zou QM, Yu PW, Zuo QF, Li N, Tang B, Liu KY, et al. Plasma microRNAs, miR-223, miR-21 and miR-218, as novel potential biomarkers for gastric cancer detection. PLoS One. 2012;7:e41629. https://doi.org/10.1371/journal.pone.0041629.
79. Zhou H, Xiao B, Zhou F, Deng H, Zhang X, Lou Y, Gong Z, Du C, Guo J. MiR-421 is a functional marker of circulating tumor cells in gastric cancer patients. Biomarkers. 2012;17:104–10. https://doi.org/10.3109/1354750X.2011.614961.
80. Jiang Z, Guo J, Xiao B, Miao Y, Huang R, Li D, Zhang Y. Increased expression of miR-421 in human gastric carcinoma and its clinical association. J Gastroenterol. 2010;45:17–23. https://doi.org/10.1007/s00535-009-0135-6.
81. Zhang WH, Gui JH, Wang CZ, Chang Q, Xu SP, Cai CH, Li YN, Tian YP, Yan L, Wu B. The identification of miR-375 as a potential biomarker in distal gastric adenocarcinoma. Oncol Res. 2012;20:139–14. https://doi.org/10.1007/s10620-013-2970-9.
82. Xu Q, Dong QG, Sun LP, He CY, Yuan Y. Expression of serum miR-20a-5p, let-7a, and miR-320a and their correlations with pepsinogen in atrophic gastritis and gastric cancer: a case-control study. BMC Clin Pathol. 2013;13:11. https://doi.org/10.1186/1472-6890-13-11.
83. Tsujiura M, Ichikawa D, Komatsu S, Shiozaki A, Takeshita H, Kosuga T, Konishi H, Morimura R, Deguchi K, Fujiwara H, Okamoto K, Otsuji E. Circulating microRNAs in plasma of patients with gastric cancers. Br J Cancer. 2010;102:1174–9. https://doi.org/10.1038/sj.bjc.6605608.
84. Huang YK, Yu JC. Circulating microRNAs and long noncoding RNAs in gastric cancer diagnosis: an update and review. World J Gastroenterol. 2015;21:9863–86. https://doi.org/10.3748/wjg.v21.i34.9863.
85. Tang R, Yang C, Ma X, Wang Y, Luo D, Huang C, Xu Z, Liu P, Yang L. MiR-let-7a inhibits cell proliferation, migration, and invasion by down-regulating PKM2 in gastric cancer. Oncotarget. 2016;7:5972–84. https://doi.org/10.18632/oncotarget.6821. https://doi. org/10.3748/wjg.v21.i34.9863.
86. Pichler M, Calin GA. MicroRNAs in cancer: from developmental genes in worms to their clinical

application in patients. Br J Cancer. 2015;113:569–73. https://doi.org/10.1038/bjc.2015.253.
87. Riquelme I, Letelier P, Riffo-Campos AL, Brebi P, Roa JC. Emerging role of miRNAs in the drug resistance of gastric cancer. Int J Mol Sci. 2016;17:424. https://doi.org/10.3390/ijms17030424.
88. Wang R, Ma J, Wu Q, Xia J, Miele L, Sarkar FH, Wang Z. Functional role of miR-34 family in human cancer. Curr Drug Targets. 2013;14:1185–91. https://doi.org/10.2174/13894501113149990191.
89. Misso G, Di Martino MT, De Rosa G, Farooqi AA, Lombardi A, Campani V, Zarone MR, Gulla A, Tagliaferri P, Tassone P, Caraglia M. Mir-34: a new weapon against cancer? Mol Ther Nucleic Acids. 2014;3:e194. https://doi.org/10.1038/mtna.2014.47.
90. Zhang DG, Zheng JN, Pei DS. P53/microRNA-34-induced metabolic regulation: new opportunities in anticancer therapy. Mol Cancer. 2014;13:115. https://doi.org/10.1186/1476-4598-13-115.
91. Tsai MM, Wang CS, Tsai CY, Huang HW, Chi HC, Lin YH, Lu PH, Lin KH. Potential diagnostic, prognostic and therapeutic targets of microRNAs in human gastric cancer. Int J Mol Sci. 2016;17 https://doi.org/10.3390/ijms17060945.
92. Akers JC, Gonda D, Kim R, Carter BS, Chen CC. Biogenesis of extracellular vesicles (EV): exosomes, microvesicles, retrovirus-like vesicles, and apoptotic bodies. J Neuro-Oncol. 2013;113(1):1–11. https://doi.org/10.1007/s11060-013-1084-8.
93. Shi T, Gao G, Cao Y. Long noncoding RNAs as novel biomarkers have a promising future in cancer diagnostics. Dis Markers. 2016, 9085195:10. https://doi.org/10.1155/2016/9085195
94. Reis EM, Verjovski-Almeida S. Perspectives of long non-coding RNAs in cancer diagnostics. Front Genet. 2012;3(32):32. https://doi.org/10.3389/fgene.2012.00032.
95. Shao Y, Ye M, Jiang X, et al. Gastric juice long noncoding RNA used as a tumor marker for screening gastric cancer. Cancer. 2014;120(21):3320–8. https://doi.org/10.1002/cncr.28882.
96. Silva A, Bullock M, Calin G. The clinical relevance of long non-coding RNAs in cancer. Cancer. 2015;7(4):2169–82. https://doi.org/10.3390/cancers7040884.
97. Zhang K, Shi H, Xi H, et al. Genome-wide lncRNA microarray profiling identifies novel circulating lncRNAs for detection of gastric cancer. Theranostics. 2017;7(1):213–27. https://doi.org/10.7150/thno.16044.
98. Zhou X, Yin C, Dang Y, Ye F, Zhang G. Identification of the long non-coding RNA H19 in plasma as a novel biomarker for diagnosis of gastric cancer. Sci Rep. 2015;5:11516. https://doi.org/10.1038/srep11516.
99. Arita T, Ichikawa D, Konishi H, et al. Circulating long non-coding RNAs in plasma of patients with gastric cancer. Anticancer Res. 2013;33(8):3185–93. Available on: http://ar.iiarjournals.org/content/33/8/3185.long
100. Trajkovic K, Hsu C, Chiantia S, et al. Ceramide triggers budding of exosome vesicles into multivesicular endosomes. Science (New York, NY). 2008;319(5867):1244–7. https://doi.org/10.1126/science.1153124.
101. Johnstone RM. Exosomes biological significance: a concise review. Blood Cells Mol Dis. 2006;36(2):315–21. https://doi.org/10.1016/j.bcmd.2005.12.001.
102. Huang X, Yuan T, Tschannen M, et al. Characterization of human plasma-derived exosomal RNAs by deep sequencing. BMC Genomics. 2013;14(1):319. https://doi.org/10.1186/1471-2164-14-319.
103. Li Q, Shao Y, Zhang X, et al. Plasma long noncoding RNA protected by exosomes as a potential stable biomarker for gastric cancer. Tumour Biol. 2015;36(3):2007–12. https://doi.org/10.1007/s13277-014-2807-y.
104. Ren S, Wang F, Shen J, et al. Long non-coding RNA metastasis associated in lung adenocarcinoma transcript 1 derived miniRNA as a novel plasma-based biomarker for diagnosing prostate cancer. Eur J Cancer (Oxford, England: 1990). 2013;49(13):2949–59. https://doi.org/10.1016/j.ejca.2013.04.026.
105. Arroyo JD, Chevillet JR, Kroh EM, et al. Argonaute2 complexes carry a population of circulating microRNAs independent of vesicles in human plasma. Proc Natl Acad Sci U S A. 2011;108(12):5003–8. https://doi.org/10.1073/pnas.1019055108.
106. Wang K, Zhang S, Weber J, Baxter D, Galas DJ. Export of microRNAs and microRNA-protective protein by mammalian cells. Nucleic Acids Res. 2010;38(20):7248–59. https://doi.org/10.1093/nar/gkq601.

Immunomodulation and Immunotherapy for Gastric Cancer

12

Riccardo Dolcetti and Valli De Re

Introduction

Although surgery is a curative treatment for early-stage gastric cancer (GC), the median overall survival for patients diagnosed in a metastatic stage is less than 1 year [1]. New treatment options are therefore urgently needed. Recently, immunotherapy has emerged as one of the most promising strategies in cancer treatment, with outstanding results in several tumor types [2–4]. The clinical successes of immune checkpoint inhibitors have revolutionized cancer treatment clearly indicating that targeting the host immune system rather than the tumor may be more effective than conventional therapies. Although encouraging, the results so far obtained in GC patients are however still unsatisfactory, and the majority of novel immunotherapies in this setting are still in early-phase clinical investigation [5, 6]. Several complex factors are limiting the development of effective immunotherapeutic strategies for GC, including the heterogeneous immunogenicity among and within tumor subtypes and the different and still poorly defined immunosuppressive mechanisms that may hamper the effective control of the tumor by host immune cells. A deeper genetic and immunologic characterization of GC is required to allow for a more precise identification of patients who could benefit from modalities of immune intervention, as monotherapy or more likely within combination schedules. Here we will highlight the immunologic characteristics of different GC subsets, with particular focus on the tumor microenvironment, as a potential basis to improve tailoring of (immune) therapies. We will also review the state of the art of the various strategies of immunotherapy and immunomodulation investigated in the preclinical and clinical settings of GC.

Antitumor Immune Responses

The critical role of host immunity in controlling cancer is now well recognized. Available evidence supports the concept that our immune system is able to prevent cancer development through a process termed immune surveillance [7]. Dying cancer cells may express and release tumor-specific and tumor-associated antigens that can be taken up and processed by tissue-resident dendritic

R. Dolcetti (✉)
Immunopathology and Biomarker Unit/Bio-proteomics Facility, Department of Research and Advanced Tumor Diagnostics, IRCCS, CRO Aviano, National Cancer Institute, Aviano, PN, Italy

Translational Research Institute, University of Queensland Diamantina Institute, Brisbane, QLD, Australia
e-mail: r.dolcetti@uq.edu.au

V. De Re
Immunopathology and Tumor Biomarkers Unit/Bio-proteomics Facility, Department of Research and Advanced Tumor Diagnostics, IRCCS, CRO Aviano, National Cancer Institute, Aviano, PN, Italy
e-mail: vdere@cro.it

© Springer Nature Switzerland AG 2019
V. Canzonieri, A. Giordano (eds.), *Gastric Cancer In The Precision Medicine Era*, Current Clinical Pathology, https://doi.org/10.1007/978-3-030-04861-7_12

cells, which then maturate in antigen-presenting cells in the presence of an appropriate microenvironment, usually enriched in activator molecules, the so-called danger-associated molecular patterns (DAMPs) [7]. Induction of effective anticancer immunity requires that mature antigen-presenting cells efficiently present tumor antigens in the form of peptides to CD8⁺ T lymphocytes through major histocompatibility complex (MHC) class I molecules and to CD4⁺ T lymphocytes through MHC class II molecules. The strongest tumor antigens are those provided by nonself or mutated proteins, such as those encoded by viruses or generated by somatic mutations occurring in genes expressed by tumor cells. For an efficient activation of the CD8⁺ T cells, both antigen presentation (first signal) and the presence of costimulatory molecules (second signal) are needed [7]. After activation, T lymphocytes proliferate and infiltrate the tumor bed; promote the recruitment of other immune cells, including natural killer (NK) cells and M1 macrophages; and directly kill cancer cells through the release of cytokines, perforin, and granzymes [7]. Of relevance in the light of clinical application of immunotherapeutic strategies is the notion that not all conventional cytotoxic chemotherapeutic drugs are immunosuppressive. Recent evidence clearly indicates that certain commonly used drugs, including doxorubicin, mitoxantrone, bortezomib, oxaliplatin, and cyclophosphamide, can kill tumor cells also by an immunogenic cell death pathway, which activates robust innate and adaptive antitumor immune responses [8]. The immunogenic cell death is the consequence of the activation of adaptive responses in dying cells, which ultimately result in the exposure or secretion of immunostimulatory molecules commonly referred to as "damage-associated molecular patterns" [8]. Radiotherapy is also capable of rendering tumor cells immunogenic by modifying their phenotype and the surrounding microenvironment [9]. After treatment, danger signals are locally released resulting in maturation of dendritic cells and priming of cytotoxic T cells as well as in activation of NK cells. Despite being a local therapy characterized by an impressively high degree of spatial accuracy, radiotherapy can elicit systemic immune effects, which occasionally lead to regression and rejection of nonirradiated, distant tumor lesions, the so-called abscopal effect [10]. On these grounds, the present challenge is to better understand the potential immunomodulatory properties of currently used chemo- or radiotherapeutic regimens, in order to maximize the efficacy of their combination with immunotherapeutic strategies.

Tumor Microenvironment and Immunogenicity of GC

Immunogenic Subtypes of GC

Recently, the Cancer Genome Atlas (TGCA) classified GC into four main molecularly defined subgroups: (1) Epstein-Barr virus (EBV)-positive GCs (~9% of all GC), which frequently carry PIK3CA mutations, PD-L1/PD-L2 overexpression, and extreme DNA hypermethylation; (2) microsatellite instability (MSI) tumors (15–30% of all GC), which are frequently hypermutated; (3) chromosomal instability (CIN) tumors (50%, mainly junctional), which show a high rate of copy number variations, TP53 mutations, and receptor tyrosine kinase-Ras activation; and (4) genomically stable (GS) GCs (20%), which show altered motility and mutations in adhesion molecules [11]. These findings stimulated a great interest to tailor therapeutic approaches according to the features of each GC subset. This may be particularly relevant for immunotherapeutic purposes, considering the different level of immunogenicity shown by the four TGCA subsets.

A meta-analysis demonstrated that patients with EBV-associated GC have a better prognosis as compared to those with an EBV-unrelated GC [12]. Although the underlying mechanisms are not clear, the extensive lymphocyte infiltration, particularly of CD8⁺ T cells, which characterizes this GC subset suggests that antitumor immune responses triggered by viral antigens may have a role in determining a better clinical outcome [13, 14]. In EBV⁺ GC, genes involved in cytokine/chemokine pathways are frequently deregulated [15], and programmed cell death ligand 1 (PD-L1) expression is markedly increased via multiple mechanisms [16].

MSI is characterized by alterations in length within short repeated DNA sequences (microsatellites), which are the consequence of inactivating mutations or epigenetic silencing of DNA mismatch repair genes (e.g., *MSH1*, *MSH2*, *MSH3*, and *MLH1*) [17]. These mutations include frameshift mutations in coding regions that can drive oncogenesis by inactivating tumor-suppressor genes or disrupting noncoding regulatory sequences. GCs with high frequency of mutations within microsatellite markers (MSI-high) are characterized by older age, mostly female, distal location, and better survival [18]. The defect in the DNA mismatch repair system of these tumors generates thousands of mutations which may result in a high load of neo-antigens that can be recognized by immune cells [19]. In particular, about 30% of GC was shown to carry a burden of non-synonymous mutations, suggesting that this subgroup of tumors may be particularly responsive to immunotherapy [19]. Of note, MSI-high GC usually shows a prominent lymphocytic infiltrate that is the likely consequence of the high immunogenicity of this subset of GC. The T-cell responses elicited by MSI-high cancers are frequently directed against tumor-specific new carboxy-terminal epitopes originating from short insertion/deletion mutations in coding genes, although frameshift mutations frequently also result in premature arrest of the protein production (stop codon) (Fig. 12.1) [20]. Nevertheless, the same mutator phenotype characterizing the MSI GCs reduces the rates of neo-antigen presentation to the immune system by generating alterations also in genes encoding for MHC class I molecules [21].

Integrated genomic analysis also showed that the two other molecular subtypes of GC, the CIN and GS, are characterized by less evident immune signatures [11, 22], suggesting an inherently reduced responsiveness to immunotherapeutic approaches.

Tumor-Infiltrating Lymphocytes

The composition of the immune microenvironment differs among patients and cancers of the

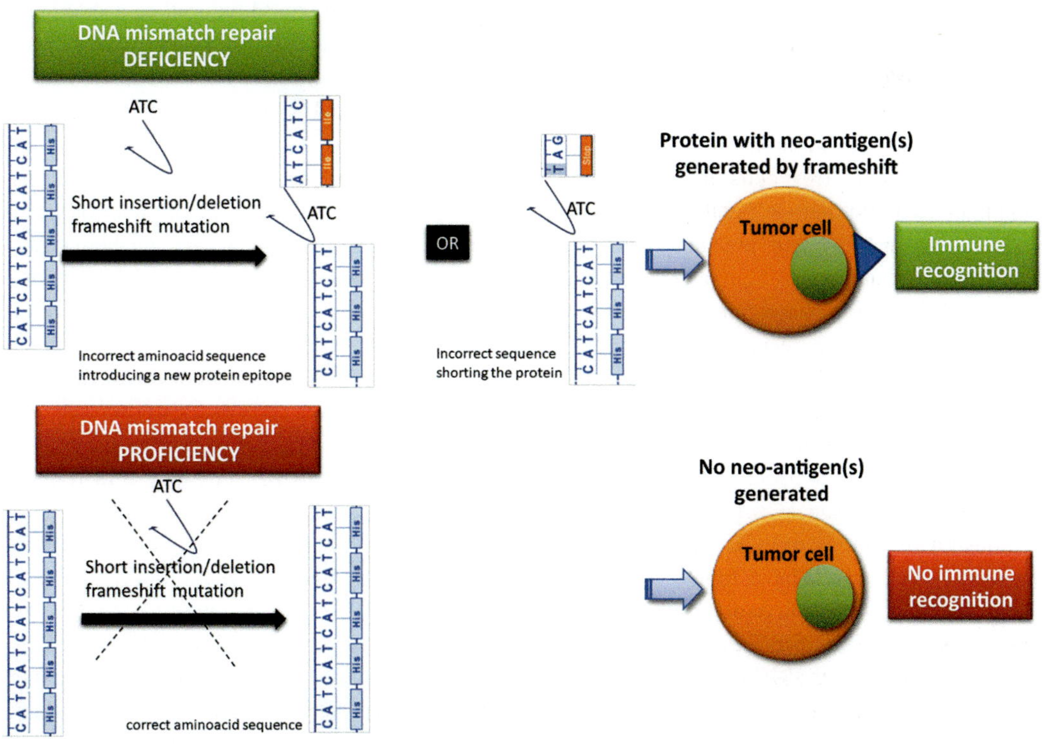

Fig. 12.1 Continuous generation of immunogenic neo-antigens by frameshift mutations not repaired by a deficient DNA mismatch repair machinery, as in the case of MSI-high GC

same type. The nature, number, and spatial distribution of immune cells within the tumor define the host immune background. Several lines of evidence indicate that tumor-infiltrating lymphocytes (TILs) may have an important role in influencing the clinical course of various tumors, also including GC [23]. A higher density of both intratumoral cytotoxic $CD8^+$ TILs and $FoxP3^+$ regulatory T cells (Treg) was associated with good prognosis, and this is particularly true for MSI GC, including those *H. pylori*- or EBV-positive [24, 25]. A recent meta-analysis of 31 observational studies including 4185 GC patients investigated the significance of the prognostic role of specific T-cell subsets, focusing on overall survival and disease-free survival [26]. In particular, the study concluded that the number of $CD8^+$, $FoxP3^+$, $CD3^+$, $CD57^+$, $CD20^+$, $CD45RO^+$, granzyme B^+, and T-bet$^+$ infiltrating lymphocytes was significantly associated with improved survival ($p < 0.05$). Notably, the amount of $CD3^+$ TILs in intratumoral compartment was the most significant prognostic marker (pooled HR = 0.52; 95% CI = 0.43–0.63; $P < 0.001$). Infiltrating FoxP3+ Treg cells showed bidirectional prognostic roles, which had positive effect in the intratumoral compartment and negative effect in extra-tumoral compartment [26]. There is an increasing interest in Tregs as one of the major components of the immune-suppressive tumor microenvironment. Treg cells inhibit cytotoxic lymphocytes and/or helper T-cell activity as well as NK cell function, and physiologically they play an important role in maintaining immunological tolerance to self-antigens and in suppressing excessive immune responses that would be deleterious to the host. Tregs have also been identified as the major regulatory component of the adaptive immune response in *H. pylori*-related inflammation, GC, and bacterial persistence [27] as well as in EBV-related GC [25]. A recent study demonstrated that $Foxp3^+CD4^+ICOS^+$ effector Tregs (eTregs), which have highly suppressive functions, were more abundant in late-stage GCs [28]. These TILs exhibited the ability to produce IL-10 but not IFN-γ, TNF-α, or IL-17 and to inhibit the proliferation of responder $CD8^+$ T cells. The expression of ICOS on Treg cells was

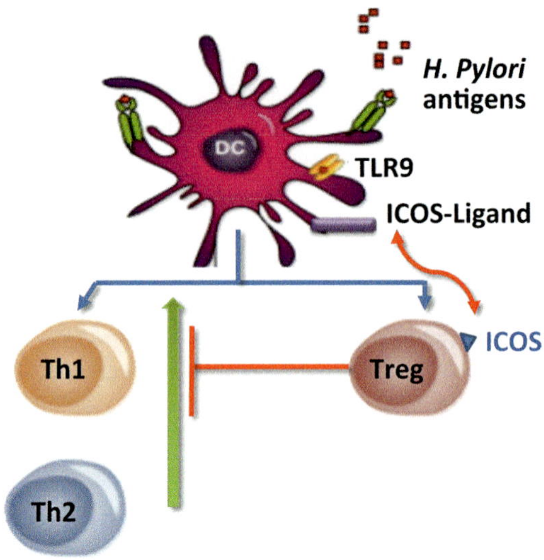

Fig. 12.2 Treg cells expressing ICOS may inhibit the activation of plasmacytoid dendritic cells expressing ICOS-ligand and TLR9 in the setting of *H. pylori* infection. These findings suggest that ICOS could be used as a promising target to eradicate *H. pylori* and treat GC

found closely related to plasmacytoid dendritic cells expressing ICOS-ligand and TLR9 as well as *H. pylori* infection (Fig. 12.2). These findings suggest that ICOS could be used as a promising target to GC and to eradicate *H. pylori* by an indirect immune therapy [27].

Tumor infiltration by lymphoid cells is mediated by various mechanisms, including the release of CXCR3 ligands, which behave as chemotactic cytokines whose major function is the recruitment and homing of specific hematopoietic cellular subsets during homeostatic, inflammatory, and neoplastic conditions. CXCR3 is predominantly expressed on activated T lymphocytes, NK cells, inflammatory dendritic cells, macrophages, and B cells and also on tumor and vascular cells. CXCR3 is rapidly induced on naive T cells following activation and remains highly expressed on $CD4^+$ type-1 helper (Th1) T cells, effector CD8+ T cells, and innate-type lymphocytes, such as NK and natural killer T (NKT) cells [29]. CXCR3 expression in GC tissues was significantly higher than in normal adjacent tissues and higher CXCR3 expression correlated with increased dendritic cell and both $CD8^+$ and $CD4^+$ TIL infiltration. By contrast, low levels of

CXCR3 expression were associated with a deeper tumor invasion, III/IV TNM stage, lymph node metastasis, and poorly differentiated tumor cells in GC patients. Notably, univariate and multivariate analyses indicated that CXCR3 expression was an independent prognostic factor for overall survival [30]. Further prospective studies are however required to assess the clinical relevance of CXCR3 overexpression as biomarker of favorable prognosis and therapeutic target in GC.

With regard to other tumor-infiltrating lymphoid populations, it has been reported that in patients with adenocarcinoma of the esophagogastric junction, a high density of tumor-infiltrating B cells, as well as plasma cells, was significantly correlated with better overall survival compared to patients with no infiltrates. B-cell infiltration was as an independent prognostic factor in this study [31].

Overall, the results obtained so far by TILs studies not only support a critical interplay between host immunity and GC but also indicate that the extent and the quality of infiltrating immune cells may have predictive and prognostic significance. As discussed below, ex vivo isolation and expansion of TILs may also constitute a valuable immunotherapeutic approach for GC.

Mechanisms of Immune Evasion in GC

Active cancer immunosurveillance is the ability of host immune system to recognize tumor cells and eliminate them before the development of an overt malignancy [32]. This complex process functions through a mechanism of "immunoediting," which consists of three sequential phases: (1) the *elimination phase*, growing tumors are effectively recognized and eliminated by the concerted action of innate and adaptive immune responses that also recognize remodeling of stroma and changes in the microenvironment. (2) The *equilibrium phase* during which antigen-presenting cells, tumor cells, and $CD8^+$ T cells remain in a state of dynamic balance, and the surviving tumor cells remain quiescent under the pressure of immune cells. In this long phase, the immune system of the host sculpts the immunogenicity of genetically unstable tumor clones, allowing for the selection of resistant tumor cells, thus leading to (3) the *escape phase*, favored by Treg cells and immunosuppressive cytokines including transforming growth factor-β (TGF-β), TNF-α, and IL-10. The immune effector cells in this phase may undergo apoptosis [33].

Tumor cells may activate a variety of mechanisms that help them to interfere with the immune system and avoid detection and killing by immune effector cells. Defects in antigen presentation occur at high frequency in tumors of various origins, including GC, and are a feature of immune evasion that renders cancer cells invisible to cytotoxic T lymphocytes [34]. Selective loss or reduced expression levels of MHC-I or of components of the antigen-processing machinery (APM) are generally associated with disease progression and reduced patient survival [34]. The molecular mechanisms underlying the defect in antigen presentation are diverse and include either irreversible structural alterations or reversible deregulatory processes of APM components [34]. While mutations, deletions, and/or loss of heterozygosity may occur in up to 30% of cases, the expression of APM components in tumors is more frequently deregulated by transcriptional, epigenetic, or posttranscriptional mechanisms [34]. The local microenvironment generated by tumor cells during malignant progression has a major contributory role in functionally impairing antitumor immune responses by promoting the polarization of infiltrating immune cells toward less cytotoxic and pro-inflammatory subsets of T cells (e.g., TH2, TH17, and Treg cells). This process is extremely complex and involves a large number of different cytokines and multiple cellular and stromal cell interactions. In GC microenvironment, the tumor-associated macrophages (TAMs) represent one of the most abundant immune cell populations. These cells can exert antitumor activities or have pro-tumorigenic effects supporting cancer initiation and malignant progression according to differentiation patterns into M1 or M2 subtypes [35]. While M1 TAMs may contribute to tumor control through the release of pro-inflammatory cytokines (IL-1, IL-6, IL-23, TNF-α), M2 TAMs may drive local immune suppression by producing IL-10 and TGF-β[35]. Indeed, TAM infiltration was shown to functionally inhibit T cells in GC [36, 37] and may represent a biomarker of poor prognosis [38, 39]. Myeloid-derived suppressor cells (MDSCs) are a heterogeneous population of immature myeloid cells able to inhibit both innate and adaptive immune responses against tumors [40]. The numbers of MDSCs are increased in the blood of GC patients compared with healthy individuals, and this increase was associated with adverse clinical outcomes [41]. Preclinical evidence indicates that CD40 expression upregulates the chemokine receptor CXCR5 and promotes MDSC migration toward and accumulation within GC tissues [42]. More recently, a multiparametric flow cytometry characterization of $CD45^{+}CD11b^{+}$ $CD14^{+}$ $HLA\text{-}DR^{-}$ MDSCs infiltrating GC disclosed that high numbers of these cells correlated with decreased overall survival and were an independent prognostic factor for overall survival [43].

Another possible immune evasive mechanism is related to the demonstration that GC expresses Fas ligand (FasL) irrespective of tumor stages. This property allows tumor cells to induce a Fas receptor-mediated apoptosis of activated lymphocytes, thus inhibiting antitumor immune responses [44].

Tumor cells may also induce T-cell suppressive signaling pathways to successfully evade immune-mediated elimination. The inhibitory signals to suppress T-cell activity are mediated by a variety of "immune checkpoint" molecules (inhibitory ligands and their cognate receptors), including the CD28/cytotoxic T-lymphocyte antigen 4 (CTLA-4) axis and PD-L1/PD-1 which have emerged as promising druggable targets (Fig. 12.3). Other checkpoint molecules such as TIM3, B7H3, VISTA, LAG3, and TIGIT are currently being evaluated as potential targets for cancer immunotherapy [45, 46]. Pathways involving these regulatory molecules are crucial for maintaining tolerance against self-antigens and to modulate the duration and amplitude of immune responses against nonself or mutated antigens in order to reduce collateral tissue damage [45]. Immune checkpoint molecules play their roles when the immune system recognizes and responds to antigens, mainly provided by infectious agents or cancer cells, and are regulated by ligand/receptor interactions. When these negative regulatory proteins are blocked, the inhibition of immune effector cells is released,

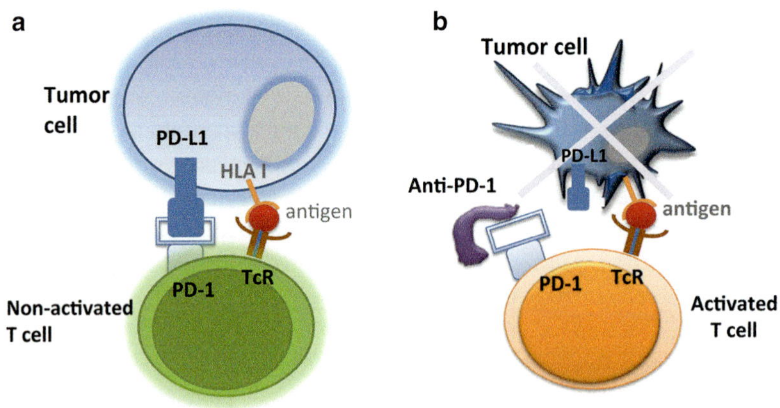

Fig. 12.3 Antibodies/agents against PD-1 receptor on T cells and/or PD-L1 ligand on antigen-presenting cells or tumor cells reactivate pre-existing antitumor T cells that can induce tumor cell killing. Recognition of the human leukocyte antigen (HLA) class I/peptide antigen complex by the T-cell receptor present on T cells is required to induce the tumor cell killing. (**a**) PD-1/PD-L1 interaction is not blocked, and the tumor cell is not killed. (**b**) PD-1 receptor is blocked by an anti-PD-1 antibody, and the T cell is activated and thus able to kill the tumor cell

and these cells regain their ability to become activated and kill tumor cells [47].

About the expression of immune checkpoint molecules in GC, there are variations in methodologies and antibody clones used in immunohistochemistry, clearly pointing to the need to develop and validate standardized approaches [48]. Data collected so far indicate that PD-L1 is expressed in up to 65% of GC tissues, whereas it was undetectable in normal gastric mucosa of healthy individuals [48–50]. A comprehensive immunohistochemical analysis carried out in a series of 127 GCs from Caucasian patients showed that PD-L1 and CTLA-4 were expressed in 44.9% and 86.6% of the cases analyzed, respectively. The load of somatic mutations did not reveal any correlation with the expression of these molecules on tumor cells. Notably, positive tumor cell staining for PD-L1 or CTLA-4 was associated with inferior overall survival. The study also showed that TILs expressed PD-1, PD-L1, and CTLA-4 at significantly higher levels compared to peripheral blood. In addition, PD-1 and PD-L1 were expressed far higher by TILs than CTLA-4 [51]. Despite the efforts carried out so far, the value of PD-L1 in predicting responses of GC patients to anti-PD-1/PD-L1 immunotherapy is controversial. A recent study investigated the expression of PD-L1, PD-L2, and PD-1 as well as $CD8^+$ T-cell density in primary tumors and lymph nodes from patients with stage $T_{1-4}N_+M_0$ GC. In multivariate analysis, PD-L1 expression, PD-L2 expression, a low density of $CD8^+$ T cells in primary tumors, and PD-1 expression on $CD8^+$ T cells in primary tumors were associated with poor prognosis. In the series analyzed, however, the expression of PD-L1 was heterogeneous in primary tumors and in metastatic lymph nodes, which might explain the inconsistent results in assessing the prognostic value of PD-L1 expression in previous studies [52]. A recent meta-analysis carried out on 15 studies including 3291 GC patients showed that the expression level of PD-L1 in tumor cells significantly correlated with a worse overall survival. In addition, subgroup analysis showed that GC patients with deeper tumor infiltration, positive lymph node metastasis, positive venous invasion, EBV infection, or MSI are more likely to express PD-L1. These findings suggest that GC patients, specifically those with EBV^+ and MSI tumors, may be preferred candidates for PD-1-targeting therapies [53]. Several studies focused on the possible pathogenic and prognostic role of the PD-1/PD-L1 pathway specifically in the subset of EBV-associated GC. Expression of PD-L1 was frequently detected in cancer cells of these GC, usually associated with a stromal infiltration of $PD\text{-}L1^+$ immune cells. Both expression of PD-L1 in cancer cells and $PD\text{-}L1^+$ immune cell infiltration was significantly correlated with diffuse histology. PD-L1 expression in tumor cells correlated with poor outcomes in both overall survival and disease-specific survival. FISH analysis demonstrated gene amplification of PD-L1 in 11% of cases [54, 55]. These results are consistent with the possibility that PD-L1 expression in tumor cells and their microenvironment may contribute to the progression of EBV-associated GC, and gene amplification occurs as clonal evolution during progression.

Expression of PD-L1 by T lymphocytes infiltrating GC may be also of potential prognostic relevance, as shown by a large study carried out on 240 GC patients that found a significantly shorter 5-year overall survival in patients with positive PD-L1 expression on TILs [56]. Expression of PD-1 on NK cells was correlated with a functional hyperresponsiveness of these immune effector cells. PD-1 was found highly expressed on peripheral and tumor-infiltrating NK cells from patients with digestive cancers including esophageal, liver, colorectal, gastric, and biliary cancer. The increased PD-1 expression on NK cells was associated with a shorter survival in esophageal and liver cancers. Functional studies carried out in vitro revealed that blocking PD-1/PD-L1 signaling markedly enhanced cytokine production and degranulation and suppressed apoptosis of NK cells. Intriguingly, treatment with a PD-1 blocking antibody significantly inhibited the growth of xenografts in nude mice, an effect that was completely abrogated by NK depletion [57]. These findings strongly suggested that PD-1 is an inhibitory regulator of NK cells in digestive cancers and indicated that PD-1 blockade might be an efficient strategy in NK cell-based tumor immunotherapy.

With regard to new immune checkpoint molecules, VISTA appears of particular interest. It encodes for a type I membrane protein and is expressed predominantly on myeloid, granulocytic, and T cells. Although the ligands for VISTA are not yet known, available evidence indicates that VISTA may serve both as a ligand (for antigen-presenting cells) and as a receptor (for T cells) and that VISTA suppresses T-cell activation [58]. In preclinical models, VISTA inhibition increased the number and activation of intratumoral T cells resulting in enhanced antitumor immunity. Of note, VISTA-induced T-cell activation seems to be non-redundantly from the PD-1/PD-L1 pathway [59], suggesting a combined VISTA/PD-1 blockade might be a promising new immunotherapeutic option. Analysis of a large cohort of 464 therapy-naive GC samples and 14 corresponding liver metastases disclosed that VISTA expression in tumor cells was detected in 41 GCs (8.8%) and 2 corresponding liver metastases (14.3%). Moreover, VISTA expression in immune cells was detected in 83.6% of GCs and 42.9% liver metastases. VISTA expression was associated with the Laurén phenotype, tumor localization, Epstein-Barr virus infection, KRAS- and PIK3CA-mutational status, and PD-L1 expression. However, no significant correlation with patient outcome was observed. The concomitant VISTA and PD-L1 expression indicates a dual immune evasion mechanism of GC tumor cells and support the rationale for combination therapies targeting these two immune checkpoint inhibitors in this setting [60].

Tim-3, a member of the TNF family, is a negative regulator of CD4+ helper 1 and CD8+ cytotoxic T cells [61]. The observation that Tim-3 is highly expressed on exhausted or functionally impaired CD8+ T cells suggested a possible correlation between PD-1 and Tim-3 expression and immune evasion in patients with GC [62]. It has been reported that Tim-3 expression defines a subpopulation of PD-1$^+$ exhausted NY-ESO-1-specific CD8$^+$ T cell and that PD-1$^+$Tim-3$^+$ CD8$^+$ T cells represented the largest subset of NY-ESO-1-specific CD8$^+$ T cells in GC patients. Functional analyses disclosed that CD8$^+$PD-1$^+$Tim-3$^+$ T cells were more impaired in IFN-γ, TNF-α, and IL-2 production as compared with PD-1$^+$Tim-3$^-$ or PD-1$^-$Tim-3$^-$ subsets. Concomitant inhibition of Tim-3 and PD-1 during T-cell priming efficiently enhanced proliferation and cytokine production by NY-ESO-1-specific CD8$^+$ T cells, providing thus the rationale for combination immunotherapy targeting these two checkpoint inhibitory molecules [63].

Cancer Vaccines

The therapeutic potential of cancer vaccines is due to their ability to activate and boost antitumor immune responses mainly mediated by T lymphocytes specifically recognizing tumor-associated antigens. The ideal vaccine should be simple and not expensive to produce, easy to administer, safe, and able to induce prolonged protection with a long-lasting memory response. Dendritic cells are professional antigen-presenting cells that play a pivotal role in orchestrating and coordinating antitumor immune responses, being able to activate NK cells, B lymphocytes, and naïve and memory T cells [64]. Tumor antigens processed by DC are loaded in the form of small peptides onto MHC class I molecules for presentation to the cytotoxic CD8$^+$ T cells or to MHC class II molecules for presentation to CD4$^+$ helper T lymphocytes. These functional properties stimulated the development of various strategies aimed at exploiting DC for cancer immunotherapy. Despite these premises, however, the use of DC-based vaccines in the clinical setting is limited by the short life span of these cells in vivo. In GC patients, a higher number of DCs infiltrating the tumor were shown to correlate with lower lymph node metastases and lymphatic invasion and better 5-year survival rates [65–67]. Various tumor-associated antigens were used so far to load DC cells to vaccinate GC patients. Advanced gastrointestinal tumor patients were treated with four injections of autologous DCs pulsed with melanoma-associated antigen (MAGE) A3 peptides showing the induction of peptide-specific T-cell responses and a minor tumor regression in a proportion of patients [68]. No correlation was however observed between the clinical outcome and the induction of tumor antigen-specific immune responses [68]. An immunogenic HLA-A2 epitope peptide derived from the HER2/neu oncogene was used in a phase 1 clinical trial to pulse autologous DCs and treat a small number of patients with advanced or recurrent GC overexpressing HER2/neu. No severe toxicity was observed, and HER2/neu peptide-specific T-cell recognition could be demonstrated in six of nine patients after immunization. One of the patients underwent a partial clinical response concurrent with a decrease in the blood levels of the carcinoembryonic antigen tumor marker, whereas a stabilization of disease for 3 months was observed in another patient [69]. Peptide-based vaccination strategies for GC have been also investigated in combination with chemotherapy obtaining encouraging results. One study evaluated the effect of adjuvant immunochemotherapy with the use of BCG (bacille Calmette-Guerin) and FAM (5-fluorouracil, Adriamycin, mitomycin C) chemotherapy on the survival of patients with locally advanced resectable GC. In radically resected stage III/IV GC, adjuvant immunochemotherapy significantly prolonged the overall 10-year survival (47.1%) as compared to FAM (30%) or surgery alone (15.2%) [70]. In a multicenter phase II trial, patients with advanced GC or gastroesophageal junction carcinomas were treated with the gastrin-17 diphtheria toxoid (G17DT, Aphton) vaccine targeting gastrin peptide in combination with cisplatin and 5-fluorouracil. Immune responders (61% of the total 94 patients) were identified based on increased levels of anti-gastrin antibody levels on two consecutive tests and showed a significantly longer time to progression and a longer median survival rate compared to non-responders [71]. Recently, the safety and immunogenicity of peptide vaccination with HLA-A*2402-restricted URLC10-A24-177 and VEGFR1-A12-9 1084 epitope peptides were investigated in a phase I clinical trial of patients with advanced GC who were refractory to chemotherapy. No patient had a severe treatment-related adverse event, and specific cytotoxic T-cell responses were detected in 62.5% and 50% of patients for URLC10 and VEGFR1, respectively [72]. To personalize the choice of peptides to be used as vaccines in individual GC patients, pre-vaccination peripheral blood mononuclear cells (PBMCs) were screened for their reactivity in vitro to each of 14 peptides on HLA-A24 or 16 peptides on -A2 allele, and then only the reactive peptides (maximum 4) were administered in vivo. Delayed-type hypersensitivity (DTH) to the vaccinated peptides was observed in four patients, whereas increased cellular and humoral immune responses to the vaccinated peptides were observed in postvaccination PBMCs from four of eight patients and in postvaccination sera of eight of ten patients tested, respectively. Prolonged survival was observed in patients showing cellular and humoral immune responses to the peptides included in the vaccine in the postvaccination samples [73]. The same approach of personalized choice of vaccination peptides was adopted in combination with oral administration of a 5-fluorouracil derivative (TS-1) in a small series of advanced GC. An increase in peptide-specific IgG after the sixth vaccinations was observed in most patients irrespective of the dose of TS-1 used, whereas an increase in peptide-specific interferon-gamma production by T cells was most evident in patients who were administered the highest dose of TS-1. These results indicated that administration of the standard dose (80 mg/m^2/day) of TS-1 in combination with a personalized peptide vaccination does not necessarily hamper immunological responses in GC patients and could maintain or enhance them [74]. Encouraging clinical results were recently obtained by a study in which patients with advanced or recurrent GC were vaccinated with HLA-A24-restricted vascular endothelial growth factor receptor 1 (VEGFR1)-1084 and VEGFR2-169 peptides combined with S-1 and cisplatin chemotherapy. Most patients (82%) showed the induction of VEGFR1-specific cytotoxic T-lymphocyte responses, 12 patients (55%) showed partial response, and 10 had stable disease after two cycles of the combination therapy.

Notably, patients showing VEGFR-specific T-cell responses had significantly overall survival and time to progression, indicating that cancer vaccination combined with standard chemotherapy warrants further analysis as a promising strategy for the treatment of advanced GC [75]. More recently, a cocktail vaccine including multiple peptides (DEPDC1, FOXM1, KIF20, URLC10, and VEGFR1) combined with S-1 chemotherapy was administered as postoperative adjuvant therapy in a series of pathologically stage III advanced GC patients. The treatment was well tolerated, and the optimal relative dose intensity of S-1 was achieved in combination group, paving the way for further studies aiming at assessing the efficacy of this therapeutic strategy [76].

Adoptive Cell Therapy

The tumor-killing properties of T cells and NK cells provide opportunities to treat cancer. Adoptive cell therapies (ACT) are harnessing this potential by exploiting these effectors, particularly by endowing a functionally diverse repertoire of T cells with genetically modified, tumor-specific recognition receptors [77]. This form of immunotherapy involves the isolation and ex vivo expansion and manipulation of tumor-specific T cells or NK cells, which are then reinfused into cancer patients to combat the disease. This process is applicable to the vast majority of cancer patients who are unable to mount an effective anticancer immunity prior to intervention and therefore at least theoretically will not respond to immune checkpoint inhibitors. Notably, ACT has multiple advantages compared with other forms of cancer immunotherapy that rely on the active in vivo development of sufficient numbers of antitumor immune cells. In vitro activation allows such cells to be released from the inhibitory factors that exist in vivo and that are among the most relevant factors limiting the efficacy of cancer immunotherapy. Moreover, ACT enables the manipulation of the host (e.g., T-cell-depleting chemotherapy) before cell transfer to provide a more favorable microenvironment to efficiently support antitumor immunity. There are several different forms of ACT being used for cancer treatment; most of them have been or are being investigated in the clinical setting for their potential efficacy in GC patients.

Tumor-Infiltrating Lymphocytes (TILs)

Several studies have evaluated the predictive and prognostic relevance of TILs in GC [78]. These cells can infiltrate stroma and tumor cells and are considered the expression of the spontaneous host immune response against the tumor. TILs can recognize cancer antigens that are considered foreign to the body, such as (1) viral proteins, (2) mutated proteins uniquely expressed by tumors (neo-antigens), and (3) cancer germline antigens or fetal proteins that may be aberrantly re-expressed by tumor cells. About GC, MHC class I-restricted T cells specifically recognizing GC antigens were successfully isolated from primary tumors, metastatic lymph nodes, and ascites from a series of GC patients [79]. The different antigen recognition pattern of TILs generated from different sites may have implication for TIL-based adoptive immunotherapy. Although this immunotherapeutic strategy showed promising results in preclinical models, less encouraging findings were observed in the clinical setting except for the treatment of melanoma patients [78]. Indeed, the feasibility of this approach has some important limitations including the limited proportion (about 40%) of biopsies yielding satisfactory T-cell populations and the time (about 6 weeks) required to generate adequate numbers of cells for infusion [78]. Cytotoxic T-cell lines specific for the MAGE tumor antigen and able to recognize and kill GC cells in a HLA-A2-restricted fashion were successfully generated from the spleen of GC patients [80]. These findings suggest that the spleen may have an important role in either clinical tumor vaccination or the treatment of cancer patients by adoptive immunotherapeutic approaches using the tumor-specific peptides [80]. One study reported 13% of complete remissions and 21.7% of partial responses in a series of 23 patients with non-operable advanced GC treated with autologous TILs after in vitro culture with recombinant IL-2 and administered with the same cytokine [81]. The effects of ACT were also investigated in combination with chemotherapy. Patients with GC were treated with expanded activated autologous lymphocytes obtained from peripheral blood after stimulation with anti-CD3 antibody and IL-2. The group receiving this ACT regimen in addition to conventional treatment showed a significantly longer overall survival (27.0 vs. 13.9 months, $p = 0.028$) as compared to patients receiving standard treatment alone [82]. A randomized controlled study investigated the efficacy of T-activated lymphocytes generated from GC patients with IL-2 and administered either intraperitoneally or intravenously in combination with low-dose cisplatin and 5-fluorouracil. The overall survival of patients receiving ACT was significantly better than that of patients treated with chemotherapy alone [83]. A promising strategy to improve the feasibility and efficacy of T-cell based ACT is to use T lymphocytes taken directly from the patient's blood after they have received a cancer vaccine. It has been shown that "priming" rare tumor antigen-specific T cells first, with active immunization, is associated with a more effective expansion of tumor-specific T cells, which can be obtained in greater numbers for therapeutic infusion [78].

Natural Killer (NK) Cells

NK cells have cytotoxic activity against solid tumors and are particularly relevant to prevent the metastatic dissemination of cancer cells. The cytotoxic activity of NK cells is finely regulated through a balance of activating and inhibitory receptors that prevent killing of healthy cells while maintaining effective cytotoxic capacity against neoplastic cells. Therefore, these immune effectors have garnered immense attention as a promising immunotherapeutic agent for treating cancers [84]. Available evidence indicates that individuals with high levels of NK cell cytotoxicity have reduced incidence of cancer and that the infusion of human NK cells into tumor patients may induce significant clinical responses [84]. In a large cohort of GC patients, it has been shown that a high intratumoral infiltration of NK cells, identified by the expression of CD57, correlated with smaller tumors, limited lymph node involvement, and a better 5-year overall survival rate [65]. The positive prognostic significance of NK cell infiltration was confirmed in an independent series of GCs [85]. In keeping with these findings is the observation that a high number of apoptotic NK cell-expressing Fas correlated with cancer progression in GC patients [86]. Among the different approaches attempted so far to exploit NK cells for cancer immunotherapy, the use of in vitro expanded allogeneic NK cells appears particularly promising. Compared to autologous NK cells, allogeneic NK cells are more suitable for quality controls and large-scale production and have the advantage of not being inhibited by self-histocompatibility antigens [84]. NK cells can be successfully expanded from peripheral blood mononuclear cells of healthy donors, in the presence of K562 cells expressing membrane-bound IL-15 and 4-1BB Ligand, and from patients with different solid tumors, including GC [87]. Nevertheless, current approaches of NK cell-based immunotherapy need to be improved to make clinical application more feasible. In this respect, it has been recently shown that PD-1, the well-known immune checkpoint of T cells is highly expressed on peripheral and tumor-infiltrating NK cells from patients with digestive cancers including GC. Blocking PD-1/PD-L1 signaling markedly enhanced cytokine production and degranulation and suppressed apoptosis of NK cells in vitro. Notably, treatment of nude mice carrying tumor xenografts with a PD-1-blocking antibody significantly suppressed tumor growth, an effect that was completely abrogated by NK depletion [57]. These findings strongly suggested that PD-1 is an inhibitory regulator of NK cells in digestive cancers and indicated that PD-1 blockade might be an efficient strategy in NK cell-based tumor immunotherapy.

Cytokine-Induced Killer Cells

Cytokine-induced killer cells (CIK) are a heterogeneous population of immune effector cells that can be easily developed from peripheral blood lymphocytes after stimulation with interferon-γ (IFN-γ), monoclonal antibody against CD3, and interleukin (IL)-2 [88]. These cells exert a potent, non-major histocompatibility complex (MHC)-restricted cytotoxicity mainly through expansion of $CD3^+CD8^+CD56^-$ cells to CD56-positive natural killer (NK) T cells [88]. CIK cell cytotoxicity is mediated by perforin release and dependent on NKG2D recognition and signaling [88] (Fig. 12.4). Notably, CIK cells have also been shown to be effective against multidrug-resistant and FasL-positive malignant cells [85, 89]. Moreover, CIK cells can regulate and increase host cellular immune function in vivo by secretion of cytokines, such as IFN-γ, and several chemokines, including RANTES, MIP-1α, and MIP-1β [85]. Because of their safety and inherently high antitumor activity, CIK cells represent one of the promising cellular immunotherapies. Preclinical studies indicated that CIK cells can exert strong antiproliferative and pro-apoptotic effects in the MGC-803 GC cell line [90] and the MKN74 human GC cell line, mainly releasing IFN-γ and TNFα. In addition, available evidence indicates that ACT in general and therapy with CIK cells in particular benefit from the combination with chemotherapy, which may at least in part overcome the limited GC stroma infiltration of transferred cells [91, 92]. Combination with chemotherapy may also have the advantage of benefitting from the ability of several drugs, including doxorubicin, mitoxantrone, oxaliplatin, and cyclophosphamide, to induce an immunogenic cell death [93]. Indeed, the combination of CIK with oxaliplatin showed superior antitumor effects as compared to monotherapy against drug-resistant GC cells both in vitro and in vivo [94]. Several clinical trials have been carried out so far to investigate the safety and efficacy of CIK therapy in GC patients. A series of 53 patients with stage II–III GC was treated after gastrectomy with autologous CIK cells combined with chemotherapy, and the results were compared with those obtained in 112 GC patients receiving chemotherapy alone. The CIK group showed a significantly improved 5-year OS rate (56.6% vs. 26.8%, $p = 0.014$) and PFS rate (49.1% vs. 24.1%, $p = 0.026$) compared to the control group, and no serious side effect was observed in the CIK group. These results suggested that immunotherapy with CIK cells may serve as an adjuvant treatment to prolong the survival of patients with stage II–III gastric carcinoma [95]. Another study carried out in the adjuvant setting included 151 patients with stage III/IV (M0) GC who had undergone gastrectomy (R0/D2) and who were treated with 6 cycles of adjuvant 5-FU, followed by at least 3 cycles of autologous CIK cells. In the whole series, CIK immunotherapy was associated with a significant improvement in 5-year disease-free survival

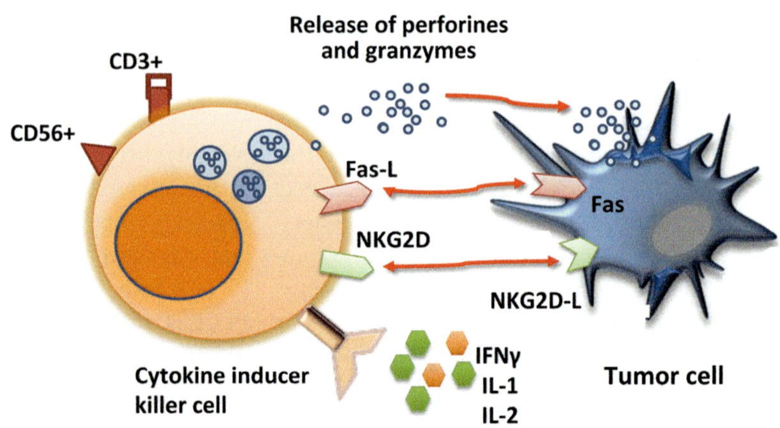

Fig. 12.4 Cytokine-inducer killer (CIK) cells are CD3+ CD56+ cells with a HLA-unrestricted NK cell cytotoxicity. They release perforins and granzymes that kill tumor cells after the recognition of altered cells by a still unknown mechanism. Interaction between NKG2 with its cognate ligand seems to be required for CIK activation and killing

(DFS) rates (28.3% vs. 10.4%; $p = 0.044$), although the difference in overall survival (OS) rates was only of borderline significance. Notably, for patients with intestinal-type GC, the 5-year OS and DFS rates were significantly higher in the CIK group (OS, 46.8% vs. 31.4%; $p = 0.045$; DFS, 42.4% vs. 15.7%; $p = 0.023$). In addition, patients treated with immunotherapy showed increased numbers of $CD3^+$ and $CD4^+$ T cells and increased $CD4^+/CD8^+$ ratio suggesting a reshuffling of T-lymphocyte subset distribution. These findings add further support to the possible clinical benefit provided by CIK cell adjuvant therapy and suggest that intestinal-type GCs could be selected as an important indication for this type of therapy [96]. The efficacy of CIK cell immunotherapy was also investigated in combination with FOLFOX4 in 51 GC patients after gastrectomy. A significant improvement in immune functions was observed in patients treated with CIK and FOLFOX4 compared with the functions of the patients who received FOLFOX4 treatment alone ($P < 0.05$). Notably, the group of patients also receiving CIK treatment showed significantly reduced GC recurrence rates and enhanced survival rates [97]. A meta-analysis considering six relevant clinical trials with case-control studies concluded that CIK cell therapy significantly increased 5-year survival rate compared to conventional chemotherapy among GC patients, thus providing statistical evidence supporting the activation of large-scale clinical trials with CIK cell therapy [98]. The observation that the combination of DCs and CIKs leads to a remarkable increase in cytotoxic activity [99] stimulated the execution of several studies in which this treatment was combined with different chemotherapy regimens. A recent meta-analysis included 1735 GC patients treated with chemotherapy in combination with CIK/DC-CIK within 17 different trials. The analysis showed that the combination therapy significantly increased the OS and DFS rates compared with those of patients treated with chemotherapy alone. The overall response rate ($P = 0.002$), disease control rate ($P = 0.0007$), and quality-of-life improved rate ($P = 0.0008$) were also significantly improved in patients who received the combined treatment. Interestingly, the percentage of lymphocyte subsets ($CD3^+$, $CD4^+$ and $CD3^-CD56^+$, $CD3^+CD56^+$; $P < 0.01$) and the levels of IL-12 and IFN-γ, which reflect immune function, were significantly increased ($P < 0.05$) after the CIK/DC-CIK therapy [101]. Some studies have attempted to identify markers predictive to the response to CIK cell therapy. Of particular interest in this respect is the observation that cell signaling through MHC-I-related chain A (MICA)-natural killer group 2, member D (NKG2D) results in CIK cell activation leading to cytolytic activities against tumor cells [88]. In a cohort of GC patients receiving adjuvant chemotherapy plus CIK or chemotherapy alone, MICA high-expression was found in 36.6% of tumors. Notably, MICA expression significantly correlated with the stage, and there was a borderline association with histological grade ($P = 0.054$). In the adjuvant chemotherapy plus CIK group, GC patients with high MICA expression had longer DFS (46.0 vs. 41.0 months, $p = 0.027$) and OS (48.0 vs. 42.0 months, $p = 0.031$). In multivariate analysis, CIK therapy alone and the interaction of MICA status with CIK therapy were independent prognostic factors for DFS and OS [100]. Although promising, the possible value of MICA status in the clinical decision-making process warrants adequate validation in prospective clinical trials. A particularly attractive perspective for the clinical exploitation of CIK cells is their combination with monoclonal antibodies [101, 102]. Indeed, preclinical evidence has been provided indicating that CIK cells combined with a monoclonal antibody against epidermal growth factor receptor (EGFR) enhanced the antitumor ability of CIK cells both in vitro and in vivo [103].

Chimeric Antigen Receptor T (CAR-T) Cells

To broaden the applicability and enhance the efficacy of adoptive cell therapy, techniques were recently developed to introduce antitumor receptors into normal T cells that could be used for therapy. The specificity of T cells can be redirected by the integration of genes encoding either conventional alpha-beta TCRs or CARs [104]. The TCR recognition process requires antigen presentation via the major histocompatibility (MHC) complex. However, a significant proportion of tumors downregulate MHC expression to escape immune surveillance [105]. Engineering T lymphocytes with CARs have the advantage to bypass the need for MHC interaction [104]. A CAR T cell can be viewed as the combination of an antibody and a TCR. Its extracellular part is a ligand-binding domain composed of a B-cell receptor-derived single-chain variable fragment, whereas the signaling domain is composed of CD3ζ and one or more intracellular costimulatory domains. Thus, CAR function is independent of MHC presentation or any additional costimulatory signaling [104]. Adoptive transfer of CAR-T cells has so far demonstrated promising antitumor effects in advanced hematologic cancers, such as relapsed or refractory acute lymphoblastic leukemia, chronic lymphocytic leukemia, and non-Hodgkin lymphoma [104]. Nevertheless, in patients with solid tumors, CAR-T cells were able to provide only limited benefit, due to heterogeneous antigen expression, immunosuppressive networks in the tumor microenvironment limiting CAR T-cell function and persistence, and suboptimal trafficking to solid tumors [104]. In a preclinical model of GC, treatment with a humanized chA21 single-chain fragmented antibody (scFv)-based CAR-T targeting HER2 induced a marked regression of HER2-overexpressing tumor and prolonged survival of tumor-bearing mice while spared the progression of HER2 low-expressing tumor [106]. Another CAR-T construct harboring the CD137 and CD3ζ moieties and targeting HER2 exhibited considerably enhanced tumor inhibition ability, promoted long-term survival and homing to targets, compared with those of non-transduced T cells. The sphere-forming ability and in vivo tumorigenicity of patient-derived GC stem-like cells expressing HER2 and the CD44 protein, were also inhibited [107]. To enhance the antitumor activity and in vivo persistence of CAR-T cells, lymphocytes were transduced with a scFv specific for the carcinoembryonic antigen (CEA) in combination with a fusion protein of IL-2. In comparison with free IL-2, the combination of peripheral blood mononuclear cells expressing this CAR and the fusion protein containing IL-2 significantly enhanced the antitumor activity against the human GC cell line MKN-45 cells [108]. This novel combination therapy of CAR and a fusion protein consisting of a functional cytokine and a fully human scFv may be a promising approach for adoptive cancer immunotherapy. Several clinical trials are ongoing to assess the safety and efficacy of CAR-T cells targeting CEA (NCT02349724, NCT02850536, NCT02416466), HER2 (NCT02713984), EpCAM (NCT02725125, NCT03013712), or MUC1 (NCT02617134) in GC patients.

Immune Checkpoint Inhibition

Immune checkpoint inhibitors are certainly the real game changers of modern oncology. The anti-CTLA-4 ipilimumab and the anti-PD-1 antibodies, pembrolizumab and nivolumab, were firstly approved by the US FDA for the treatment of patients with metastatic melanoma in 2011 and 2014, respectively [2, 109]. This class of drugs offers a promising avenue also for GC patients. Data accumulated so far indicate that while anti-CTLA-4 compounds (tremelimumab, ipilimumab) have produced unsatisfactory results, PD-1/PD-L1 inhibitors are showing more promising results.

Anti-CTLA-4 Antibodies

Preclinical and clinical data indicate that drugs targeting the immune checkpoint molecule CTLA-4 function not only by blocking inhibitory signals from reaching effector T cells but also by depleting the Treg cell populations present within the tumor microenvironment [110]. Initial studies in mouse models demonstrated that anti-CTLA-4 antibodies were active in inhibiting tumor growth without inducing serious immune adverse effects [111–113]. The therapeutic efficacy of these drugs was however more limited, if any, in mice bearing tumors with low immunogenicity.

Notably, combination of CTLA-4 blockade with a cellular vaccine transduced with granulocyte-macrophage colony-stimulating factor significantly inhibited the growth of tumors with low immunogenic profile [112]. These findings suggested that CTLA-4 inhibition may be more effective in tumors inherently able to mount a spontaneous antitumor immune response.

Tremelimumab is a fully human IgG2 monoclonal antibody able to inhibit the binding of B7-1 and B7-2 to CTLA-4. A phase II study investigated the efficacy of tremelimumab as second-line therapy in a small cohort of GC patients [114]. The ORR of 5% and the median survival of 4.8 months were quite disappointing, although like those expected with other chemotherapies in GC. Interestingly, patients with a posttreatment carcinoembryonic antigen proliferative response had median survival of 17.1 months compared with 4.7 months for non-responders ($p = 0.004$). These findings support the rationale for combinations of CTLA-4 blockade with vaccines targeting GC antigens. Similar results were observed in a randomized phase II study in which ipilimumab was compared to best supportive care in pre-treated patients with metastatic or locally advanced GC or carcinomas of gastroesophageal junction (GEJ): the survival outcome was similar between the two arms [115].

Pembrolizumab

In the KEYNOTE-012 phase Ib study, single-agent pembrolizumab, a PD-1 inhibitor, was administered to patients with PD-L1^{+} recurrent or metastatic adenocarcinoma of the stomach/GEJ until progression or intolerable adverse events [116]. Available data indicate that a partial response rate of 22% (8 of 36 evaluable patients) was observed for this group of heavily pre-treated patients, more than 75% of whom had received two or more prior therapies in the metastatic setting. The toxicity observed was manageable, with 13% of patients experiencing grade 3-4 toxicity, and no discontinuation of the therapy due to treatment-related adverse event was recorded.

The KEYNOTE-028 phase Ib study investigated the role of pembrolizumab administered every 2 weeks up to 2 years or until progression in PD-L1^{+} advanced solid tumors including esophageal/GEJ cancers (adenocarcinoma and squamous cell cancer) [117]. Twenty-three patients were enrolled (the majority of patients were Asian; $n = 12$), with a median follow-up duration of 7 months. Overall response rate (ORR) was 30% (95% CI, 13–53%) and the median duration of response was 15 months (range, 6–26 months). Analysis of a six-gene IFN-γ gene expression signature (*CXCL9*, *CXCL10*, *IDO1*, *IFNG*, *HLA-DRA*, and *STAT1*) analysis suggested that patients with low signature score (non-inflamed) GCs generally had lower response rates and did not show delays in progression. By contrast, delays in progression and increased ORR tended to occur among patients with higher immune gene signature scores [117].

With the aim to improve clinical response rates, PD-1 inhibitors are currently being investigated in combination with chemotherapy in a variety of tumors, including GC. The clinical data of these studies are eagerly awaited after the positive results from a lung cancer trial of pembrolizumab plus chemotherapy [118]. In the KEYNOTE-059 first-line HER2-phase II study, patients with advanced gastric/GEJ adenocarcinoma were treated with pembrolizumab plus 5-FU fluorouracil (or capecitabine in Japan) plus cisplatin every 3 weeks for six cycles, followed by pembrolizumab plus 5-FU/capecitabine maintenance for up to 2 years or until progression [119]. Notably, patients were mainly recruited from the USA (47.9%), only 13.1% from East Asia, and 39.0% from the rest of the world. PDL-1 expression was positive in 57.1% of tumors, and although PD-L1 positivity was associated with a higher ORR of 15.5%, responses were also observed in patients with PD-L1-negative tumors (ORR 6.4%). Indeed, comparable rates of complete responses were seen in the PD-L1 positive (2.0%) and the PD-L1 negative cohort (2.8%). Best responses were seen in patients with MSI-high tumors (four out of seven patients). Overall, treatment with pembrolizumab resulted in an ORR of 11.6% and the reduction in tumor in 42.4% of patients [119].

KEYNOTE-061 is an ongoing phase III open-label trial evaluating pembrolizumab versus paclitaxel for patients with advanced gastric/GEJ cancer whose tumors have progressed after first-line therapy with a platinum/fluoropyrimidine combination [120]. Treatment will continue until the disease progresses or the drug is no longer tolerated. PFS and OS for patients with PD-L1$^+$ tumors are the primary efficacy endpoints. In the KEYNOTE-062 trial, the efficacy and safety of pembrolizumab alone or in combination with cisplatin plus 5-FU will be compared with chemotherapy alone (cisplatin +5-FU) as first-line therapy for PD-L1$^+$/HER2$^-$ advanced GC or GEJ adenocarcinoma. Primary endpoints are OS and progression-free survival (PFS).

Nivolumab

Like pembrolizumab, nivolumab is a humanized IgG4 monoclonal antibody against PD-1 with activity in multiple tumor types. The phase 1/2 CheckMate 032 trial compared the combination of nivolumab and ipilimumab to nivolumab monotherapy in 160 patients with advanced/metastatic gastric or gastroesophageal cancer [121]. Patients receiving the combination nivolumab and ipilimumab had an ORR of 24%, compared with 12% in patients receiving nivolumab alone. Of interest, ORR in the combination arms seemed to be dependent on dosing, as only 8% patients who received the alternate dosing (nivolumab 3 mg/kg and ipilimumab 1 mg/kg) responded. Responses were observed regardless of PD-L1 expression. As expected from other combination studies, nivolumab + ipilimumab therapy was associated with higher serious toxicity (43%) as compared to nivolumab alone (10%) [121].

ONO-12 (ATTRACTION-2) was a multicenter, double-blind, randomized phase III study of nivolumab for patients with unresectable advanced or recurrent gastric or GEJ cancer refractory to or intolerant of two or more prior chemotherapy regimens (NCT02267343). This was the first randomized, placebo-controlled, phase III trial of immune checkpoint blockade in gastrointestinal cancers. The study showed for the first time that PD-1 inhibition can improve the OSS for patients with heavily pre-treated gastric or gastroesophageal cancer [122]. The observed median OS was 5.32 months (95% CI, 4.63–6.41) with nivolumab vs. 4.14 months (95% CI, 3.42–4.86) with placebo, and the 12-month OS rate was 26.6% (95% CI, 21.1–32.4%) versus 10.9% (HR 0.63; 95% CI, 6.2%–17%; $p < 0.0001$). In addition, median PFS was 1.61 months with nivolumab versus 1.45 months with placebo (HR 0.60; $p < 0.0001$). The ORR rate was 11.2% with nivolumab versus 0% with placebo, and the median duration of response to nivolumab was 9.53 months (95% CI, 6.14–9.82 months) [122]. Patients treated with nivolumab showed a favorable safety profile with treatment-related adverse events (grade 3 or 4) occurring in 34 (10%) of 330 patients, with a frequency similar to those with placebo [122]. It should be considered, however, that the ATTRACTION-2 enrolled only patients from Asian countries, and therefore the results observed might not be applicable to European and North American populations. Recent evidence has suggested the existence of distinct gene signatures associated with inflammation and immunity in GC from Asian and non-Asian patients [123]. A study carried out on a large cohort of more than 1600 GC patients showed that non-Asian GCs were significantly enriched in signatures related to T-cell biology, including CTLA-4 signaling, whereas the immunosuppressive T-regulatory cell marker FOXP3 was significantly enriched in Asian populations.

Avelumab

Avelumab, an anti-PD-L1 IgG1 antibody, is currently being assessed in the JAVELIN trial (NCT01772004) with expansion cohorts for selected tumor types, including gastric/GEJ who had at least one prior therapy or who received avelumab as switch maintenance after chemotherapy [124]. Patients received 10 mg/kg of avelumab every 2 weeks, and preliminary data show a 9.7% response rate and 6.0 weeks of PFS in the second-line setting. For Japanese patients who had progressed while receiving prior chemotherapy, the reported overall response rate was 15% (3/20 patients), with the proportion of patients' progression-free survival at 12 weeks being 43.3% [125]. The JAVELIN Gastric 300 trial is currently recruiting patients with recurrent, locally advanced, or metastatic gastric/GEJ tumors in an open-label study comparing avelumab to best supportive care in the third-line setting (NCT02625623). Maintenance immunotherapy is being assessed in the JAVELIN Gastric 100 study, which compares single-agent avelumab (10 mg/kg every 2 weeks) to continuation of first-line chemotherapy (NCT02625610) [126]. One recently reported case of metastatic GC who experienced a strong clinical benefit from treatment with avelumab prompted a further characterization of the tumor. The analysis showed no evidence of high mutation burden or mismatch repair defect but disclosed a strong positivity for EBV-encoded RNA. Analysis of The Cancer Genome Atlas GC data (25 EBV^+, 80 MSI, 310 microsatellite-stable, MSS) showed that EBV-positive tumors were MSS and had low-mutation burden but stronger evidence of immune infiltration compared with MSI tumors. Notably, EBV-positive GC had higher expression of immune checkpoint pathway (PD-1, CTLA-4) genes in RNA-seq data and higher lymphocytic infiltration by histology compared with MSS tumors [127]. These findings suggest that EBV-positive low-mutation burden GC are a subset of MSS tumors that may respond to immune checkpoint therapy.

Durvalumab

Durvalumab is a selective, high-affinity, human IgG1κ monoclonal antibody that blocks PD-L1 binding to CD80 and PD-1. Available data indicate that 10 mg/kg of single-agent durvalumab given intravenously every 2 weeks for 12 months showed potential clinical activity in gastroesophageal cancers [128]. Treatment-related adverse events occurred in 33% of patients, with 7% of grade 3 toxicities. A phase IB/II study is currently enrolling patients with GEJ or gastric adenocarcinomas in the second- and third-line metastatic settings for treatment with single-agent durvalumab, single-agent tremelimumab, or combination durvalumab and tremelimumab (anti-CTLA-4) [129].

Combination Strategies Including Immune Checkpoint Blockade

The efficacy of immunotherapies targeting the PD-1/PD-L1 has stimulated the activation of combination studies with other active targeted biologic agents or immune-modulating treatments. The rationale supporting combination immunotherapy is supported by several preclinical data indicating that targeting only one of the complex steps required for the generation of an effective antitumor immune responses is often insufficient. Particularly challenging is the appropriate targeting of the immunosuppressed tumor microenvironment. Preclinical evidence demonstrated that inhibition of the PD-1/PD-L1 axis positively synergizes with antibodies blocking the vascular endothelial growth factor (VEGF)/VEGF receptor (VEGFR) pathway [130]. A recent phase Ia/Ib study investigated the safety and efficacy of the combination of anti-PD-L1 (durvalumab) and anti-VEGFR2 ramucirumab antibodies in patients with refractory GC/GEJ tumors [131]. Preliminary efficacy data showed clinical responses in 3 of 40 (7.5%) patients a 45% disease control rate. Median PFS was 2.10 months for patients treated with ramucirumab 8 mg/kg on days 1 and 2.60 months for patients treated with the same drug given at 10 mg/kg on day 1 only. Ten (25%) patients had grade 3–4 toxicities, most commonly colitis (7.5%) and hypertension (7.5%) [131].

Taking into account the ability of some chemotherapeutic drugs to induce immunogenic cell death, therapeutic approaches combining immunotherapy and chemotherapy are being actively investigated. Based on the promising results obtained with pembrolizumab and considering that PD-L1 is a predictive biomarker for pembrolizumab in lung cancer, a phase II study, KEYNOTE-059, was developed to further evaluate pembrolizumab in GC. The multilevel study design included three cohorts: (1) 259 patients with metastatic GC who received pembrolizumab alone, after pre-treatment with two or more lines of chemotherapy; (2) 25 patients with newly diagnosed metastatic GC who received a combination of pembrolizumab and chemotherapy (5-fluorouracil and cisplatin); and (3) 31 patients with newly diagnosed metastatic GC who received pembrolizumab alone. The primary endpoints were safety (all three cohorts) and objective response rate (cohorts one and three) [132]. After a median follow-up of 6 months, an overall objective response rate of 12% was observed in the pre-treated patients (cohort one) who received pembrolizumab alone. Expression of PD-L1 was associated with an increase likelihood to obtain a response (objective response rates of 16% vs. 6%). Many of the responses were durable. Grade 3 to 5 treatment-related adverse events occurred in 18% of patients in cohort one, and 3% had to discontinue treatment as a result [133]. These results are particularly encouraging considering that the expected response rate in these heavily pre-treated patients was close to zero. Based on these promising results, the randomized, phase III KEYNOTE-062 study (NCT02494583) was designed to compare the efficacy and safety of pembrolizumab alone or in combination with cisplatin + a fluoropyrimidine with those of cisplatin + a fluoropyrimidine as first-line therapy for PD-L1+/HER2– advanced GC/GEJ adenocarcinoma. The primary study hypotheses are that pembrolizumab in combination with chemotherapy is superior to chemotherapy alone in terms of progression-free survival and overall survival and that pembrolizumab monotherapy is as good as or better than chemotherapy alone in terms of overall survival.

The promising results of these combination studies in advanced disease prompted the activation of multiple trials in patients with earlier-stage disease, including the adjuvant nivolumab phase III trial in resected esophageal and GEJ (CheckMate-577) and a phase I neoadjuvant trial of nivolumab and ipilimumab in stage II–III patients (NCT03044613) [134].

Combination therapies with immune checkpoint inhibitors have also targeted the subset of HER2-overexpressing tumors, which almost invariably become resistant to trastuzumab-containing regimens and progress. Preclinical evidence supports the rationale for combining trastuzumab and inhibitors of the PD-1/PD-L1 axis. In fact, it has been demonstrated that HER2 inhibition can promote T-cell activation and trafficking, enhance IFNγ production by NK cells, and boost antibody-dependent cellular toxicity which may efficiently synergize with inhibition of the PD-1/PD-L1 pathway [135]. A phase Ib/II, open-label, dose-escalation study is investigating the novel anti-HER2 mAb margetuximab in combination with pembrolizumab in patients with advanced HER2-amplified GC who are refractory to standard trastuzumab-based combination chemotherapy (NCT02689284) [136]. A variety of other combinations is being investigated in which, on the backbone of inhibitors of PD-1/PD-L1 axis, other drugs target additional nodes in the cancer immunity cycle [137]. These latter include agents inhibiting other immune checkpoints (TIM3, LAG3), T-cell costimulatory agonist antibodies (GITR, OX40, 4-1BB), enzymatic inhibitors (IDO-1), as well as radiation and other cytotoxic drugs. Additionally, the combination of nivolumab and GS-5745, a matrix metalloproteinase-9 inhibitor, is also being investigated in patients with unresectable or recurrent GC/GEJ adenocarcinoma (NCT02864381). Combination with radiotherapy represents a promising therapeutic opportunity, although still poorly explored in the setting of GC. Single-dose and fractionated radiotherapy can upregulate tumor PD-L1 expression in various preclinical models. Administration of anti-PD-1 antibody concurrently with radiotherapy can overcome the adaptive upregulation of PD-L1 and restore long-term tumor control. Moreover, combination radiotherapy and PD-1/PD-L1 axis blockade demonstrated synergistic antitumor activity and reduce tumor-infiltrating myeloid-derived suppressor cells [138]. An intriguing possibility is that radiotherapy could be used to increase both the necessary antigen recognition machinery (MHC-I expression) and the magnitude of anti-PD-L1 antibodies binding to tumor cells [138]. Clinical trials involving GC patients are ongoing including studies combining pembrolizumab with palliative radiotherapy in the metastatic setting, as well as with neoadjuvant chemoradiotherapy for GEJ and gastric cardia cancers in earlier-stage resectable disease (NCT02730546) [139].

Concluding Remarks and Future Perspectives

Over the last decade, our understanding of the mechanisms underlying immune modulation has greatly improved, allowing for the development of multiple therapeutic approaches that are revolutionizing the treatment of cancer. Immunotherapy for GC is still in early phases but is rapidly evolving. The challenges moving forward are to put much effort in biologic and immunologic explorations in the GC setting to fine-tune and tailor more precisely the various immunotherapeutic approaches available or emerging. In addition, we must learn how to appropriately integrate immunotherapeutic strategies active against GC with molecularly targeted agents, chemotherapy, and radiotherapy. Rational combinations of different but complementary immune-based approaches should be also carefully investigated with the final goal to offer to each individual the most effective schedule/regimen in relation to the clinico-pathologic, genetic, virologic and immunologic features of his/her own tumor. In this respect, it will be necessary to design large prospective trials to validate reliable predictive factors allowing for the selection of GC patients with the highest chance to benefit from immunotherapy.

References

1. Bilici A. Treatment options in patients with metastatic gastric cancer: current status and future perspectives. World J Gastroenterol. 2014;20(14):3905–15.
2. Larkin J, Chiarion-Sileni V, Gonzalez R, Grob JJ, Cowey CL, Lao CD, et al. Combined nivolumab and ipilimumab or monotherapy in untreated melanoma. N Engl J Med. 2015;373(1):23–34.
3. Motzer RJ, Escudier B, McDermott DF, George S, Hammers HJ, Srinivas S, et al. Nivolumab versus everolimus in advanced renal-cell carcinoma. N Engl J Med. 2015;373(19):1803–13.
4. Reck M, Rodríguez-Abreu D, Robinson AG, Hui R, Csőszi T, Fülöp A, et al. Pembrolizumab versus chemotherapy for PD-L1-positive non-small-cell lung cancer. N Engl J Med. 2016;375(19):1823–33.
5. Bonotto M, Garattini SK, Basile D, Ongaro E, Fanotto V, Cattaneo M, et al. Immunotherapy for gastric cancers: emerging role and future perspectives. Expert Rev Clin Pharmacol. 2017;10(6):609–19.
6. Procaccio L, Schirripa M, Fassan M, Vecchione L, Bergamo F, Prete AA, et al. Immunotherapy in gastrointestinal cancers. Biomed Res Int. 2017;2017:4346576.
7. Finn OJ. A believer's overview of cancer immunosurveillance and immunotherapy. J Immunol. 2018;200(2):385–91.
8. Galluzzi L, Buqué A, Kepp O, Zitvogel L, Kroemer G. Immunogenic cell death in cancer and infectious disease. Nat Rev Immunol. 2017;17(2):97–111.
9. Frey B, Derer A, Scheithauer H, Wunderlich R, Fietkau R, Gaipl US. Cancer cell death-inducing radiotherapy: impact on local tumour control, tumour cell proliferation and induction of systemic anti-tumour immunity. Adv Exp Med Biol. 2016;930:151–72.
10. Brix N, Tiefenthaller A, Anders H, Belka C, Lauber K. Abscopal, immunological effects of radiotherapy: narrowing the gap between clinical and preclinical experiences. Immunol Rev. 2017;280(1):249–79.
11. Bass AJ, Thorsson V, Shmulevich I, Reynolds SM, Miller M, Bernard B, et al. Comprehensive molecular characterization of gastric adenocarcinoma. Cancer genome atlas research network. Nature. 2014;513(7517):202–9.
12. Camargo MC, Kim WH, Chiaravalli AM, Kim KM, Corvalan AH, Matsuo K, et al. Improved survival of gastric cancer with tumour Epstein-Barr virus positivity: an international pooled analysis. Gut. 2014;63(2):236–43.
13. van Beek J, zur Hausen A, Snel SN, Berkhof J, Kranenbarg EK, van de Velde CJ, et al. Morphological evidence of an activated cytotoxic T-cell infiltrate in EBV-positive gastric carcinoma preventing lymph node metastases. Am J Surg Pathol. 2006;30(1):59–65.
14. Song HJ, Srivastava A, Lee J, Kim YS, Kim KM, Ki Kang W, et al. Host inflammatory response predicts survival of patients with Epstein-Barr virus-associated gastric carcinoma. Gastroenterology. 2010;139(1):84–92.
15. Kim SY, Park C, Kim HJ, Park J, Hwang J, Kim JI, et al. Deregulation of immune response genes in patients with Epstein-Barr virus-associated gastric cancer and outcomes. Gastroenterology. 2015;148:137–47.

16. Derks S, Liao X, Chiaravalli AM, Xu X, Camargo MC, Solcia E, et al. Abundant PD-L1 expression in Epstein-Barr Virus-infected gastric cancers. Oncotarget. 2016;7(22):32925–32.
17. Hause RJ, Pritchard CC, Shendure J, Salipante SJ. Classification and characterization of microsatellite instability across 18 cancer types. Nat Med. 2016;22(11):1342–50.
18. Yamamoto H, Perez-Piteira J, Yoshida T, Terada M, Itoh F, Imai K, et al. Gastric cancers of the microsatellite mutator phenotype display characteristic genetic and clinical features. Gastroenterology. 1999;116(6):1348–57.
19. Colli LM, Machiela MJ, Myers TA, Jessop L, Yu K, Chanock SJ. Burden of nonsynonymous mutations among TCGA cancers and candidate immune checkpoint inhibitor responses. Cancer Res. 2016;76(13):3767–72.
20. Schwitalle Y, Kloor M, Eiermann S, Linnebacher M, Kienle P, Knaebel HP, et al. Immune response against frameshift-induced neopeptides in HNPCC patients and healthy HNPCC mutation carriers. Gastroenterology. 2008;134(4):988–97.
21. Bernal M, García-Alcalde F, Concha A, Cano C, Blanco A, Garrido F, et al. Genome-wide differential genetic profiling characterizes colorectal cancers with genetic instability and specific routes to HLA class I loss and immune escape. Cancer Immunol Immunother. 2012;61(6):803–16.
22. Wang M, Busuttil RA, Pattison S, Neeson PJ, Boussioutas A. Immunological battlefield in gastric cancer and role of immunotherapies. World J Gastroenterol. 2016;22(28):6373–84.
23. Badalamenti G, Fanale D, Incorvaia L, Barraco N, Listì A, Maragliano R, et al. Role of tumor-infiltrating lymphocytes in patients with solid tumors: can a drop dig a stone? Cell Immunol. 2018;S0008-8749(18):30014–5.
24. Kim KJ, Lee KS, Cho HJ, Kim YH, Yang HK, Kim WH, et al. Prognostic implications of tumor-infiltrating FoxP3+ regulatory T cells and CD8+ cytotoxic T cells in microsatellite-unstable gastric cancers. Hum Pathol. 2014;45:285–93.
25. Kang BW, Seo AN, Yoon S, Bae HI, Jeon SW, Kwon OK, et al. Prognostic value of tumor-infiltrating lymphocytes in Epstein-Barr virus-associated gastric cancer. Ann Oncol. 2016;27:494–501.
26. Zheng X, Song X, Shao Y, Xu B, Chen L, Zhou Q, et al. Prognostic role of tumor-infiltrating lymphocytes in gastric cancer: a meta-analysis. Oncotarget. 2017;8(34):57386–98.
27. Kandulski A, Malfertheiner P, Wex T. Role of regulatory T-cells in H. pylori-induced gastritis and gastric cancer. Anticancer Res. 2010;30:1093–103.
28. Nagase H, Takeoka T, Urakawa S, Morimoto-Okazawa A, Kawashima A, Iwahori K, et al. ICOS+Foxp3+ TILs in gastric cancer are prognostic markers and effector regulatory T cells associated with Helicobacter pylori. Int J Cancer. 2017;140(3):686–95.
29. Groom JR, Luster AD. CXCR3 ligands: redundant, collaborative and antagonistic functions. Immunol Cell Biol. 2011;89(2):207–15.
30. Chen F, Yin S, Niu L, Luo J, Wang B, Xu Z, et al. Expression of the chemokine receptor CXCR3 correlates with dendritic cell recruitment and prognosis in gastric cancer. Genet Test Mol Biomarkers. 2018;22(1):35–42.
31. Knief J, Reddemann K, Petrova E, Herhahn T, Wellner U, Thorns C. High density of tumor-infiltrating B-lymphocytes and plasma cells signifies prolonged overall survival in adenocarcinoma of the esophagogastric junction. Anticancer Res. 2016;36(10):5339–45.
32. Matsueda S, Graham DY. Immunotherapy in gastric cancer. World J Gastroenterol. 2014;20(7):1657–66.
33. Mittal D, Gubin MM, Schreiber RD, Smyth MJ. New insights into cancer immunoediting and its three component phases – elimination, equilibrium and escape. Curr Opin Immunol. 2014;27:16–25.
34. Garrido F, Perea F, Bernal M, Sánchez-Palencia A, Aptsiauri N, Ruiz-Cabello F. The escape of cancer from T cell-mediated immune surveillance: HLA class I loss and tumor tissue architecture. Vaccines (Basel). 2017;5(1):7.
35. Murray PJ, Allen JE, Biswas SK, Fisher EA, Gilroy DW, Goerdt S, et al. Macrophage activation and polarization: nomenclature and experimental guidelines. Immunity. 2014;41(1):14–20.
36. Ishigami S, Natsugoe S, Tokuda K, Nakajo A, Okumura H, Matsumoto M, Miyazono F, Hokita S, Aikou T. Tumor-associated macrophage (TAM) infiltration in gastric cancer. Anticancer Res. 2003;23(5A):4079–83.
37. Mitchem JB, Brennan DJ, Knolhoff BL, Belt BA, Zhu Y, Sanford DE, et al. Targeting tumor-infiltrating macrophages decreases tumor-initiating cells, relieves immunosuppression, and improves chemotherapeutic responses. Cancer Res. 2013;73(3):1128–41.
38. Wu MH, Lee WJ, Hua KT, Kuo ML, Lin MT. Macrophage infiltration induces gastric cancer invasiveness by activating the β-Catenin pathway. PLoS One. 2015;10(7):e0134122.
39. Park JY, Sung JY, Lee J, Park YK, Kim YW, Kim GY, et al. Polarized CD163+ tumor-associated macrophages are associated with increased angiogenesis and CXCL12 expression in gastric cancer. Clin Res Hepatol Gastroenterol. 2016;40(3):357–65.
40. Bronte V, Brandau S, Chen SH, Colombo MP, Frey AB, Greten TF, et al. Recommendations for myeloid-derived suppressor cell nomenclature and characterization standards. Nat Commun. 2016;7:12150.
41. Choi BD, Gedeon PC, Herndon JE, Archer GE, Reap EA, Sanchez-Perez L, et al. Human regulatory T cells kill tumor cells through granzyme-dependent cytotoxicity upon retargeting with a bispecific antibody. Cancer Immunol Res. 2013;1:163.
42. Ding Y, Shen J, Zhang G, Chen X, Wu J, Chen W. CD40 controls CXCR5-induced recruitment of

myeloid-derived suppressor cells to gastric cancer. Oncotarget. 2015;6(36):38901–11.
43. Choi HS, Ha SY, Kim HM, Ahn SM, Kang MS, Kim KM, et al. The prognostic effects of tumor infiltrating regulatory T cells and myeloid derived suppressor cells assessed by multicolor flow cytometry in gastric cancer patients. Oncotarget. 2016;7(7):7940–51.
44. Bennett MW, O'connell J, O'sullivan GC, Roche D, Brady C, Kelly J, et al. Expression of Fas ligand by human gastric adenocarcinomas: a potential mechanism of immune escape in stomach cancer. Gut. 1999;44(2):156–62.
45. Sharma P, Allison JP. Immune checkpoint targeting in cancer therapy: toward combination strategies with curative potential. Cell. 2015;161(2):205–14.
46. Wilson RAM, Evans TRJ, Fraser AR, Nibbs RJB. Immune checkpoint inhibitors: new strategies to checkmate cancer. Clin Exp Immunol. 2018;191(2):133–48.
47. Topalian SL, Drake CG, Pardoll DM. Immune checkpoint blockade: a common denominator approach to cancer therapy. Cancer Cell. 2015;27:450–61.
48. Tran PN, Sarkissian S, Chao J, Klempner SJ. PD-1 and PD-L1 as emerging therapeutic targets in gastric cancer: current evidence. Gastrointest Cancer. 2017;7:1–11.
49. Böger C, Behrens HM, Mathiak M, Krüger S, Kalthoff H, Röcken C. PD-L1 is an independent prognostic predictor in gastric cancer of Western patients. Oncotarget. 2016;7(17):24269–83.
50. Kim JW, Nam KH, Ahn SH, Park DJ, Kim HH, Kim SH, et al. Prognostic implications of immunosuppressive protein expression in tumors as well as immune cell infiltration within the tumor microenvironment in gastric cancer. Gastric Cancer. 2016;19(1):42–52.
51. Schlößer HA, Drebber U, Kloth M, Thelen M, Rothschild SI, Haase S, et al. Immune checkpoints programmed death 1 ligand 1 and cytotoxic T lymphocyte associated molecule 4 in gastric adenocarcinoma. Oncoimmunology. 2015;5(5):e1100789.
52. Gao Y, Li S, Xu D, Chen S, Cai Y, Jiang W, et al. Prognostic value of programmed death-1, programmed death-ligand 1, programmed death-ligand 2 expression, and CD8(+) T cell density in primary tumors and metastatic lymph nodes from patients with stage T1-4N+M0 gastric adenocarcinoma. Chin J Cancer. 2017;36(1):61.
53. Gu L, Chen M, Guo D, Zhu H, Zhang W, Pan J, et al. PD-L1 and gastric cancer prognosis: a systematic review and meta-analysis. PLoS One. 2017;12(8):e0182692.
54. Saito R, Abe H, Kunita A, Yamashita H, Seto Y, Fukayama M. Overexpression and gene amplification of PD-L1 in cancer cells and PD-L1+ immune cells in Epstein-Barr virus-associated gastric cancer: the prognostic implications. Mod Pathol. 2017;30(3):427–39.
55. Seo AN, Kang BW, Kwon OK, Park KB, Lee SS, Chung HY, et al. Intratumoural PD-L1 expression is associated with worse survival of patients with Epstein-Barr virus-associated gastric cancer. Br J Cancer. 2017;117(12):1753–60.
56. Fang W, Chen Y, Sheng J, Zhou T, Zhang Y, Zhan J, et al. Association between PD-L1 expression on tumour-infiltrating lymphocytes and overall survival in patients with gastric cancer. J Cancer. 2017;8(9):1579–85.
57. Liu Y, Cheng Y, Xu Y, Wang Z, Du X, Li C, et al. Increased expression of programmed cell death protein 1 on NK cells inhibits NK-cell-mediated anti-tumor function and indicates poor prognosis in digestive cancers. Oncogene. 2017;36(44):6143–53.
58. Nowak EC, Lines JL, Varn FS, Deng J, Sarde A, Mabaera R, et al. Immunoregulatory functions of VISTA. Immunol Rev. 2017;276(1):66–79.
59. Liu J, Yuan Y, Chen W, Putra J, Suriawinata AA, Schenk AD, et al. Immune-checkpoint proteins VISTA and PD-1 nonredundantly regulate murine T-cell responses. Proc Natl Acad Sci U S A. 2015;112(21):6682–7.
60. Böger C, Behrens HM, Krüger S, Röcken C. The novel negative checkpoint regulator VISTA is expressed in gastric carcinoma and associated with PD-L1/PD-1: a future perspective for a combined gastric cancer therapy? Oncoimmunology. 2017;6(4):e1293215.
61. Du W, Yang M, Turner A, Xu C, Ferris RL, Huang J, et al. TIM-3 as a Target for Cancer Immunotherapy and Mechanisms of Action. Int J Mol Sci. 2017;18(3):645.
62. Takano S, Saito H, Ikeguchi M. An increased number of PD-1+ and Tim-3+ CD8+ T cells is involved in immune evasion in gastric cancer. Surg Today. 2016;46(11):1341–7.
63. Lu X, Yang L, Yao D, Wu X, Li J, Liu X, et al. Tumor antigen-specific CD8+ T cells are negatively regulated by PD-1 and Tim-3 in human gastric cancer. Cell Immunol. 2017;313:43–51.
64. Palucka K, Banchereau J. Cancer immunotherapy via dendritic cells. Nat Rev Cancer. 2012;12(4):265–77.
65. Ishigami S, Natsugoe S, Tokuda K, Nakajo A, Xiangming C, Iwashige H, et al. Clinical impact of intratumoral natural killer cell and dendritic cell infiltration in gastric cancer. Cancer Lett. 2000;159(1):103–8.
66. Ananiev J, Gulubova MV, Manolova IM. Prognostic significance of CD83 positive tumor-infiltrating dendritic cells and expression of TGF-beta 1 in human gastric cancer. Hepato-Gastroenterology. 2011;58(110–111):1834–40.
67. Niccolai E, Taddei A, Prisco D, Amedei A. Gastric cancer and the epoch of immunotherapy approaches. World J Gastroenterol. 2015;21(19):5778–93.
68. Sadanaga N, Nagashima H, Mashino K, Tahara K, Yamaguchi H, Ohta M, et al. Dendritic cell vaccination with MAGE peptide is a novel therapeutic approach for gastrointestinal carcinomas. Clin Cancer Res. 2001;7(8):2277–84.

69. Kono K, Takahashi A, Sugai H, Fujii H, Choudhury AR, Kiessling R, et al. Dendritic cells pulsed with HER-2/neu-derived peptides can induce specific T-cell responses in patients with gastric cancer. Clin Cancer Res. 2002;8(11):3394–400.
70. Popiela T, Kulig J, Czupryna A, Szczepanik AM, Zembala M. Efficiency of adjuvant immunochemotherapy following curative resection in patients with locally advanced gastric cancer. Gastric Cancer. 2004;7(4):240–5.
71. Ajani JA, Hecht JR, Ho L, Baker J, Oortgiesen M, Eduljee A, Michaeli D. An open-label, multinational, multicenter study of G17DT vaccination combined with cisplatin and 5-fluorouracil in patients with untreated, advanced gastric or gastroesophageal cancer: the GC4 study. Cancer. 2006;106(9):1908–16.
72. Higashihara Y, Kato J, Nagahara A, Izumi K, Konishi M, Kodani T, et al. Phase I clinical trial of peptide vaccination with URLC10 and VEGFR1 epitope peptides in patients with advanced gastric cancer. Int J Oncol. 2014;44(3):662–8.
73. Sato Y, Shomura H, Maeda Y, Mine T, Une Y, Akasaka Y, et al. Immunological evaluation of peptide vaccination for patients with gastric cancer based on pre-existing cellular response to peptide. Cancer Sci. 2003;94(9):802–8.
74. Sato Y, Fujiwara T, Mine T, Shomura H, Homma S, Maeda Y, et al. Immunological evaluation of personalized peptide vaccination in combination with a 5-fluorouracil derivative (TS-1) for advanced gastric or colorectal carcinoma patients. Cancer Sci. 2007;98(7):1113–9.
75. Masuzawa T, Fujiwara Y, Okada K, Nakamura A, Takiguchi S, Nakajima K, et al. Phase I/II study of S-1 plus cisplatin combined with peptide vaccines for human vascular endothelial growth factor receptor 1 and 2 in patients with advanced gastric cancer. Int J Oncol. 2012;41(4):1297–304.
76. Fujiwara Y, Sugimura K, Miyata H, Omori T, Nakano H, Mochizuki C, et al. A pilot study of postoperative adjuvant vaccine for advanced gastric cancer. Yonago Acta Med. 2017;60(2):101–5.
77. Yang JC, Rosenberg SA. Adoptive T-cell therapy for cancer. Adv Immunol. 2016;130:279–94.
78. Kang BW, Kim JG, Lee IH, Bae HI, Seo AN. Clinical significance of tumor-infiltrating lymphocytes for gastric cancer in the era of immunology. World J Gastrointest Oncol. 2017;9(7):293–9.
79. Kono K, Ichihara F, Iizuka H, Sekikawa T, Matsumoto Y. Differences in the recognition of tumor-specific CD8+ T cells derived from solid tumor, metastatic lymph nodes and ascites in patients with gastric cancer. Int J Cancer. 1997;71(6):978–81.
80. Fujie T, Tanaka F, Tahara K, Li J, Tanaka S, Mori M, et al. Generation of specific antitumor reactivity by the stimulation of spleen cells from gastric cancer patients with MAGE-3 synthetic peptide. Cancer Immunol Immunother. 1999;48(4):189–94.
81. Xu X, Xu L, Ding S, Wu M, Tang Z, Fu W, et al. Treatment of 23 patients with advanced gastric cancer by intravenously transfer of autologous tumor-infiltrating lymphocytes combined with rIL-2. Chin Med Sci J. 1995;10(3):185–7.
82. Zhang GQ, Zhao H, Wu JY, Li JY, Yan X, Wang G, et al. Prolonged overall survival in gastric cancer patients after adoptive immunotherapy. World J Gastroenterol. 2015;21(9):2777–85.
83. Kono K, Takahashi A, Ichihara F, Amemiya H, Iizuka H, Fujii H, et al. Prognostic significance of adoptive immunotherapy with tumor-associated lymphocytes in patients with advanced gastric cancer: a randomized trial. Clin Cancer Res. 2002;8(6):1767–71.
84. Malmberg KJ, Carlsten M, Björklund A, Sohlberg E, Bryceson YT, Ljunggren HG. Natural killer cell-mediated immunosurveillance of human cancer. Semin Immunol. 2017;31:20–9.
85. Rigueiro MP, Kassab P, Ilias EJ, Castro OA, Novo NF, Lourenço LG. Correlation of natural killer cells with the prognosis of gastric adenocarcinoma. Rosso D, Arq Bras Cir Dig. 2012;25(2):114–7.
86. Saito H, Takaya S, Osaki T, Ikeguchi M. Increased apoptosis and elevated Fas expression in circulating natural killer cells in gastric cancer patients. Gastric Cancer. 2013;16(4):473–9.
87. Voskens CJ, Watanabe R, Rollins S, Campana D, Hasumi K, Mann DL. Ex-vivo expanded human NK cells express activating receptors that mediate cytotoxicity of allogeneic and autologous cancer cell lines by direct recognition and antibody directed cellular cytotoxicity. J Exp Clin Cancer Res. 2010;29:134.
88. Guo Y, Han W. Cytokine-induced killer (CIK) cells: from basic research to clinical translation. Chin J Cancer. 2015;34:6.
89. Verneris MR, Kornacker M, Mailander V, Negrin RS. Resistance of ex vivo expanded CD3+ CD56+ T cells to Fas-mediated apoptosis. Cancer Immunol Immunother. 2000;49:335–45.
90. Sun S, Li XM, Li XD, Yang WS. Studies on inducing apoptosis effects and mechanism of CIK cells for MGC-803 gastric cancer cell lines. Cancer Biother Radiopharm. 2005;20(2):173–80.
91. Bourquin C, von der Borch P, Zoglmeier C, Anz D, Sandholzer N, Suhartha N, et al. Efficient eradication of subcutaneous but not of autochthonous gastric tumors by adoptive T cell transfer in an SV40 T antigen mouse model. J Immunol. 2010;185(4):2580–8.
92. Thompson J, Epting T, Schwarzkopf G, Singhofen A, Eades-Perner AM, van Der Putten H, et al. A transgenic mouse line that develops early-onset invasive gastric carcinoma provides a model for carcinoembryonic antigen-targeted tumor therapy. Int J Cancer. 2000;86(6):863–9.
93. Wu J, Waxman DJ. Immunogenic chemotherapy: dose and schedule dependence and combination with immunotherapy. Cancer Lett. 2018;419:210–21.
94. Zhao Q, Zhang H, Li Y, Liu J, Hu X, Fan L. Antitumor effects of CIK combined with oxaliplatin in human oxaliplatin-resistant gastric cancer

cells in vivo and in vitro. J Exp Clin Cancer Res. 2010;29:118.
95. Zhao H, Fan Y, Li H, Yu J, Liu L, Cao S, et al. Immunotherapy with cytokine-induced killer cells as an adjuvant treatment for advanced gastric carcinoma: a retrospective study of 165 patients. Cancer Biother Radiopharm. 2013;28(4):303–9.
96. Shi L, Zhou Q, Wu J, Ji M, Li G, Jiang J, et al. Efficacy of adjuvant immunotherapy with cytokine-induced killer cells in patients with locally advanced gastric cancer. Cancer Immunol Immunother. 2012;61(12):2251–9.
97. Liu H, Song J, Yang Z, Zhang X. Effects of cytokine-induced killer cell treatment combined with FOLFOX4 on the recurrence and survival rates for gastric cancer following surgery. Exp Ther Med. 2013;6(4):953–6.
98. Liu K, Song G, Hu X, Zhou Y, Li Y, Chen Q, et al. A positive role of cytokine-induced killer cell therapy on gastric cancer therapy in a Chinese population: a systematic meta-analysis. Med Sci Monit. 2015;21:3363–70.
99. Mao Q, Li L, Zhang C, Sun Y, Liu S, Cui S. Clinical effects of immunotherapy of DC-CIK combined with chemotherapy in treating patients with metastatic breast cancer. Pak J Pharm Sci. 2015;28(3 Suppl):1055–8.
100. Chen Y, Zhou Z, Wei-feng Z, Chen G, Shi Y, Lin W, et al. Tumor mica status predicts the efficacy of immunotherapy with cytokine-induced killer cells for patients with gastric cancer. J Immunother Cancer. 2015;3(Suppl 2):P61.
101. Mu Y, Zhou CH, Chen SF, Ding J, Zhang YX, Yang YP, et al. Effectiveness and safety of chemotherapy combined with cytokine-induced killer cell /dendritic cell-cytokine-induced killer cell therapy for treatment of gastric cancer in China: a systematic review and meta-analysis. Cytotherapy. 2016;18(9):1162–77.
102. Introna M, Correnti F. Innovative Clinical Perspectives for CIK Cells in Cancer Patients. Int J Mol Sci. 2018;19(2):358.
103. Zhang L, Zhao G, Hou Y, Zhang J, Hu J, Zhang K. The experimental study on the treatment of cytokine-induced killer cells combined with EGFR monoclonal antibody against gastric cancer. Cancer Biother Radiopharm. 2014;29(3):99–107.
104. Mirzaei HR, Rodriguez A, Shepphird J, Brown CE, Badie B. Chimeric antigen receptors T cell therapy in solid tumor: challenges and clinical applications. Front Immunol. 2017;8:1850.
105. Leone P, Shin EC, Perosa F, Vacca A, Dammacco F, Racanelli V. MHC class I antigen processing and presenting machinery: organization, function, and defects in tumor cells. J Natl Cancer Inst. 2013;105:1172–87.
106. Han Y, Liu C, Li G, Li J, Lv X, Shi H, et al. Antitumor effects and persistence of a novel HER2 CAR T cells directed to gastric cancer in preclinical models. Am J Cancer Res. 2018;8(1):106–19.
107. Song Y, Tong C, Wang Y, Gao Y, Dai H, Guo Y, et al. Effective and persistent antitumor activity of HER2-directed CAR-T cells against gastric cancer cells in vitro and xenotransplanted tumors in vivo. Protein Cell. 2018;9(10):867–78.
108. Shibaguchi H, Luo N, Shirasu N, Kuroki M, Kuroki M. Enhancement of antitumor activity by using a fully human gene encoding a single-chain fragmented antibody specific for carcinoembryonic antigen. Onco Targets Ther. 2017;10:3979–90.
109. Robert C, Schachter J, Long GV, Arance A, Grob JJ, Mortier L, et al. Pembrolizumab versus ipilimumab in advanced melanoma. N Engl J Med. 2015;372(26):2521–32.
110. Simpson TR, Li F, Montalvo-Ortiz W, Sepulveda MA, Bergerhoff K, Arce F, et al. Fc-dependent depletion of tumor-infiltrating regulatory T cells co-defines the efficacy of anti-CTLA-4 therapy against melanoma. J Exp Med. 2013;210(9):1695–710.
111. Leach DR, Krummel MF, Allison JP. Enhancement of antitumor immunity by CTLA-4 blockade. Science. 1996;271(5256):1734–6.
112. van Elsas A, Hurwitz AA, Allison JP. Combination immunotherapy of B16 melanoma using anti-cytotoxic T lymphocyte-associated antigen 4 (CTLA-4) and granulocyte/macrophage colony-stimulating factor (GM-CSF)-producing vaccines induces rejection of subcutaneous and metastatic tumors accompanied by autoimmune depigmentation. J Exp Med. 1999;190(3):355–66.
113. Quezada SA, Simpson TR, Peggs KS, Merghoub T, Vider J, Fan X, et al. Tumor-reactive CD4(+) T cells develop cytotoxic activity and eradicate large established melanoma after transfer into lymphopenic hosts. J Exp Med. 2010;207(3):637–50.
114. Ralph C, Elkord E, Burt DJ, O'Dwyer JF, Austin EB, Stern PL, et al. Modulation of lymphocyte regulation for cancer therapy: a phase II trial of tremelimumab in advanced gastric and esophageal adenocarcinoma. Clin Cancer Res. 2010;16(5):1662–72.
115. Bang YJ, Cho JY, Kim YH, Kim JW, Di Bartolomeo M, Ajani JA, et al. Efficacy of sequential ipilimumab monotherapy versus best supportive care for unresectable locally advanced/metastatic gastric or gastroesophageal junction cancer. Clin Cancer Res. 2017;23(19):5671–8.
116. Muro K, Chung HC, Shankaran V, Geva R, Catenacci D, Gupta S, et al. Pembrolizumab for patients with PD-L1-positive advanced gastric cancer (KEYNOTE-012): a multicentre, open-label, phase 1b trial. Lancet Oncol. 2016;17(6):717–26.
117. Doi T, Piha-Paul SA, Jalal SI, Saraf S, Lunceford J, Koshiji M, et al. Safety and antitumor activity of the anti-programmed death-1 antibody pembrolizumab in patients with advanced esophageal carcinoma. J Clin Oncol. 2018;36(1):61–7.
118. Langer CJ, Gadgeel SM, Borghaei H, Papadimitrakopoulou VA, Patnaik A, Powell SF, et al. Carboplatin and pemetrexed with or without pembrolizumab for advanced, non-squamous

non-small-cell lung cancer: a randomised, phase 2 cohort of the open-label KEYNOTE-021 study. Lancet Oncol. 2016;17(11):1497–508.
119. Fuchs CS, Doi T, Jang RW-J, Muro K, Satoh T, Machado M, et al. KEYNOTE-059 cohort 1: efficacy and safety of pembrolizumab (pembro) monotherapy in patients with previously treated advanced gastric cancer. J Clin Oncol. 2017;35(15_suppl):4003.
120. Ohtsu A, Tabernero J, Bang YJ, et al. Pembrolizumab (MK-3475) versus paclitaxel as second-line therapy for advanced gastric or gastroesophageal junction (GEJ) adenocarcinoma: phase 3 KEYNOTE-061 study. J Clin Oncol. 2016;34(suppl 4S):abstr TPS183.
121. Janjigian YY, Ott PA, Calvo E, Kim JW, Ascierto PA, Sharma P, et al. Nivolumab ± ipilimumab in pts with advanced (adv)/metastatic chemotherapy-refractory (CTx-R) gastric (G), esophageal (E), or gastroesophageal junction (GEJ) cancer: CheckMate 032 study. J Clin Oncol. 2017;35(15_suppl):4014.
122. Kang YK, Boku N, Satoh T, Ryu MH, Chao Y, Kato K, et al. Nivolumab in patients with advanced gastric or gastro-oesophageal junction cancer refractory to, or intolerant of, at least two previous chemotherapy regimens (ONO-4538-12, ATTRACTION-2): a randomised, double-blind, placebo-controlled, phase 3 trial. Lancet. 2017;390(10111):2461–71.
123. Lin SJ, Gagnon-Bartsch JA, Tan IB, Earle S, Ruff L, Pettinger K, et al. Signatures of tumour immunity distinguish Asian and non-Asian gastric adenocarcinomas. Gut. 2015;64(11):1721–31.
124. Kelly K, Patel MR, Infante JR, et al. Avelumab (MSB0010718C), an anti-PD-L1 antibody, in patients with metastatic or locally advanced solid tumors: assessment of safety and tolerability in a phase I, open-label expansion study. J Clin Oncol. 2015;33(suppl):abstr 3044.
125. Nishina T, Shitara K, Iwasa S, et al. Safety, PD-L1 expression, and clinical activity of avelumab (MSB0010718C), an anti-PD-L1 antibody, in Japanese patients with advanced gastric or gastroesophageal junction cancer. J Clin Oncol. 2016;34(suppl 4S):abstr 168.
126. Moehler MH, Taïeb J, Gurtler JS, et al. Maintenance therapy with avelumab (MSB0010718C; anti-PD-L1) vs continuation of first-line chemotherapy in patients with unresectable, locally advanced or metastatic gastric cancer: the phase 3 JAVELIN Gastric 100 trial. J Clin Oncol. 2016;34(suppl):abstr TPS4134.
127. Panda A, Mehnert JM, Hirshfield KM, Riedlinger G, Damare S, Saunders T, et al. Immune activation and benefit from avelumab in EBV-positive gastric cancer. J Natl Cancer Inst. 2017;110(3):316–20.
128. Segal NH, Antonia SJ, Brahmer JR, et al. Preliminary data from a multi-arm expansion study of MEDI4736, an anti-PD-L1 antibody. J Clin Oncol. 2014;32(5s(suppl)):abstr 3002.
129. Kelly RJ, Chung K, Gu Y, et al. Phase Ib/II study to evaluate the safety and antitumor activity of durvalumab (MEDI4736) and tremelimumab as monotherapy or in combination, in patients with recurrent or metastatic gastric/gastroesophageal junction adenocarcinoma. J Immunother Cancer. 2015;3(suppl 2):P157.
130. Voron T, Marcheteau E, Pernot S, Colussi O, Tartour E, Taieb J, Terme M. Control of the immune response by pro-angiogenic factors. Front Oncol. 2014;4:70.
131. Chau I, Bendell J, Calvo E, Santana-Davila R, Ahnert J, Penel N. Interim safety and clinical activity in patients (pts) with advanced gastric or gastroesophageal junction (G/GEJ) adenocarcinoma from a multicohort phase 1 study of ramucirumab (R) plus pembrolizumab (P). J Clin Oncol. 2017;35:102.
132. Fuchs CS, Denker AE, Tabernero J, et al. KEYNOTE-059: Phase 2 study of pembrolizumab (MK-3475) for recurrent or metastatic gastric or gastroesophageal junction adenocarcinoma. J Clin Oncol. 2015;33(15suppl):TPS4135.
133. Bang Y-J, Muro K, Fuchs CS, et al. KEYNOTE-059 cohort 2: Safety and efficacy of pembrolizumab (pembro) plus 5-fluorouracil (5-FU) and cisplatin for first-line (1L) treatment of advanced gastric cancer. J Clin Oncol. 2017;35(suppl):4012.
134. Janjigian YY, Adenis A, Aucoin J-S, et al. Checkmate 649: a randomized, multicenter, open-label, phase 3 study of nivolumab (Nivo) plus ipilimumab (Ipi) versus oxaliplatin plus fluoropyrimidine in patients (Pts) with previously untreated advanced or metastatic gastric (G) or gastroesophageal junction (GEJ) cancer. J Clin Oncol. 2017;35(4 suppl):TPS213.
135. Vanneman M, Dranoff G. Combining immunotherapy and targeted therapies in cancer treatment. Nat Rev Cancer. 2012;12(4):237–51.
136. Catenacci DVT, Kim SS, Gold PJ, et al. A phase 1b/2, open label, dose-escalation study of margetuximab (M) in combination with pembrolizumab (P) in patients with relapsed/refractory advanced HER2+ gastroesophageal (GEJ) junction or gastric (G) cancer. J Clin Oncol. 2017;35(suppl 4S):abstract TPS219.
137. Chen DS, Mellman I. Oncology meets immunology: the cancer-immunity cycle. Immunity. 2013;39(1):1–10.
138. Ngwa W, Irabor OC, Schoenfeld JD, Hesser J, Demaria S, Formenti SC. Using immunotherapy to boost the abscopal effect. Nat Rev Cancer. 2018;18(5):313–22.
139. Chao J, Chen Y-J, Frankel PH, et al. Combining pembrolizumab and palliative radiotherapy in gastroesophageal cancer to enhance antitumor T-cell response and augment the abscopal effect. J Clin Oncol. 2017;35(suppl 4S):abstract TPS220.

Nanomedicine in Gastric Cancer

13

Nayla Mouawad, Maguie El Boustani, Vincenzo Canzonieri, Isabella Caligiuri, and Flavio Rizzolio

Introduction

Gastric cancer (GC), a multifactorial disease, is the fourth most common cancer and the second leading cause of cancer death worldwide. According to geographic areas and sociocultural and economic entities, the distribution of GC varies widely, with the highest rates in East Asia, particularly China, Japan, and South Korea [1]. Many factors are involved in this disease, including infectious, environmental, or host-related factors (age, gender, family history, diet, obesity, tobacco, alcohol, and race). Until now, different therapeutic approaches have already been incorporated to address GC [2]. Current treatment options for GC include a combination of surgery, radiation therapy, and chemotherapy.

Over the past decade, increased knowledge of the tumour microenvironment has facilitated the ability to design new treatments for cancer. Cancer tissue is composed of two compartments: the noncellular (i.e. vascular and interstitial) and cellular compartments surrounded by the normal tissue, which is challenging for local delivery of drugs to tumour cells. Within the noncellular compartment of tumour tissue, regions of fast-dividing cells of the tumour possess a high vascular density, while regions that display tumour necrosis receive little blood supply. Moreover, the tumour cells away from blood vessels have a decreased amount of oxygen. New blood vessels are synthesized by tumours in a process known as angiogenesis.

N. Mouawad
Pathology Unit, Department of Translational Research, IRCCS, CRO Aviano, National Cancer Institute, Aviano, PN, Italy

Department of Pharmacy, University of Pisa, Pisa, Italy

M. El Boustani
Pathology Unit, Department of Translational Research, IRCCS, CRO Aviano, National Cancer Institute, Aviano, PN, Italy

Doctoral School in Molecular Biomedicine, University of Trieste, Trieste, Italy

V. Canzonieri
Pathology Unit, IRCCS, CRO Aviano, National Cancer Institute, Aviano, PN, Italy

Department of Medical, Surgical and Health Sciences, University of Trieste, Trieste, Italy

CRO Biobank, IRCCS, CRO Aviano, National Cancer Institute, Aviano, PN, Italy

Department of Biology, Temple University, Philadelphia, PA, USA

I. Caligiuri (✉)
Pathology Unit, Department of Translational Research, IRCCS, CRO Aviano, National Cancer Institute, Aviano, PN, Italy

F. Rizzolio (✉)
Pathology Department, IRCCS, CRO Aviano, National Cancer Institute, Aviano, PN, Italy

Department of Molecular Sciences and Nanosystems, Ca' Foscari University of Venice, Venice, Italy

Department of Biology, Temple University, Philadelphia, PA, USA
e-mail: flavio.rizzolio@unive.it

© Springer Nature Switzerland AG 2019

V. Canzonieri, A. Giordano (eds.), *Gastric Cancer In The Precision Medicine Era*, Current Clinical Pathology, https://doi.org/10.1007/978-3-030-04861-7_13

These vessels are abnormal, with increased numbers of proliferating endothelial cells and vessel tortuosity, deficient pericytes, and abnormalities in the basement membrane with large gaps [3, 4]. Furthermore, the upregulation of vascular endothelial growth factor, bradykinin, prostaglandins, and nitric oxide contributes to the hyperpermeable nature of tumours. Unlike normal tissues, the environment surrounding tumour cells has high interstitial pressure and the absence of a functioning lymphatic network [5]. The combination of deficient lymphatic drainage with increased vascular permeability is responsible for the enhanced permeability and retention (EPR) effect that facilitates the delivery of chemotherapeutic agents to well-vascularized parts of the tumour [6, 7]. However, the drugs may not reach the poorly vascularized regions, thus preventing some cancer cells from receiving cytotoxic treatment. This effect is due to the low microvascular pressure in these regions, which reduces the extravasation of drugs. In addition, the decreased amount of oxygen due to the lack of vasculature results in hypoxic regions of tumours. These regions have a decreased supply of nutrients, such as glucose and essential amino acids. In fact, tumour cells use glycolysis to convert glucose into lactate and obtain the energy that they need to survive and proliferate. In these regions, the formation of lactic acid via anaerobic glycolysis results in an acidic microenvironment. The acidic pH confers resistance against ionized basic drugs. In fact, molecules diffuse passively across the cell membrane most often in the uncharged form. Because the extracellular pH in tumours is low and the intracellular pH of tumour cells is neutral to alkaline, ionized basic drugs that have an acid dissociation constant of 7.5–9.5 are protonated and display decreased cellular uptake [8].

Within the cellular compartment of tumour tissue, there are at least two distinct populations of cells. The first population is made up of a large population of rapidly proliferating cells that form the majority of the tumour mass. The second population is composed of a small rare and quiescent population known as cancer stem cells (CSCs), which are able to regenerate the tumour and retain their genetic programmes for cell migration (i.e. invasion and metastasis) and self-protection differently from non-CSCs that do not have the capacity to self-sustain or metastasize. Most therapeutic treatments target non-CSCs, leaving the CSCs behind, which can then regenerate the tumour, explaining in part why tumours often recur after treatment. Hence, new treatments are being designed to specifically target CSCs, which are now believed to be the critical therapeutic target to prevent local recurrence and metastasis [9]. Inside cancer cells, there are biochemical and metabolic changes that contribute to the cellular mechanisms of drug resistance. Furthermore, the non-specific systemic biodistribution of many chemotherapeutic drugs, resulting in systemic cytotoxicity and lower concentrations of drug delivered directly to the tumour, has limited the full therapeutic benefit of these chemotherapeutic drugs [10].

To overcome these obstacles, new therapies are being designed to deliver chemotherapeutic drugs to the tumour at higher concentrations with a minimal damage to normal tissues using targeting agents conjugated with drugs. However, studies have shown some limitations in their administration to the target sites in vivo, with similar limitations noted for molecular imaging agents [10–12].

New strategies have emerged using nanoparticles (NPs) for drug delivery (therapy), imaging (diagnosis and prognosis), or theranostics for cancer patients [13]. Because of their unique biological properties including their small size, NPs have a high surface area-to-volume ratio, which allows them to bind, absorb, and carry other compounds, such as small molecule drugs, DNA, RNA, proteins, and probes. In addition, their tunable size, shape, and surface characteristics enable them to have high stability, a high carrier capacity, the ability to incorporate both hydrophilic and hydrophobic substances, and compatibility with different administration routes, thereby making them a valuable tool in many aspects of medicine. However, the lack of biodegradation and slow dissolution rates of some NPs raises concern over their safety, especially for long-term administration [14]. NPs can be categorized into those made from biological-like materials (i.e. phospholipids, lipids, dextran, and chitosan), carbon-based materials (i.e. carbon dots), and inorganic NPs (i.e. those based on metals, metal oxides, and metal sulphides), which also include semiconductor NPs (i.e. quantum dots [QDs]).

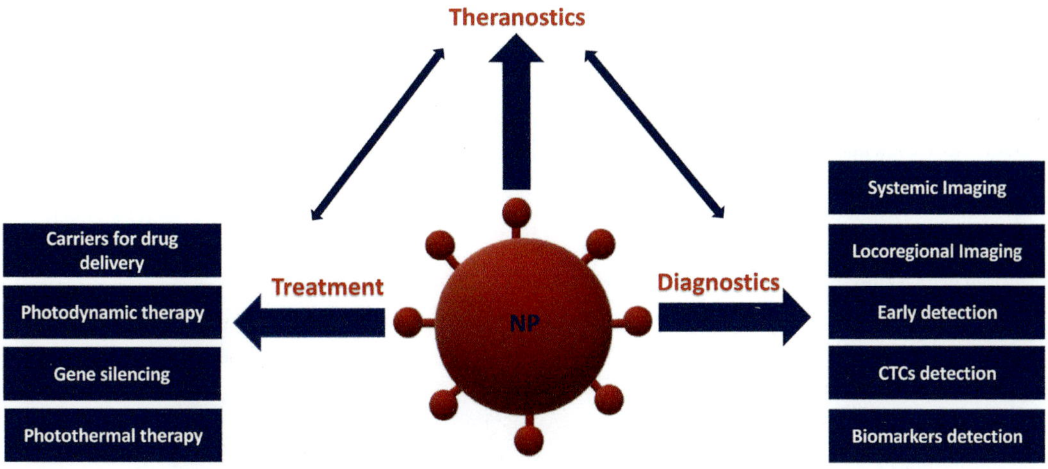

Fig. 13.1 Application of nanoparticles in the treatment, diagnostics, and theranostics of gastric cancer

Depending on the composition, their interaction with cells will be quite different.

In this book chapter, we will discuss the application of NPs in three different fields: treatment, diagnostics, and theranostics of GC (Fig. 13.1). First, we will discuss how NPs are able to function as carriers of chemotherapeutic drugs to increase their therapeutic index and how they can function as therapeutic agents in photodynamic, gene, and thermal therapies. Second, we will discuss the importance of NPs as imaging agents to be applied in systemic and locoregional imaging, early detection and biomarkers, and uncovering circulating tumor cells (CTC). Third, we will describe how NPs could combine diagnosis and therapy as theranostic agents.

Nanoparticles as Carriers for Drug Delivery in GC

The use of nanotechnology in medicine and more specifically drug delivery is helping to revolutionize the treatment of cancer, which includes GC. The NP-drug complex consists of two main components: the NP used as carrier agent and the chemotherapeutic drug [11]. The drug can be adsorbed, dissolved, dispersed, or attached into or onto a nano-matrix. In comparison to conventional formulations, the NP formulation has shown greater bioavailability and a longer sustainable therapeutic time [15]. In addition, the NP formulation overcomes issues, which include low water solubility and severe side effects of drugs. To be effective carriers of chemotherapeutic drugs, NP-drug complexes must fulfil certain criteria:

- The NPs should bind or contain the drug(s).
- The NP-drug complex must remain stable in the serum to accomplish systemic delivery of the drug.
- The NP-drug complex must be delivered only to tumour cells either by receptor-mediated interactions or via the EPR effect.
- The NPs must release the drug once at the tumour site.
- The residual NP must be made of a biological or biologically inert material with a limited lifespan to be safely degraded. If a non-biodegradable material is used, it must be proven to be safe at the doses needed or eliminated from the subject.

After administration into the systemic circulation, NPs loaded with anticancer drugs help to target specifically the tumour either passively or actively and get rid of them without altering or hampering the surrounded non-cancerous tissues [16] (Fig. 13.2). In passive delivery, the EPR effect enables the drug to leave the systemic circulation and enter the extravascular space, where they can accumulate around tumour cells. In active delivery, surface modifications of NPs (i.e. the addition of ligands, such as peptides, small molecules, oligo-

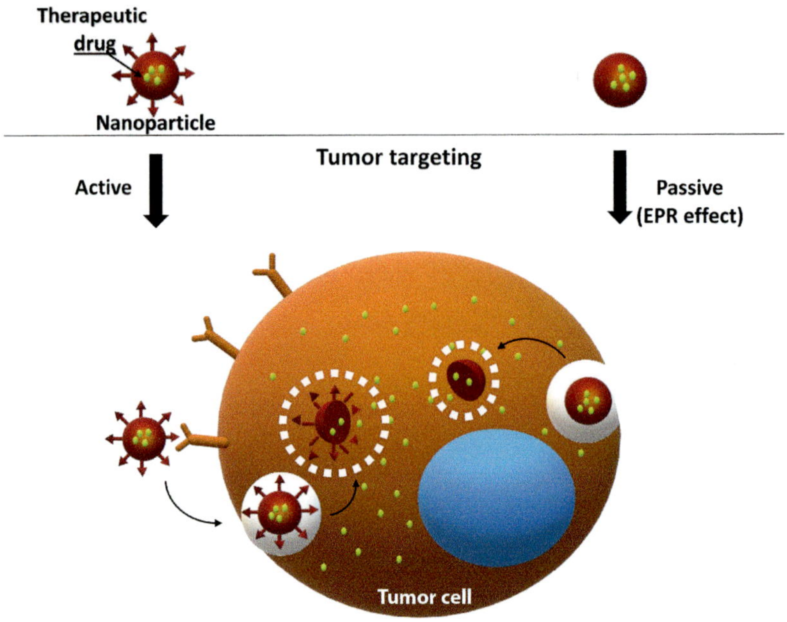

Fig. 13.2 Passive and active targeting approaches of nanoparticles in drug delivery in cancer therapy. Passive tumour targeting (right) is achieved by extravasation of nanoparticles through increased permeability of the tumour vasculature and ineffective lymphatic drainage (EPR effect). Active tumour targeting (left) can be achieved by functionalization of nanoparticles with targeting ligands that promote cell-specific recognition and binding

saccharides, antibodies, and affibodies) allow the NPs to recognize and bind to complementary target molecules on the surface of tumour cells that are overexpressed compared with healthy cells.

Different chemotherapeutic agents have been used to treat GC. According to the National Comprehensive Cancer Network (NCCN) guidelines, 5-fluorouracil (5-FU), cisplatin, and epirubicin continue to be availed as the first-line therapy [17]. Other chemotherapeutic agents have been emerging, including taxanes (docetaxel and paclitaxel), oral fluoropyrimidines (capecitabine and S-1), as well as oxaliplatin and irinotecan [18]. Table 13.1 shows a list of some drugs that are or could be used in GC treatment.

These drugs may work as an individual anticancer drug or in combination [17, 18, 32]. Despite their anticancer properties, these agents still show several side effects in humans [34]. In addition, their delivery method is sometimes difficult. Therefore, the use of NPs has become practical as they could reduce side effects and improve the efficacy of the treatment.

A wide range of studies have already been performed by different researchers to demonstrate the effectiveness of NPs as carriers for drug delivery to treat GC. Table 13.2 shows a list of some NPs that are used for drug delivery in GC treatment.

Camptothecin (CPT) is an effective anticancer drug that is used in multiple types of cancer and has shown remarkable anticancer activity in animal tumour models [35]. It is a DNA topoisomerase 1 inhibitor [36, 37]. However, its clinical utility is limited by its poor solubility and high systemic toxicity. The analogues of CPT, e.g. irinotecan (IRN) and topotecan (TPT), overcome some of its limitations, but they still have suboptimal toxicity profiles and pharmacokinetics. For this purpose, a NP combination, CRLX101, containing a cyclodextrin-based polymer and CPT, was evaluated [38]. The results showed that in a xenograft mouse model utilizing the GC cell line BGC823, CRLX101 is safe, effective, and more bioavailable than the parental drug. Another anticancer drug, docetaxel (DOC), has been reported to exhibit radio-enhancement efficacy in different cancers, including GC [39–41]. However, its applicability remains to be improved because of its non-specific distribution that demonstrates several side effects, such as myelosuppression, neurotoxicity, and musculoskeletal toxicity [42]. To solve this problem, DOC-loaded poly(ethylene glycol) (PEG)-poly(ε-caprolactone) (PCL) NPs were targeted with gelatinase to a radioresistant cell population. Comparing the radiosensitization effect on GC between DOC-NPs and DOC

Table 13.1 Drugs for gastric cancer treatment

Class	Name	Target	Action	Administration route	References
Glutamic acid derivatives	Raltitrexed	Thymidylate synthase	Inhibitor	IV	[19, 20]
	Pemetrexed	Thymidylate synthase	Inhibitor	IV	[19, 21]
		Bifunctional purine biosynthesis protein PURH	Inhibitor		
		Dihydrofolate reductase	Inhibitor		
		Trifunctional purine biosynthetic protein adenosine-3	Inhibitor		
	Leucovorin	Folic acid targets	Folic acid analogue	IV	[22]
	Methotrexate	Dihydrofolate reductase	Inhibitor	IV	[23]
Platinum derivatives	Cisplatin	DNA	Cross-linking/alkylation	IV	[23, 24]
	Carboplatin	DNA	Cross-linking/alkylation	IV	[24]
	Oxaliplatin	DNA	Cross-linking/alkylation	IV	[23, 24]
Anthracyclines	Doxorubicin	DNA	Intercalation	IV	[25]
		DNA topoisomerase 2-alpha	Inhibitor		
	Epirubicin	Chromodomain-helicase-DNA-binding protein 1	Antagonist	Oral	[25, 26]
		DNA topoisomerase 2-alpha	Inhibitor		
		DNA	Intercalation		
Mitomycins	Mitomycin	DNA	Antagonist Cross-linking/alkylation	IV	[27]
Camptothecins	Irinotecan	DNA topoisomerase I	Inhibitor	IV	[28]
	Topotecan	DNA	Intercalation	IV	[28]
Fluoropyrimidines	5-FU	Thymidylate synthase	Inhibitor	IP	[23, 29]
		DNA/RNA	Incorporation into and destabilization		
	Capecitabine	Thymidylate synthase	Inhibitor	Oral	[29]
		DNA/RNA	Incorporation into and destabilization		
	S-1	Thymidylate synthase	Inhibitor	Oral	[29]
		DNA/RNA	Incorporation into and destabilization		
	Doxifluridine	Thymidylate synthase	Inhibitor	Oral	[30]
		DNA/RNA	Incorporation into and destabilization		
	UFT	Thymidylate synthase	Inhibitor	Oral	[31]
		DNA/RNA	Incorporation into and destabilization		

(continued)

Table 13.1 (continued)

Class	Name	Target	Action	Administration route	References
Taxanes derivatives	Paclitaxel	Apoptosis regulator Bcl-2	Inhibitor	IV	[32]
		Tubulin beta-1 chain	Inhibitor		
		Nuclear receptor subfamily 1 group I member 2	Inducer		
	Docetaxel	Nuclear receptor subfamily 1 group I member 2	Binder	IV	[32]
Matrix Metalloproteinase Inhibitors	Marimastat	Matrix metalloproteinase	Inhibitor	Oral	[19]
Tyrosine kinase inhibitors	Lapatinib	Epidermal growth factor receptor	Antagonist	Oral	[33]
		Receptor tyrosine-protein kinase erbB-2	Antagonist		
	Foretinib	Vascular endothelial growth factor receptor 2	Antagonist	Oral	[33]
		Hepatocyte growth factor	Antagonist		
	Sunitinib	Platelet-derived growth factor receptors	Inhibitor	Oral	[33]
		Vascular endothelial growth factor receptors	Inhibitor		
		stem cell factor receptor	Inhibitor		
		Fms-like tyrosine kinase-3	Inhibitor		
		Colony-stimulating factor receptor type 1	Inhibitor		
		Glial cell line-derived neurotrophic factor receptor	Inhibitor		
Monoclonal antibodies	Ramucirumab	Vascular endothelial growth factor receptor 2	Antagonist	IV	[33]
	Pertuzumab	Receptor tyrosine-protein kinase erbB-2	Antibody	IV	[33]
	Trastuzumab	Receptor tyrosine-protein kinase erbB-2	Antibody	IV	[33]

I.V. Intravenous, *I.P.* Intraperitoneal

Table 13.2 Nanoparticles for drug delivery in GC treatment

Type of nanoparticle	Use	Anticancer strategy	Stage of development	References
Cyclodextrin-based polymeric NPs	Carrier	CPT	In vivo/in vitro	[38]
Gelatinase-stimuli PEG-Pep-PCL NPs	Carrier	DOC	In vivo/in vitro	[43]
γ-PGA-based NPs	Carrier	Co-loading of CET and DOC	In vivo/in vitro	[48]
HA-modified layer-by-layer NPs	Carrier	Co-loading of IRN and 5-FU	In vivo/in vitro	[49]
Amphiphilic mPEG-PCL block copolymer NPs	Carrier	UA	In vitro	[53]
Liposomes	Carrier	Poly(I:C)	In vivo/in vitro	[59]
Lipid-coated nanodiamond	Carrier	Sorafenib	In vivo	[65]
Copolymer PMMA-AA encapsulated ZnO NPs	Carrier	Cur	In vitro	[69]
CO NPs	Anticancer agent	Upregulation of DHX15 protein	In vivo/in vitro	[70]
CH NPs	Anticancer agent	Proliferation inhibition	In vitro	[72]
CH-HA-coated SWNTs	Carrier	SAL	In vitro	[84]
Beta-casein NPs	Carrier	PTX	In vitro	[85]
PLGA NPs coated with hCTLs membranes	Biomimetic delivery system	PTX	In vivo/ex vivo	[93]

in vitro and in vivo revealed a significant increase in the radiosensitivity of DOC-NPs in all three gelatinase-overexpressing GC cells (BGC823, SGC7901, and MKN45 cell lines) compared with normal mucosa cells. In addition, the radiosensitization efficacy of DOC-NPs was more prominent than DOC by intravenous injection in a xenograft. Thus, gelatinase-mediated nanoscale delivery system could serve as a potential strategy to increase the radiosensitization and the specificity of DOC as well as to reduce its side effects [43].

The epidermal growth factor receptor (EGFR), which is upregulated in GC patients, is an oncogene that has reported to be an indicator of a poor prognostic outcome and, in turn, an important therapeutic target [44]. Cetuximab (CET) is a chimeric IgG monoclonal antibody (MAb) directed against EGFR. It was approved by the US Food and Drug Administration (FDA) for the use in colorectal carcinoma, and it has also shown clinical benefit towards advanced/metastatic gastric adenocarcinoma in combination with other chemotherapeutic agents as a first-line treatment [45–47]. To enhance the therapeutic efficiency of conventional chemotherapeutics, a study reported the development of CET-conjugated DOC-loaded poly(γ-glutamic acid) (γ-PGA) NPs (CET-DOCT- γ-PGA-NPs) [48]. Compared with non-targeted and free drug formulations, CET-DOC- γ-PGA-NPs showed EGFR-specific cellular internalization and significant cancer cell death in vitro induced by active targeting. In addition, this system showed improved systemic circulation and enhanced tumour accumulation by passive targeting due to the EPR effect of the tumour environment and EGFR-mediated cellular internalization, enhancing the drug availability at the tumour site and resulting in tumour growth inhibition in vivo in the MKN-28 GC xenograft model. Thus, the combination of the targeting agent CET and the therapeutic agent DOC, with the γ-PGA nano-matrix, was found to be an effective targeted nanoformulation for EGFR-overexpressing GCs.

To target GC, hyaluronic acid (HA)-modified layer-by-layer NPs were used for the co-loading of IRN and 5-FU to improve anticancer treatment efficacy and reduce side effects [49]. A polymer-chitosan (CH)-HA hybrid formulation (HA-CH-

IRN/5-FU NPs) consisting of poly(lactic-co-glycolic acid) (PLGA) and IRN as the core, CH and 5-FU as a shell, and HA as the outermost layer was prepared. Human gastric carcinoma cells (MGC803 cells) and cancer-bearing mice were used to test the in vitro cytotoxicity and in vivo antitumour efficiency of HA-CH-IRN/5-FU NPs. The results demonstrated that this targeted drug delivery system has an impressive antitumour activity in vitro and in vivo.

Cyclooxygenase-2 (COX-2), an inducible isoform of cyclooxygenase, is regulated by cytokines and growth factors, such as IL1β, IL6, or TNFα. This isoform is overexpressed during inflammation, constitutively expressed in GC, and associated with tumour progression [50]. It has been shown that ursolic acid (UA) can induce apoptosis of cancer cells by inhibiting the expression of COX-2 [51, 52]. UA is relatively nontoxic, but its clinical application is limited due to several problems, including poor water solubility leading to low bioavailability and poor pharmacokinetics, subsequently restricting its effectiveness and its non-specific distribution throughout the body when administered intravenously. To overcome these limitations, UA-loaded NPs (UA-NPs) were prepared using amphiphilic methoxypolyPEG-PCL (mPEG-PCL) block copolymers as drug carriers. This nano-drug delivery system effectively transported UA into SGC7901 cells and increased cell apoptosis to improve the anticancer efficiency of UA [53].

Several immunoagents have been developed as anticancer drugs. Among them, poly(inosinic-cytidylic) acid or poly(I:C), a synthetic analogue of double-stranded RNA (dsRNA), has been found to trigger apoptosis in a variety of cancers [54–58]. However, there have been few studies on GC. A study has shown that intracellular delivery of poly(I:C) by liposomes has a pro-apoptotic effect on human gastric adenocarcinoma cells in vitro and significantly inhibits xenograft tumour growth of human gastric adenocarcinoma in nude mice [59].

Approximately 80–90% of patients diagnosed with GC present metastasis [60–62]; in turn, it is a great challenge to improve the survival rate. Sorafenib is an oral molecular targeting agent with anti-proliferative and antiangiogenic activities. It is a potential agent for the treatment of metastatic GC [63]. However, it is almost insoluble in water, and its oral bioavailability is extremely low, which greatly restricts its therapeutic efficacy towards cancer metastasis. Nanodiamond, a member of the carbon NP family, is characterized by a large surface area, high adsorption capacity, and good biocompatibility, which makes it attractive for drug delivery and cellular imaging [64]. A study has shown that lipid-coated nanodiamonds loaded with sorafenib can increase the oral bioavailability of the drug and its efficacy in the suppression of GC metastasis in tumour xenograft models [65].

Curcumin (Cur) is a well-known phytochemical that demonstrates antitumour activity in many human cancers including GC. It can induce cell apoptosis, especially in malignant cells, by causing DNA damage. Cur is safe even at high doses, but its utility is limited due to poor aqueous solubility and oral bioavailability and multidrug resistance [66, 67]. Thus, creating a drug delivery system with enhanced drug solubility leading to improved bioavailability and efficacy is an exigency. ZnO NPs with a tunable size and shape have many advantages to construct such drug delivery systems due to their reduced toxicity and stability towards the environment [68]. ZnO itself is nontoxic, but after decomposition, Zn^{2+} ions are cytotoxic. A study successfully developed a copolymer, PMMA-AA encapsulated ZnO NPs, for the loading of Cur and tested it in AGS GC cell lines in vitro [69]. Compared with free Cur, Cur/PMMA-AA/ZnO NPs enhanced cellular uptake and reduced the cytotoxicity of Cur; rapid release of the payload was observed at a low pH and with high bioavailability. Therefore, the Cur/PMMA-AA/ZnO NPs constitute an alternative method to enhance the anticancer activity and delivery of hydrophobic anticancer drugs with biocompatible and pH-sensitive nano-vehicles.

Another well-known anticancer agent, cerium oxide NP (CO NP), has been tested in human GC cell lines (MKN28 and BGC823) and GC xenografts. In fact, research data have shown diverse abilities of CO NPs, including antioxidant capabilities and cancer cell sensitization to radiation therapy and chemotherapy. The results suggest that CO NPs have an inhibitory effect on cell migration and proliferation both in vitro and in vivo by increasing the expression of putative ATP-dependent RNA helicase DEAH (Asp-Glu-Ala-His) box helicase 15 (DHX15). This protein can activate the p38 MAPK signal pathway and in turn inhibit proliferation and metastasis. The inhibitory effect of CONPs is dose-independent, whereas their effect on proliferation is dose-dependent and only a relatively high concentration of CONPs suppresses proliferation [70].

CH NPs are widely studied NPs in anticancer treatment because of many advantages, including particle size, zeta potential, morphology, safety, bioavailability, and biocompatibility [71]. A study aiming to identify the effects of these NPs on the proliferation of the human GC cell line MGC803 in vitro has shown that after treatment with CH NPs, these NPs are cytotoxic and effectively inhibit cell proliferation through multiple mechanisms [72].

GC stem cells (CSCs) play a pivotal role in the initiation, development, relapse, and metastasis of GC because they are resistant to standard chemotherapy, and the residual CSCs are able to proliferate indefinitely [73]. Therefore, eradication of this cell population has important clinical implications in cancer therapy. Several studies have identified CD44 as a cell surface marker of gastric CSCs [74–77]. HA has been identified as a potent targeting ligand of tumours possessing CD44-overexpressing cells [78]. Several findings have strongly suggested that salinomycin (SAL), an anticancer drug, might represent a class of agent for targeting CSCs [79–82]. However, its poor aqueous solubility [83] has limited its application. Therefore, to overcome the poor solubility as well as improve the biodistribution to yield superior drug encapsulation and accumulation in tumours, a research group assembled a gastric CSC targeting drug delivery system [84]. This system is based on CH-coated single-wall carbon nanotubes (SWNTs) loaded with SAL functionalized with HA (SAL-SWNT-CH-HA), which helps to minimize the movement and intrusion of GC stem cells as well as their eradication.

Paclitaxel (PTX) is a widely used chemotherapeutic agent but with undesirable side effects during injection since it needs to be delivered intravenously. Different approaches to administer PTX orally have been attempted by using organic and synthetic delivery systems, but they remain unsuccessful. A study evaluated a potential drug delivery system composed of the hydrophobic anticancer drug PTX entrapped within beta-casein (b-CN) NPs, which can be degraded by the stomach enzyme pepsin [85]. After encapsulation and simulated digestion with pepsin, PTX maintained its cytotoxic activity towards human N-87 GC cells, whereas, without prior simulated digestion with pepsin, the b-CN-PTX NPs were non-cytotoxic. These data suggest that b-CN may protect upper gastrointestinal regions from PTX and efficiently release it in the stomach without compromising drug cytotoxicity. It has been found that this system shows promise to be useful for target-activated oral delivery of hydrophobic chemotherapeutics in the treatment of gastric carcinoma. The integration of synthetic (inorganic or organic) NPs in GC treatment has shown many advantages, including an increased chemotherapeutic drug concentration at tumour sites, decreased systemic exposure, and an EPR effect because of their passive accumulation ability and targeting ligand incorporation on their surface [86–88]. However, their short circulation time, the complexity of producing such actively targeted carriers, the difficulty of heterogeneous and varied tumour vascularization and tumour permeability with different tumour types and stages, and their unknown toxicity have limited their clinical utility. Therefore, combining synthetic NPs with natural biomaterials to create biomimetic delivery systems is becoming more attractive because of their ability to mimic many features of their source cells as a new engineering strategy [89–92].

To enhance PTX targeting in GC treatment, a study aimed to produce a biomimetic system based on human cytotoxic T lymphocyte (hCTL) membranes because of the long blood circulation time and ability to recruit and localize at tumour sites of this cell type [93]. In this platform, local low dose irradiation (LDI), which induces the expression of adhesion molecules and chemoattractants [94, 95], was used to guide PTX-loaded PLGA NPs coated with cellular membranes isolated from hCTLs. After systemic administration, this new system reduced NP phagocytosis by macrophages to 23.99% and inhibited the growth of human GC by 56.68% in Balb/c nude mice. The application of LDI at the tumour site significantly increased the tumour growth inhibition rate to 88.50%, and two mice achieved complete remission. Combining ex vivo experiments with in vivo experiments, this new drug delivery platform favoured both the long circulation time and the tumour site accumulation ability of hCTLs, while local LDI significantly enhanced tumour localization. This LDI-guided biomimetic drug delivery platform provides a promising system for cancer immunotherapy, photothermal therapy, and diagnosis in the near future.

Nanoparticles for RNAi Delivery

Gene silencing is the regulation of gene expression to prevent the expression of a certain gene. For the silencing of gene expression, antisense oligonucleotides (ASOs) and small interfering RNAs (siRNAs) are the two most widely used strategies [96]. siRNA holds great promise in cancer treatment, as numerous studies have shown that the growth and proliferation of cancer cells can be greatly inhibited by using this approach in vitro and in vivo [97–99]. In addition, different siRNAs are able to silence not only one but several oncogenes with high efficacy and specificity, allowing the simultaneous targeting of multiple pathways. Moreover, siRNA-based therapeutics have demonstrated great potential in sensitizing cancer cells to chemotherapy by silencing genes that play a role in drug resistance during chemotherapy [100, 101]. However, several limitations reduce the therapeutic efficacy of siRNA, including delivery problems, side effects due to off-target actions, and others [102]. In addition, unmodified siRNA molecules are highly unstable when delivered into the systemic circulation and are unable to enter cells due to their size and the high polyanionic charge of the phosphate backbone. Therefore, delivery systems such as NPs are currently being explored as an alternative way to safely transport siRNA (Fig. 13.3).

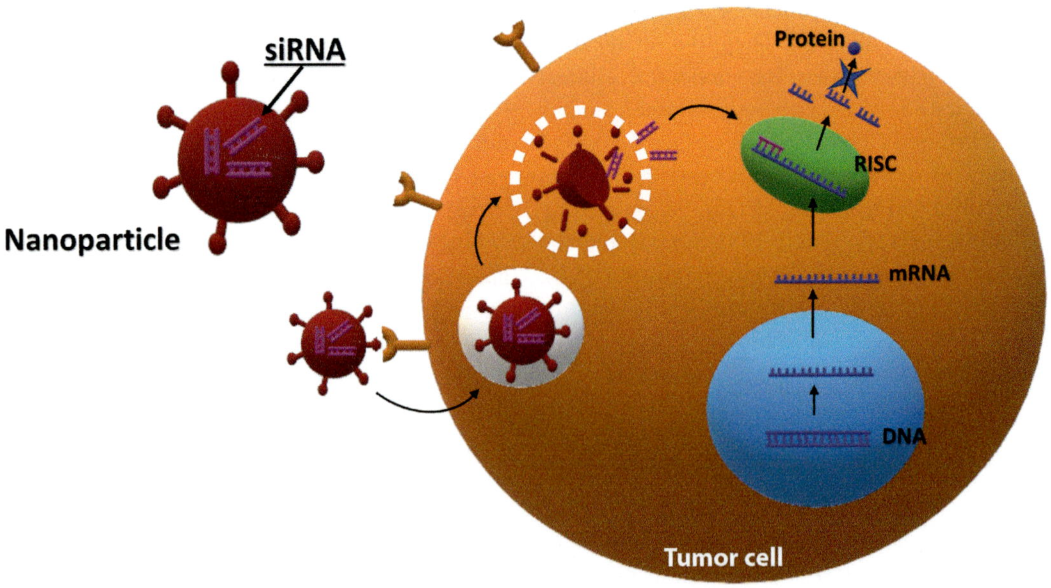

Fig. 13.3 Nanoparticles in gene therapy. Nanoparticles can deliver small interfering RNAs (siRNAs) into tumour cells, where they can interact with the translation of a targeted messenger RNA (mRNA) molecule. Delivered siRNAs are processed by specific RNA-induced silencing complex (RISC), the double-stranded RNA is unwound, and one strand is degraded, whereas the other strand binds to the targeted mRNA by complementarity, leading to its degradation by endonuclease activity and thus silencing gene expression

Table 13.3 Nanoparticles used as delivery systems for gene silencing in GC treatment

Type of nanoparticle	Use	Anticancer strategy	Stage of development	References
AMO-21-HER-PEG-PCL NPs	Carrier	MiR-21	In vivo/in vitro	[107]
Folate-conjugated 3WJ-BRCAA1 siRNA-pRNA NP system	Carrier	BRCAA1	In vivo/in vitro	[115]
PEG-modified PEI NPs	Carrier	CD44v6	In vitro	[116]
Calcium phosphate NPs	Carrier	Suicide genes	Ex vivo	[117]

NPs have a large surface area-to-volume ratio and thereby can carry and protect siRNA from degradation, specifically targeting and delivering siRNA to cancer cells after functionalization with tissue-specific ligands. In addition, NPs are efficiently taken up into cells through membrane fusion or receptor-mediated endocytosis. Table 13.3 shows some studies that utilized nanoparticles as delivery systems for gene silencing in GC treatment.

Despite the advantages of combination chemotherapy, approximately 7–34% of GC are characterized by a poor prognosis associated with amplification of the human epidermal growth factor receptor 2 gene (HER2) [103–106]. MiR-21 is a microRNA that is frequently overexpressed in GC, decreasing the sensitivity of GC cells to trastuzumab, which is a humanized MAb targeting HER2. A study used PEG-PCL NPs coated with trastuzumab to target GC cells, which overexpressed HER2 receptor using anti-miRNA-21 antisense oligonucleotides (AMO-21) [107]. The antibody conjugates significantly enhanced cellular uptake of NPs. The HER-PEG-PCL NPs effectively suppressed miRNA expression in GC cells, resulting in enhancing sensitivity of HER2-expressing GC cells to trastuzumab. The biological and clinical potential of targeted AMO-21 delivery using modified trastuzumab for GC treatment have been shown by comparing the antitumour effects of AMO-21-HER-PEG-PCL NPs with trastuzumab in xenograft GC mice.

As mentioned before, it remains very difficult to effectively cure GC patients because most of them present advanced stages of the disease. Advanced and metastatic cases do not respond to chemo- or radiation therapies [108, 109]. Resistance to chemotherapy-induced apoptosis is a major cause for the failure of conventional therapies [110, 111]. The current prognosis of GC is very poor, with 5-year survivals of less than 24% [112]. Therefore, how to recognize, track or kill early GC cells is a great challenge for patients with early GCI. Breast cancer-associated antigen 1 (BRCAA1) is overexpressed in GC with no expression in normal control gastric mucous tissues [113, 114], strongly suggesting that BRCAA1 antigen may be selected as a potential target for early GC. A research group has successfully designed a folate-conjugated three-way junction (3WJ)-BRCAA1 siRNA-packaging RNA (pRNA) NP system [115]. RNA NPs can enter the cytoplasm specifically via folic acid (FA) receptor-mediated endocytosis and inhibit BRCAA1 expression in GC to induce GC MGC803 cells and reduce the burden of tumour xenografts in vivo. Therefore, RNA nanotechnology provides a promising strategy that can overcome conventional cancer therapeutic limitations due to the specific delivery of therapeutics to stomach cancer without damaging normal cells, reduce toxicity and side effects, and improve the therapeutic effect.

siRNA is an efficient tool to suppress the activity of CD44v6, a protein involved in the progression of GC. However, its potential for clinical therapy has been limited due to its instability and low transfection efficiency. To bypass these limitations, a research group studied and synthesized poly(ethylene glycol)-poly(ethyleneimine) (PEG-PEI) NPs, a non-viral carrier of siRNA targeting CD44v6 in SGC7901 human gastric carcinoma cells. This non-viral carrier may be a promising system for altering gene expression in the treatment of GC, exhibiting many advantages, such as a relatively high gene transfection efficiency and low cytotoxicity [116].

In another gene therapy in vivo approach, calcium phosphate NPs were combined with suicide genes, e.g. bCD (bacterial cytosine deaminase), to test the efficacy of these NPs against GC [117]. The expression of suicide genes delivered by these NPs in specific GC tissues inhibits gastric carcinoma growth.

Nanoparticles as Therapeutic Agents in GC treatment

Photodynamic Therapy

Photodynamic therapy (PDT) has recently emerged as an attractive approach for the treatment of several types of cancers, particularly GC [118] (Fig. 13.4).

PDT uses drugs called photosensitizers (PSs) and a particular type of light. When PSs are exposed to a specific wavelength of light, they generate cytotoxic oxygen-based molecular species that cause damage to plasma membranes and subcellular organelles, resulting in cell death either by apoptosis, necrosis, or autophagy. PSs are able to transfer the absorbed energy from light to either oxygen molecules to produce singlet oxygen or to surrounding molecules to form free radicals. The effectiveness of PDT depends on the capacity of PSs to generate singlet oxygen and their ability to be selectively delivered at therapeutic concentrations to the target tumour tissue [119]. However, there are several difficulties associated with the use of PSs in PDT, such as low accumulation in specific target cells, environmental degradation, and a short lifespan of singlet oxygen species [119–121]. To overcome these problems, various NP-based systems have been investigated. NPs used in PDT can be functionally divided into passive or active. Passive PDT NPs are carriers of PSs and can be made from either biodegradable material or non-polymer-based materials, such as ceramic and metallic NPs. Active PDT NPs can produce reactive species without the presence of PSs.

Several studies have shown that NPs could be potential carriers of PSs to improve PDT in the treatment of GC. Table 13.4 provides a list of some NPs involved in PDT for the treatment of GC.

For example, a study has focused on the development of a biodegradable NP system based on polyethylene glycol-modified gelatine (PEG-GEL) and poly(lactic acid) (PLA) biopolymers as a carrier for a potent PDT agent, cyclohexane-1,2-diamino hypocrellin B (CHA2HB), to improve its photodynamic efficacy [122]. In vitro experiments indicated that CHA2HB-loaded PEG-GEL-PLA NPs were efficiently taken up by AGS human gastric carcinoma cells and induced both apoptotic and necrotic cell death as a result of photoirradiation, suggesting that PEG-GEL/

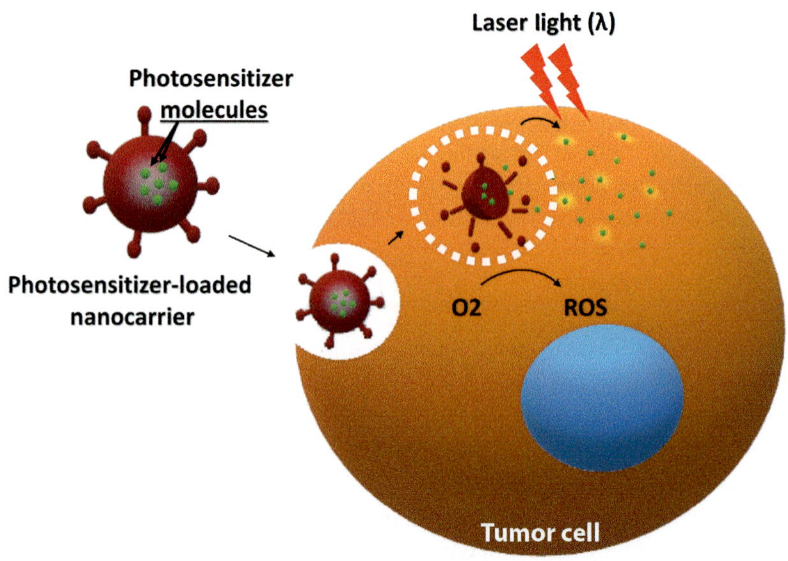

Fig. 13.4 Nanoparticles in photodynamic therapy. Nanoparticles can be used in PDT due to the delivery of light-activatable chemicals, known as photosensitizer molecules, to tumour cells. After the absorption of light, photosensitizer molecules can generate cytotoxic oxygen-based reactive species that cause cellular damage and cell death via oxidative stress

Table 13.4 Nanoparticles involved in PDT for the treatment of GC

Type of nanoparticle	Use	Photodynamic therapeutic (PDT) agent	Stage of development	References
PEG-GEL/PLA NPs	Carrier	CHA2HB	In vitro	[122]
PVP-coated rGO NPs	Carrier	Ce6	In vitro	[123]
Linolenic acid-conjugated polyhedral oligomeric silsesquioxane nanohybrids	Carrier	PPIX	In vitro	[124]
Upconversion LNPs	Carrier	PPIX	In vitro	[125, 126]
Semiconductor Pdots	Carrier	Tetraphenylporphyrin	In vivo/in vitro	[127]

PLA NPs are highly effective for the delivery and phototoxic enhancement of CHA2HB against cancer cells in vitro.

Another study successfully developed a facile surface functionalization strategy using chemically reduced graphene oxide (rGO) as a carbon NP model to allow both biocompatibility and receptor-targeted drug delivery [123]. To improve the aqueous dispersibility and biocompatibility of rGO and provide anchoring sites for RGD peptide, NPs were coated with polyvinylpyrrolidone (PVP). The nanodelivery system rGO-PVP-RGD could effectively load aromatic PS chlorin e6 (Ce6) via hydrophobic interactions and π-π stacking, as well as significantly increase the accumulation of Ce6 in the MGC803 GC cell line, improving the efficacy of PDT compared with Ce6 alone.

The poor water solubility and cellular internalization of protoporphyrin IX (PpIX), a PS used in PDT for cancer, limit its direct application. To improve this limitation, a biocompatible PpIX/linolenic acid-conjugated polyhedral oligomeric silsesquioxane (PPLA) nanohybrid was developed [124]. This nanocarrier system enhanced the intracellular uptake of PSs due to improved water solubility when evaluated using a human GC cell line (MKN-28).

Some studies describe the improvement in PDT efficiency against a human GC cell line (MKN45) using lanthanide NPs (LNPs) and 5-aminolevulinic acid (ALA) [125, 126]. In fact, PpIX is a PS that is selectively accumulated in cancer cells after oral administration of ALA. However, the low tissue penetrability resulting from blue incident lights required to excite PpIX limited its application to surface cancers. To overcome this limitation, these studies have shown how LNP could be employed as a light energy upconverter, which, upon irradiation with highly penetrative near-infrared (NIR) radiation, emits visible light to allow PpIX sensitization. An intermittent NIR irradiation of MKN45, pretreated with LNP and ALA, caused cell destruction.

A study describes the energy-transfer amplified singlet oxygen generation in semiconductor polymer dots (Pdots) for in vitro and in vivo PDT to treat GC [127]. Hydrophobic PS tetraphenylporphyrin was doped in the NPs. The antitumour effect of the Pdots was evaluated in vivo and in vitro. The in vitro studies showed that cancer cells were efficiently destroyed at a very low dose of the Pdots. Human gastric adenocarcinoma mice xenografts were significantly inhibited and eradicated in vivo.

Photothermal Therapy

Thermal therapy is a type of cancer treatment that involves heating of the tumour using radiofrequency (RF), microwaves, magnetic fields, or ultrasounds to cause irreversible cellular damage by loosening membranes and denaturing proteins, which ultimately kills cancer cells. However, thermal therapy has been limited by damage caused to surrounding normal tissue [128]. To overcome this problem, photothermal therapy (PTT) uses photothermal agents to achieve more controlled and selective heating of the target area, reducing thermal damage to the tumour (Fig. 13.5).

To be effective, photothermal agents need to have an enhanced light absorption and an efficient light-to-heat conversion. Traditional

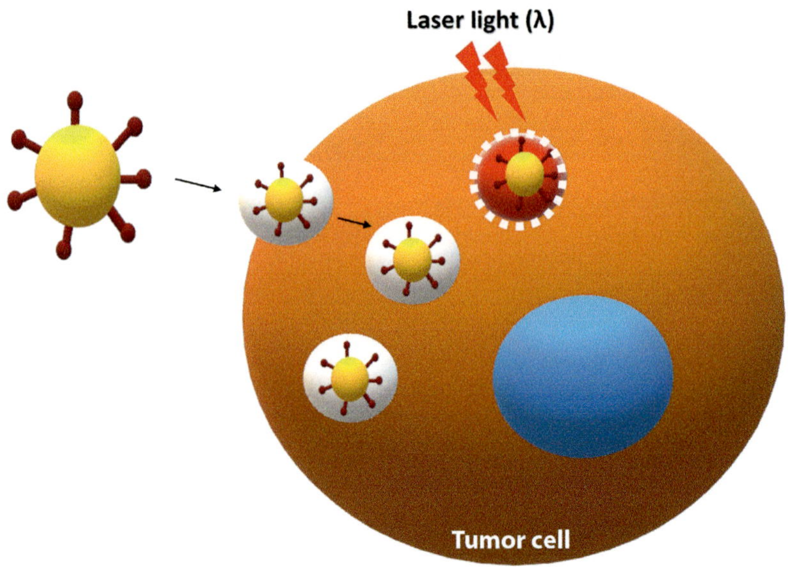

Fig. 13.5 Nanoparticles in photothermal therapy. Due to their efficient light-to-heat conversion, nanoparticles can be used in photothermal therapy. After the absorption of light, nanoparticles cause localized destruction. The controlled and selective heating of nanoparticles allows thermal damage of the target area while minimizing any damage to the surrounding normal tissue

Table 13.5 Nanoparticles involved in PTT for the treatment of GC

Type of nanoparticle	Use	Photothermal therapy (PTT) agent	Stage of development	References
GNR loaded-iPS-treated MMC	Photothermal agent	GNRs	In vivo	[130]
GNRs	Photothermal agent	GNRs	Ex vivo	[131]
Hb NPs	Carrier	Near-infrared dye IR780	In vivo	[132]
GO NPs	Photothermal agent	GO NPs	In vitro	[133]

agents suffer from low absorption, or external dyes (i.e. indocyanine green), have photobleaching limits. However, to overcome these problems, noble metal NPs (i.e. gold nanospheres, nanorods, nanoshells, and nanocages) have been developed because they have strong absorption in NIR regions of the electromagnetic spectrum due to surface plasmon resonance (SPR) [129]. This feature is advantageous because it increases the depth penetration of light into biological tissues, which exhibit minimal light absorption in this range. Table 13.5 shows a list of some NPs involved in PTT for the treatment of GC.

Gold nanorods (GNRs) have attracted substantial interest in PTT applications in the treatment of GC. In fact, despite their intrinsic tumour tropism ability, human-induced pluripotent stem cells (iPSs) are impeded in clinical applications of cancer therapy due to the formation of teratomas and their survival in normal organs. A team of researchers loaded GNRs with iPSs treated with mitomycin C (MMC) to suppress iPS proliferation as a safe delivery approach for the targeted photothermal treatment of GC [130]. The tumour cells were efficiently killed by the heat generated from the GNRs, and the iPS cells ultimately died due to the action of MMC 7 days after the photothermal treatment.

Another study aimed to find the optimal GNR concentration and laser power for inducing hyperthermic effects in tissues and test this effect on human oesophagogastric adenocarcinoma [131]. After irradiation with NIR light, a significant increase in temperature was measured in tissues incubated with an optimal concentration of

GNR solution compared with tissues not exposed to any GNRs. Thus, this method could be effective for irreversible photodestruction of oesophagogastric tumours, with minimal collateral damage expected in (healthy) tissues free from GNRs.

In contrast, a study used haemoglobin (Hb) NPs to improve the oral bioavailability of IR780, for in vivo antitumour application in PTT [132]. The HbNPs showed high stability in enzymatic and acidic conditions similar to the gastric environment and enhanced absorption of IR780 into the blood with accumulation at tumour sites. Thus, HbNPs represent a promising delivery system for improving the oral absorption of PS dye that could effectively cause a photothermal effect, resulting in tumour ablation after oral administration in tumour-bearing mice and defining new treatment modalities in GC.

Carbon-based nanomaterials have also been used in PTT for GC, particularly NPs based on graphene oxide (GO NPs). The ultrafast reduction of GO NPs with a femtosecond laser beam has been shown to create extensive microbubbling, which produces a microcavitation effect that introduces localized mechanical damage. Taking advantage of this phenomenon, GC cells labelled with GO NPs were irradiated with the laser, and the microbubbling effect greatly facilitated the destruction of cancer cells [133].

Nanoparticles for GC Diagnosis

As mentioned previously, most GC patients are diagnosed at an advanced stage. Therefore, it is difficult to cure this disease. Apart from early diagnosis, tumour staging, planning for surgical resection, and prognosis are also needed in clinical practices. In addition, GC is classified as a "localized tumour" that is slightly different from "systemic" tumours, such as breast cancer and lung cancer. "Locoregional metastasis" is the most important negative prognostic factor in GC [134–136].

Thanks to the unique properties that appear at the nanoscale, nanomedicine provides many benefits in the diagnosis of cancer [137–141]. Thereby, the "diagnosis" of GC using NPs includes the following:

1. NPs for systemic imaging
2. NPs for locoregional imaging
3. Surface-enhanced Raman spectroscopy (SERS) NPs for early detection
4. NPs used in the detection of GC-related biomarkers
5. NPs used in the detection of circulating tumour cells (CTCs)

Table 13.6 shows some studies that have made progress in these fields.

Nanoparticles Used in the Systemic Imaging of GC

Conventional imaging of GC, including computed tomography (CT), magnetic resonance imaging (MRI), positron emission computed tomography (PECT), single-photon emission computed tomography (SPECT), and PET-CT, uses imaging contrasts and tracers for the whole body scan. However, these agents suffer from a non-specific distribution throughout the body, rapid clearance, not optimal pharmacokinetics and undesirable side effects [86, 142–144]. To overcome these limitations, a variety of NPs have emerged to enhance the imaging modalities of cancer due to many advantages, including nanoscale sizes, high agent loading, tailorable surface properties, controllable release patterns, and the EPR effect [86, 142], yet the successful development of safe and effective NP-based imaging modalities for in vivo and targeted GC imaging remains a great challenge.

In general, inorganic NPs are used as CT/MRI contrasts. Super paramagnetic NPs are the most studied agents [145]. There have been limited reports about other inorganic NPs.

The overexpression of CD146 in aggressive gastric or gastroesophageal cancer cells makes it an important biomarker for early diagnosis of GC [146, 147]. This biomarker has been used to engineer successfully NPs for molecular imaging of GC that could be applicable in tumours for

Table 13.6 Nanoparticles used in GC diagnosis

Imaging modalities	Types of nanoparticles	Targeting strategy	Application field	Stage of development	References
MRI	Dextran iron oxide NPs	Trastuzumab	Systemic imaging	In vivo/in vitro	[152]
	Liposome-coated fluorescent magnetic NPs	Trastuzumab	Systemic imaging	In vitro	[153]
	SPIO NPs	Passive targeting	Locoregional imaging	Phase I Clinical Trials	[161]
NIR fluorescence imaging	Nanocolloid ICG	Passive targeting	Locoregional imaging	Phase I Clinical Trials	[163]
	Liposomal ICG	Passive targeting	Locoregional imaging	In vivo	[164]
MRI/NIR fluorescence imaging	SPIO NPs coated with SiO_2	Anti-CD146 MAb	Systemic imaging	In vivo/in vitro	[148]
	Fluorescent magnetic NPs	BRCAA1 MAb	Systemic imaging	In vivo/in vitro	[114]
CT	Silica-capped gold nanoclusters	FA	Systemic imaging	In vivo	[156]
SPECT	^{111}In-labelled polymeric micelles	GRP78	Systemic imaging	In vivo	[157]
Upconversion luminescence imaging	PEGylated upconversion NPs	MGb2 Antibody	Locoregional imaging	In vivo	[160]
Multispectral optoacoustic tomography	PEGylated liposome-ICG	MUC-1 MAb	Locoregional imaging	In vivo	[165]
SERS-based CT	Magnesium sulphate aggregated silver NPs	Circulating RNA	Biomarker detection	In vitro	[181]
SERS-based biosensor	PNA probed-gold NPs	Ct DNA	Biomarker detection	In vitro	[185]
SERS-based endoscopy	SERS -NPs	EGFR and HER-2	Biomarker detection	In vivo	[186, 187]
Microfluidic biosensor	QDs	CEA, CA125 and HER-2/Neu	Biomarker detection	In vitro	[216]
Video capsule simulator	NIR labelled NPs conjugated to A1AT-specific antibodies	A1AT	Biomarker detection	In vitro	[217]
Ultrasensitive electrochemical nanobiosensor	Gold-magnetic nanocomposite	miR-106a	Biomarker detection	In vitro	[218]
Microfluidic biosensor	TiO_2 NP	CTCs	Biomarker detection	In vitro	[230]

image-guided therapy and surgery. For this purpose, superparamagnetic iron oxide NPs (SPION) were coated with nano dense-silica (dSiO$_2$) as core-shell NPs [148] and labelled with a near-infrared fluorescence (NIRF) dye and anti-CD146 MAb for a magnetic resonance (MR)/NIRF imaging study in the MKN45 xenograft GC model. The tumours were imaged at 30 min postinjection. This is the first successful study of functional NPs for MR/NIRF imaging of the cell surface glycoprotein CD146 in a GC model, suggesting that this system will be applicable in tumours for image-guided therapy/surgery.

BRCAA1 protein is found to be overexpressed in approximately 65% of GC tissues [114]. A study predicted that BRCAA1 could be one of the potential targeting molecules for in vivo GC cells and aimed to develop BRCAA1v MAb-conjugated fluorescent magnetic NPs for in vivo targeted imaging of GC [114]. In comparison to pure fluorescent magnetic NPs, BRCAA1-conjugated fluorescent magnetic nanoprobes showed very low toxicity, lower magnetic and fluorescent intensities. They could be endocytosed by GC MGC803 cells and could target in vivo GC tissues with a diameter of 5 mm at 0.5 h and 12 h postinjection. Thus, they could be used to image GC tissues by fluorescence imaging and magnetic resonance imaging as well as local thermal therapy of early GC in the near future.

Overexpression of HER2, a tyrosine kinase receptor, is correlated to metastatic GC. Trastuzumab (Herceptin), a humanized MAb that is targeted to the extracellular domain of HER2, is used to treat this subtype of metastatic GC and is validated by the FDA [149–151]. Different studies in breast cancer have conjugated trastuzumab to different superparamagnetic NPs for imaging [149], such as dextran iron oxide NPs [152] and liposome-coated fluorescent magnetic NPs [153]. These approaches can also be used for HER2 overexpressing GCs [149, 154, 155].

Folic acid (FA) is one of the micronutrients required for normal human growth. FA depletion/deficiency has been linked to GC. A study was designed to produce FA-conjugated silica-capped gold nanoclusters/nanoprobes for dual mode fluorescent imaging and CT imaging [156]. This system was successful: it was biocompatible and could target the FA (+) MGC-803 cells in vitro and in vivo, demonstrating excellent red-emitting fluorescence and CT imaging.

For the nuclear imaging of GC, there have been some attempts to enhance the effective use of NPs. An endoplasmic reticulum protein, glucose-regulated protein 78 (GRP78), is a GC biomarker due to its overexpression on the GC cell surface. In tumour cells, GRP78 functions as a refolding protein, which translocates to the plasma membrane to protect cells from apoptosis. A study designed GRP78 binding peptide (GRBP)-guided ^{111}In-labelled polymeric micelles for nuclear imaging detection of tumours [157]. In vivo studies in a murine GC xenograft demonstrated that the radioactive intensity measured in animal tumours treated with GRP78BP polymeric micelles was statistically higher than in animals administered untargeted micelles, demonstrating that GRP78BP could enhance the accumulation of micelles to the tumour tissue and could be useful in the application of nuclear imaging for tumour diagnosis.

Nanoparticles Used in Locoregional Imaging of GC

GC is specifically characterized to be a "localized" disease with lymphatic and peritoneal metastasis as independent prognostic factors [158, 159]. The status of both lymph node (LN) and peritoneal dissemination is extremely helpful in the pretreatment stage for proper treatment planning. However, there are limited imaging modalities applicable in these areas [160], such as MRI [161], upconversion luminescence imaging [162], NIR fluorescence imaging [163, 164], and multispectral optoacoustic tomography [165].

Diagnosis of LN metastasis in GC is essential to direct the operative approach and is performed through imaging tests, such as CT and ultrasonography (US). However, the accuracy of such tests has not been adequate. Ferumoxtran-10 is a lymphotropic contrast agent for MRI with reported efficacy for the detection of metastatic LNs in various cancers. To investigate the efficacy of ferumoxtran-10-enhanced MRI for the diagnosis of metastases LN in GC, a study enrolled 17 consecutive patients who were diagnosed with a non-early stage of GC. All the patients were examined by MRI before and 24 h after IV administration of superparamagnetic iron oxide—ferumoxtran-10. LNs were more readily identified and diagnosed by MRI images 24 h after IV administration of superparamagnetic iron oxide—ferumoxtran-10, suggesting that ferumoxtran-10-enhanced MRI is useful in the diagnosis of metastatic LNs and that the use of this modality will be helpful to direct the treatment course for GC patients [161].

Another type of molecular imaging probe using core@shell-structured NaGdF4:Yb,Er@ NaGdF4 upconversion NPs coated with polyethylene glycol (PEG) has high sensitivity for the detection of lymphatic metastasis of GC [160]. These NPs improved the detection sensitivity in imaging by displaying a satisfactory signal-to-noise ratio. Lymphatic metastases smaller than 1 mm were successfully detected in a mouse model of human GC [162], revealing the important role of these NPs in a highly effective approach for regional GC diagnosis.

A new modality for cancer imaging aiming to identify tumour and regional metastases during surgical resection is called image-guided surgery, a real-time imaging technique that is very useful for the surgical planning of GC and may be optimized to provide a higher signal to background by the incorporation of fluorescent NPs [166]. For instance, indocyanine green (ICG), which is an FDA-approved fluorescent probe, has shown important potential in image-guided surgery for GC. Several types of fluorescent NPs in phase I trials have been reported, such as nanocolloid ICG [163], liposome-embedded ICG [165, 167], HA-derived ICG NPs [168], SPIO-phospholipid-PEG-ICG [169], and others.

A study on 22 GC patients, using ICG:Nanocoll (adsorption of ICG to a nanocolloid), showed that among 21 patients with at least 1 LN detected by NIR fluorescence imaging, 8 had tumour-positive LNs. This technique offers 90% accuracy [163]. NIR-fluorescent liposomal probe LP-ICG-C18, a synthesized ICG liposomal derivative, has been used to evaluate the peritoneal metastases of GC on nude mice. It can effectively target peritoneal disseminated tumours and possibly detect them by a NIR imaging system [164]. In addition, ICG-lactosomes [170] (NPs composed of poly(L-lactic acid)-based depsipeptide [171]) and ICG-PEGylated liposome-ICG [165] are also used in the diagnosis of peritoneal dissemination of GC for theranostic purposes.

NPs have also been used in the field of US, such as nanobubbles, which were used as an US contrast agent, showing an improved contrast imaging effect on GC xenografts [172]. They were able to pass through the gaps between endothelial cells in the tumour vascular system to reach the tissue space.

Nanoparticles Used in Surface-Enhanced Raman Spectroscopy for the Early Detection of GC

The detection of GC at early stages is very challenging. It requires specific biomarkers at very low concentrations with high selectively to elude false positives. In addition, conventional white-light endoscopy is the most important and effective diagnostic method for the early detection of GC, apart from occult blood tests of stools [173]. However, it offers only structural information for the gastrointestinal tract without biochemical information. Among the most promissory methods to detect biomarkers using nanotechnology and to enhance the sensitivity of endoscopy, we will highlight herein those based on metallic NP plasmons.

The collective oscillation of the conduction electrons is called the plasmon [174]. Two types of surface plasmons exist: those coming from a bulk metal and those coming from metallic NPs. The metallic NPs have localized surface plasmons. Their excitation induces optical properties that are hardly achievable in other optical materials [175]. Thus, they can be used for analytical purposes, such as plasmon-enhanced spectroscopy: enhancing the signals of Raman scattering and fluorescence spectroscopy [176]. These materials can be synthesized and modified to be conjugated to antibodies, ligands, and drugs to yield a wide range of applications in many fields, such as biotechnology, magnetic separation, preconcentration of target analytes, targeted drug delivery, and vehicles for gene and drug delivery, especially diagnostic imaging [177].

Several imaging modalities have been developed as an aid to image GC, and the most important is SERS. The detection of biomarkers with very high sensitivity plays a crucial role in GC diagnosis. Gold and silver NPs can control and manipulate light at the nanoscale. They have a localized surface plasmon, so they can act as optical antennas that capture and radiate light to their vicinity, enhancing the Raman signal of many folds. Under favourable conditions, this technique can detect single molecules [178–180]. Discovered since more than 40 years ago, SERS is now a powerful analytical tool for molecular detection and characterization. In recent years, a great deal of interest has been focused on the development of SERS biomedical applications. However, the lack of the fabrication of reproducible nanostructures and their instability and tendency to aggregate have been serious obstacles to the practical applications of SERS. Nevertheless, aggregated NPs function as hotspots where the electromagnetic enhancement is particularly high, enhancing the Raman signal. Thus, controlling the formation of the aggregation in a way as to prevent total collapse of the colloid becomes a main task for experimental SERS.

Few applications have been reported in GC. A study developed a useful clinical tool for the noninvasive screening and detection of cancer with good diagnostic sensitivity and specificity. This method is based on SERS technology to analyse RNA in the circulation to discriminate GC patients from healthy controls [181]. RNA was extracted from serum samples and then scanned for significant differences in the spectral bands. Silver NPs partially aggregated using magnesium sulphate and were used as the SERS-active substrate presenting strong SERS signals to RNA. Many other papers were published concerning this method [173, 182, 183]. Despite significant differences in the intensity of several bands between cancer patients and healthy volunteers, there were no significant frequency shifts. Thus, it becomes hard to interpret with certainty the meaning of the spectral changes. This approach may serve as a screening method before performing further diagnostic tests.

The surface of the NPs is composed of two components: one component is an antibody that endows them with more specificity for their target, and the other component, called the Raman reporter, is easily detectable with Raman spectroscopy. Thanks to the functionalization of NPs, many studies have been reported on the use of plasmon-enhanced methods, in which better targeting and less aggregation can be achieved even though the synthesis process becomes more complicated and expensive [184]. These applications have been used for different types of cancer but not for GC. The development of a very sensitive detection method is highly likely using this strategy.

Circulating tumour DNA (ctDNA) is a double-stranded DNA that represents a promising biomarker for noninvasive cancer diagnosis [185]. Mutations at two hotspots of E542K (G70271A in exon 9) and E545K (G70282A in exon 9) and methylation of ctDNA of *PIK3CA* (phosphatidylinositol 3-kinase catalytic subunit) are tumour-specific genetic and epigenetic markers of ctDNA, respectively, that are well-known in many types of cancers including breast, colon, brain, liver, stomach, and lung [185]. Therefore, a study developed a peptide nucleic acid (PNA)-based nanoplasmonic for biosensor dual biomarker detection [185]. To detect genetic markers of ctDNA, gold NPs were coupled to PNA that captures and binds specifically to ctDNA. It results in a change in the refractive index surrounding the biosensor surface, generating a distinct localized surface plasmon resonance (LSPR) peak shift in the Rayleigh light scattering pattern. For epigenetic markers of ctDNA detection, gold NPs (immunogold colloids) coupled with methylcytosine MAb that bind specifically to methylated CpG sites on the ctDNA sequence were used. The tumour-specific genetic and epigenetic markers of ctDNA were successfully detected, and the enhancement assay increased the signal reducing four times the limit of detection (LOD).

This sensitive and multiplexed platform detected ctDNA in clinical samples at a low concentration. However, compared with the more commonly used methods, such as high-performance liquid chromatography (HPLC) or absorption spectroscopy, these techniques are still expensive, but they carry a huge analytical potential. Therefore, related approaches are starting to be evaluated in clinical settings. In contrast, to enhance the sensitivity of endoscopy, a study [173] has reported a noncontact, fibre optic-based Raman spectroscopy device that has the potential to provide real-time, multiplexed functional information during routine endoscopy. This tool was adjusted to be appropriate for the detection of functionalized SERS NPs as molecular imaging contrast agents.

When conjugated to tumour-targeting ligands, SERS NPs will target tumour biomarkers and be detected using a Raman spectroscopy device [173, 184]. As a result, a certain subgroup of cells (e.g. cancer cells) can be detected. A study [186, 187] used anti-EGFR-MAb and anti-HER2-MAb SERS NPs on the luminal surface of rat oesophagus and found that the EGFR and HER2-expressing tumour cells were precisely located and that the visualization and quantification of biomarker expression were in agreement with the immunohistochemistry and flow cytometry validation data. This technique is clearly based on one or more molecules expressed on the surface of cancer cells with high specificity. For GC, such molecules include carcinoembryonic antigen (CEA), cancer-related antigen 19-9 (CA19-9), cancer-related antigen 72-4 (CA72-4), HER2, EGFR, and others. Although none of the above-mentioned markers have 100% sensitivity and specificity, the combination of routine optical endoscopy and SERS NPs will probably provide a more sensitive method for early GC detection.

Nanoparticles Used in the Early Detection of GC-Related Biomarkers

The availability of GC-related biomarkers plays an important role in the early diagnosis of disease; they offer particular properties in turn, and they could be exploited for the development of nanostructured biosensors to increase high analytical performances [188].

Certain types of NPs may be used to increase the sensitivity of a biosensor and to be more accurate, precise, and faster [188]. The application of NPs could be advantageous in optical-based nanosensors [189–192], electrical- or electrochemical-based nanosensors [188, 193–195], fluorescence-based nanosensors [196], and magnetism-based nanosensors [197–199]. Several NPs are used in nanosensors, such as gold, magnetic NP-based biosensors, and quantum dots (QDs), which are the mostly used [189, 200–206]. These NPs have been successfully used into the nanosensors for the detection of carcinoembryonic antigen (CEA) [207–210], cancer antigen 125 (CA125) [200, 211, 212], CA724 [213], and HER2 [214]. In addition, these NPs could be useful for the exploration of new biomarkers for the early detection of GC [215].

Other nanostructures, such as nano-biochips, have also been applied in this field with NPs [216]. The integration of semiconductor NP QDs into biosensors in serum and saliva led to an amplified signal of CEA, CA125, and Her2/Neu biomarkers. In that study, QD probes were used in this biosensor format to produce a signal 30 times greater than that of standard molecular fluorophores with an approximately twofold reduction in observed limits of detection relative to the enzyme-linked immunosorbent assay (ELISA). A study reported a platform with immunoassay capabilities comprising sensing and detecting compartments serving as a real-time diagnostic for the early detection of a secreted biomarker model α1-antitrypsin precursor (A1AT) of GC [217]. The detecting compartment embeds NIR fluorescently labelled NPs conjugated to A1AT-specific antibodies. The specific recognition reaction between the captured A1AT and the immuno-NPs generates profound fluorescence with an intense signal that is sufficient to be detectable by a conventional endoscope or a video capsule. Another study used a double-specific probe methodology and a gold-magnetic nanocomposite as a tracing tag to develop an ultrasensitive electrochemical nanobiosensor for the detection of miR-106a, an overexpressed microRNA in GC [218]. The results showed many advantages, including high specificity, remarkable selectivity, compliant storage stability, and great performance, in an investigation of real samples with no pretreatment or amplification, suggesting that this miRNA-nanobiosensor can be used for clinical early detection of GC and additionally to screen any miRNA sequence.

Nanoparticles Used in the Detection of Circulating Tumour Cells (CTCs) of GC

CTCs are cancer cells, deriving either from primary tumours or from metastatic sites, which separate from the tumour and circulate in the peripheral blood to cause possibly metastasis [219]. CTCs found in the blood have been investigated as potential biomarkers for the diagnosis, prognosis, and molecular testing of metastatic GC [220, 221]. The term "liquid biopsy" is related to the identification of CTCs in the peripheral blood of cancer patients. Currently, both circulating nucleic acids and extracellular vesicles are included in the term liquid biopsy. Compared with tissue biopsies, liquid biopsies can be associated with noninvasiveness and a real-time response by offering the ability to guide the choice of therapy.

However, it is challenging to develop a CTC detection method with clinically significant specificity and sensitivity. Advances in nanotechnology and new nanomaterials offer promising enhancement for the detection of CTCs [220, 222], such as NPs [220, 223], microfluidic chips [222, 224], nano-roughened structures [222], nanoVelcro chips [219], and nanofibres [225].

The NPs used for the detection and/or isolation of CTCs usually include two parts: ligands that specifically bind to a known biomarker for CTCs (e.g. antibodies, aptamers) and NPs that can produce a specified signal and can be detected out of the blood [226]. Some NPs, including gold [227], magnetic [228, 229], QDs [226], and TiO_2 [230], are capable of detecting CTCs from blood. Interestingly, some of these NPs can simultaneously detect and isolate CTCs [229].

In a recent study [227], the use of magnetic NPs in combination with gold-plated carbon nanotubes enabled the detection of CTCs from a large volume of blood in the vessels of tumour-bearing mice. However, only a few reports on the detection of gastric CTCs by NPs are available. The isolation of CTCs from peripheral blood of GC patients with a nano-film made of TiO_2 biocompatible NPs has been reported, and 50% of the captured cells detached from the substrate and could be expected for potential clinical use [230]. Other NPs have emerged to detect special markers of GC or GC stem cells and are expected to be potential candidates for CTC detection, such as CD133 [231], HER2 [153], CD44 [232], and CD146 [146, 148].

Nanoparticles as Theranostic Agents

The word "theranostics" is defined as the combination of diagnosis with therapy. Various nanocarriers of biodegradable polymers are applied to sustain, control, and target the co-delivery of diagnostic and therapeutic agents for more effective theranostics and reduced side effects, including polymer conjugates, micelles, liposomes, dendrimers, metal, inorganic NPs, and carbon NPs. The importance of these platforms lies in the diagnosis and treatment of the diseases at different tumour stages, when they are most likely curable or even not curable [233]. The diagnosis and delivery of therapy to targeted cells are enhanced theranostic nanomedicine by coupling a targeting ligand and biomarkers [234]. NPs ranging from 10 to 1000 nm in size are used in theranostic nanomedicine. They are composed of different macromolecules or polymers that are conjugated to diagnostics and therapeutic agents for simultaneous diagnosis and treatment at cellular and molecular levels [235]. The advantages of this platform include controlled release, targeted delivery, and a higher transport efficiency by endocytosis [236], as well as the induction of stimulus-responsive agent release [237]. The co-encapsulation of multiple diagnostics and therapeutic modes has allowed multimodality nanotheranostics and resulted in enhanced performances of their application [238].

Oral delivery of theranostic nanomedicine can enhance oral bioavailability. For instance, D-α-tocopheryl polyethylene glycol 1000 succinate-based nanomedicine was used for the oral delivery of chemotherapeutic agents [239].

The therapeutic agents in theranostic nanomedicine include hydrophobic organic drugs, proteins, peptides, and genetic materials. Diagnostic agents are also generally used in theranostic nanomedicine and include optical imaging agents, such as fluorescent dyes or QDs; magnetic resonance imaging agents, such as superparamagnetic metals; nuclear imaging agents, such radionuclides; and CT agents, such as heavy elements [234, 240, 241].

NPs used in theranostics are based on two strategies: first, NPs can be detected themselves by imaging modalities, and second, they support the targeted co-delivery of diagnostic and therapeutic agents. These advanced theranostic platforms provide sensitive diagnosis platforms with accurate targeting and effective delivery of materials [242].

PEG-coated Fe_3O_4 NPs were chemically produced by co-precipitation method in which PEG functions as a stabilizer and dispersant. Such Fe_3O_4 NPs with tunable magnetic properties and a favourable size have shown promising biomedical applications [243]. In GC theranostics, polyethylene glycol-grafted polyethylenimine functionalized with superparamagnetic iron oxide NPs (PEG-g-PEI-SPION) has been successfully applied.

A study using an antibody-directed non-viral vector, combining PEG-g-PEI-SPION and a GC-associated CD44v6 single-chain variable fragment ($scFv_{CD44v6}$-PEG-g-PEI-SPION), was constructed for a GC-targeting and magnetic resonance imaging (MRI)-visible nanocarrier for siRNA delivery [244]. The cell viability and siRNA transfer efficiency were effective in vitro using the human gastric carcinoma cell line SGC-7901. Fluorescence-based imaging techniques revealed the success of the cellular uptake and distribution of NPs complexed with siRNA. Additionally, the targeting efficiency against GC was verified in vivo in nude female mice by MRI and by histology analysis, revealing the crucial and promising role of the non-viral vector $scFv_{CD44v6}$-PEG-g-PEI-SPION in gene therapy and the diagnosis of GC [245].

Another study developed FA- and disulphide (SS)-polyethylene glycol-conjugated polyethylenimine complexed with the SPION (FA-PEG-SS-PEI-SPION) polyplex for siRNA delivery system for programmed death ligand-1 (PD-L1) knockdown. PD-L1 is highly expressed in GC, interacts with PD-1 receptor on T cells, and is involved in T-cell immune resistance. The characterization of FA-PEG-SS-PEI-SPIONs determined its high binding ability, minimal cytotoxicity, higher transfection efficiency, and cellular internalization of the system in the folate receptor-overexpressing GC cell line compared with a non-FA-conjugated polyplex. In diagnostics, the polyplex functioned as a T_2-weighted contrast agent for enhancing cancer MRI. At the cellular level, one of the four PD-L1 siRNAs showed effective PD-L1 knockdown in cells overexpressing PD-L1, demonstrating changes in secreted cytokines and highlighting the potential of this class of these multifunctional theranostic NPs for the treatment and diagnosis of GC [246].

PEG-coated Fe_3O_4 NPs were also used as a miRNA delivery system to modulate the drug resistance of GC cells by enhancing miRNA-16 (miR16) expression in SGC7901/ADR cells. MiR16 plays a crucial role in reducing the drug resistance of SGC7901 cell lines to Adriamycin (ADR). ADR-induced apoptosis of SGC7901/ADR was examined by MTT and TUNEL and showed that miR16 combined with PEG-coated Fe_3O_4 NPs treatment increased cell apoptosis in vitro significantly. MiR16 and PEG-coated Fe_3O_4 NPs were able to significantly suppress SGC7901/ADR tumour growth in SGC7901/ADR(fluc) tumour-bearing nude mice, possibly by increasing SGC7901/ADR cell sensitivity to ADR. This system suggested an efficient delivery of miR16 by PEG-coated Fe_3O_4 NPs for drug-resistant tumours [247].

A different effective strategy for drug delivery using polymer-coated magnetic carriers can both increase drug utilization and reduce adverse reactions. Using these carriers, sensitivity to physical stimuli, such as a magnetic field and pH, has been developed, and the drugs have been conjugated to magnetic particles to target the desired position [248]. A type of magnetic-polymer nanocarrier was attached to folate receptor targeting and pH-sensitive multifunctionalities to carry doxorubicin (DOX) for advanced GC (AGC) treatment. Folate-coupled, pH-sensitive, amphiphilic poly(β-aminoester) self-assembled with hydrophobic oleic acid-modified iron oxide NPs, resulting in hydrophobic interaction area, as a reservoir for lipophilic DOX (F-P-DOX). Using confocal microscopy, it was shown that F-P-DOX treatment could maintain higher DOX accumulation in cells than P-DOX without folate conjugation, leading to an increased efficiency of DOX internalization at pH 6.5 than at pH 7.4. Using electron microscopy and real-time polymerase chain reaction, superior efficacy of F-P-DOX than free DOX on GC was observed. The efficacy was also determined by the MTT assay and xenograft model. Moreover, the accumulation of F-P-DOX in the tumour region was detected by MRI. Together, these observations affirm F-P-DOX as a promising theranostic candidate for AGC treatment [249].

Similarly, magnetic alginate (Alg)-CH beads were loaded with albendazole (ABZ) to test their pH sensitivity and drug release characteristics. These magnetic beads showed unique pH-dependent swelling behaviours with continuous release of ABZ. The beads also showed the magnetometer measurement data, a superparamagnetic property, as well as a fast magnetic response, revealing that they might be successfully used as a magnetic drug targeting system for ABZ in the gastrointestinal tract [248]. Another successful pH-sensitive magnetic NP (MNP) for targeted anticancer drug carriers is obtained by coating MNPs with poly(acrylic acid) (PAA) to obtain PAA@MNPs. These NPs exhibit a small size within 100 nm, good stability, and superparamagnetic properties. DOX was loaded onto MNPs (MNPs-DOX) via electrostatic interactions, with good drug-loading content and efficiency. Release studies showed that MNPs-DOX had excellent pH sensitivity, with 75.6% of the loaded DOX released at pH 4.0 in 48 h. MTT assays using the HUVEC and MCF-7 cell lines (breast cancer) demonstrated that MNPs-DOX had high antitumour activity, while the PAA@MNPs were practically nontoxic. Thus, PAA@MNPs would be a candidate for biomedical applications in GC, and MNPs-DOX could be used in targeted cancer therapy [250].

As described previously, PDT is a special theranostic modality for a number of diseases, based on the systemic, local, or topical administration of a nontoxic drug or dye known as PS followed by selective fluorescence characterized by an appropriate wavelength and intensity of light. The emitted light can be employed in photodiagnosis and molecular imaging to locate diseases, known as PS fluorescence detection (PFD). Online imaging of the drug for the detection of disease, image-guided drug delivery and treatment, guidance of surgical resection, and monitoring of treatment response can be performed by organic fusion of PFD and PDT [251]. A study examined PS-conjugated magnetic NPs with a diameter of ~20 nm designed for use in GC imaging and therapy, especially to integrate tumour targeting, imaging, and selective therapy into a small single NP (<50 nm). The Ce6 PS was covalently coupled onto the surface of magnetic NPs with silane coupling agent, allowing spectroscopic and functional properties for NIR fluorescence imaging and PDT and resulting in magnetically guided drug delivery and MRI. This platform is suitable for simultaneous targeting PDT and in vivo dual-mode NIR fluorescence imaging and MRI of nude mouse model with GC or other tumours [252] given the good stability and high water dispersibility and solubility, good biocompatibility, non-cytotoxicity, enhanced PS fluorescence detection, and remarkable photodynamic efficacy upon irradiation [251].

The theranostic properties of a new drug delivery system based on the loading of NPs with ICG derivative ICG-loaded lactosome (ICGm) were also applicable in a murine draining LN metastasis model of GC. The preoperative and intraoperative diagnoses of LN metastasis in patients with GC are important for the determination of the extent of LN dissection for the establishment of individualized treatment strategies. In vivo imaging successfully revealed metastatic LNs in the ICGm-treated but not in the ICG-treated mice. PDT using ICGm-induced apoptosis inhibited the growth of metastatic LNs, representing ICGm as a novel theranostic platform for LN metastasis of GC [165, 253].

ICG has also been strongly suggested for use as a photo-absorbent fluorescent probe that has been incorporated into clinically relevant PEGylated liposomes as a nanodevice for diagnosis. PEGylated liposome-ICG was synthesized using anti-MUC-1 humanized MAbhCTM01 as a tumour-specific theranostic system. Noninvasive tumour accumulation of these MAb-targeted liposomes was observed over time in a tumour mouse model using multispectral optoacoustic tomography (MSOT). Furthermore, both targeted and nontargeted liposome-ICG formulations preferentially accumulated in the tumour.

Table 13.7 Nanoparticles used in GC theranostics

Types of nanoparticles	Imaging strategy	Anticancer strategy	Stage of development	References
PEG-g-PEI-SPION	MRI	CD44v6 siRNA	In vitro/in vivo	[244]
FA-PEG-SS-PEI-SPIONs	MRI	PD-L1	In vitro	[246]
PEG-coated Fe_3O_4 NPs	MRI	MiRNA	In vitro/in vivo	[247]
pH-sensitive magnetic-polymer NPs with folate receptor targeting	MRI	DOX	In vitro/in vivo	[249]
PS-conjugated magnetic NPs	MRI	PDT	In vivo	[251, 252]
ICGm	NIR fluorescence imaging	PDT	In vivo, ex vivo	[253]
PEGylated liposome-ICG	MSOT	DOX	In vivo	[165]

A new study has reported the co-encapsulation of the natural herbal substances chrysin (Chr) and Cur in PEGylated PLGA NPs to explore their inhibitory effect against Caco-2 colon cancer cells. The free drugs and the nanoformulation showed dose-dependent cytotoxicity in Caco-2 cells. The nanoformulation had a more anti-proliferative effect with induced growth arrest of cancer cells [254].

The high stability and sensitivity of a Gd(III) amphiphilic complex loaded in poly(lactic-co-glycolic acid) NPs (PLGA NPs) allowed their accumulation in vivo in a murine melanoma xenograft and demonstrate their promise as theranostic MRI agents, once loaded with drug and contrast agents [255].

Matrix metalloproteinase (MMP) 2/9, also known as gelatinases A/B, play a key role in cancer invasion and metastasis. The gelatinase-responsive copolymer (mPEG-PCL) was synthesized for anticancer drug delivery to make use of MMP2/9 as targets for drug delivery. The cellular uptake of GEL-NPs was correlated with the level of gelatinases, which also influenced the in vitro antitumour effect of GEL-NPs. The anticancer effect of GEL-NPs exceeded the DOC. The cytotoxicity study of primary lung cancer cells also confirmed the effectiveness of the GEL-NP targeting strategy [142]. This strategy could be applied to GC.

Finally, DOC-NPs based on the gelatinase-stimulus strategy were used to compare their radiosensitization efficacy with DOC in GC. DOC-NPs showed significant radio-enhancement compared with DOC in all three gelatinase-overexpressing GC cells, associated with G2/M arrest enhancement, reactive oxygen species (ROS) production, and apoptosis induction. In addition, the radiosensitization efficacy of DOC-NPs was more prominent than DOC by intravenous injection in the xenograft. The gelatinase-mediated nanoscale delivery system serves as a potential strategy for radiosensitizer selectivity by manipulating the common microenvironment difference between the tumour and normal tissue [43].

Table 13.7 shows a list of some nanoparticles used as theranostic agents in GC.

Toxicity of Nanoparticles

NPs possess the capacity to revolutionize medical imaging, diagnostics, as well as therapeutics of GC. However, the toxicity of NPs should also be taken into consideration. Several studies have investigated the toxicity associated with specific NPs in GC. For example, a study has demonstrated that NPs made from copper increase hydrogen and bicarbonate ions and could damage gastric tissues [256]. Another study has demonstrated that high intake of superparamagnetic NPs can lead to the accumulation of iron in a specific organ to which it is delivered and thus produce toxic effects and lead to DNA damage [257]. Several studies focusing on three categories of nanomaterials, nanometals and metal oxides, carbon-based NPs, and polymer/dendrimers, have demonstrated some toxic results of these NPs when used at a high dose. However, some in vivo studies have shown that a low dose of these NPs provides nontoxic results [258]. Platinum-based NPs show a strong response against GC cells but can still accumulate in the liver or spleen and show a cytotoxic effect. To overcome this problem, the incorporation of polymers, which are safe and easily biodegradable, could reduce the side effects of NP-based anticancer formulations, i.e. the use of hyaluronan in platinum nanoparticulate-based anticancer drugs [259]. Hence, short-term and long-term toxicity studies are also needed in both cell culture and living animal models before these agents can gain FDA approval for clinical trials.

Conclusions

Currently, cancer is still an alarming disease, and people panic when they hear about it. Like all other cancers, GC can lead to death, and it is mandatory to find new ways to address this disease as existing strategies are not sufficient. This chapter describes many different applications for which NPs are being used to fight against GC. By blending with existing treatment methodologies or creating new treatments, the use of NPs could pave the way to treat GC more easily than before. In addition, the use of NPs has increased the sensitivity and specificity of GC diagnosis modalities in systemic and locoregional imaging, led to early detection and identified biomarkers, and helped elucidating CTCs. However, there are some limitations of nanomedicine. A number of limitations that are shared among current NPs compromise their further transition into clinical use. These limitations are synonymous with the obstacles that researchers are currently trying to overcome [260, 261] and include immunogenicity, poor site-specific accumulation, production costs, inability to overcome barriers in the tumour microenvironment (high interstitial fluid pressure, interactions with collagen matrix), and inability to treat small metastases for which EPR is not evoked. By successively addressing each of these barriers, innovative design features can be rationally incorporated to create a new generation of NPs, achieving a paradigmatic shift in NP-based diagnosis and therapy.

Concerning GC treatment, unlocking the full potentiality of NPs as well as safely transferring there use into clinical trials, which would eventually lead to industrial-based production, requires further dedication and effort. Concerning GC diagnosis, the application of NPs is restricted due to the limits of the specificity of markers or ligands expressed by GC. Furthermore, a large number of studies follow similar study designs for the diagnosis of breast cancer, lung cancer, and colorectal cancer. Therefore, to promote the development of nanomedicine in the treatment and diagnosis of GC, further studies and increased collaboration and knowledge exchange between scientists are needed.

References

1. Piazuelo MB, Correa P. Gastric cáncer: overview. Colomb Med (Cali, Colomb). 2013;44:192–201.
2. Sudhakar A. History of cancer, ancient and modern treatment methods. J Cancer Sci Ther. 2009;1:1–4.
3. Folkman J, Parris EE, Folkman J. Tumor angiogenesis: therapeutic implications. N Engl J Med. 1971;285:1182–6.
4. Folkman J, Shing Y. Angiogenesis. J Biol Chem. 1992;267:10931–4.
5. Jain RK. Transport of molecules in the tumor interstitium: a review. Cancer Res. 1987;47:3039–51.
6. Koo H, Huh MS, Sun I-C, Yuk SH, Choi K, Kim K, Kwon IC. In vivo targeted delivery of nanoparticles for theranosis. Acc Chem Res. 2011;44:1018–28.
7. Maeda H. The enhanced permeability and retention (EPR) effect in tumor vasculature: the key role of tumor-selective macromolecular drug targeting. Adv Enzym Regul. 2001;41:189–207.
8. Trédan O, Galmarini CM, Patel K, Tannock IF. Drug resistance and the solid tumor microenvironment. J Natl Cancer Inst. 2007;99:1441–54.
9. Niederhuber JE. Developmental biology, self-renewal, and cancer. Lancet Oncol. 2007;8:456–7.
10. Wang X, Yang L, Chen ZG, Shin DM. Application of nanotechnology in cancer therapy and imaging. CA Cancer J Clin. 2008;58:97–110.
11. Ferrari M. Cancer nanotechnology: opportunities and challenges. Nat Rev Cancer. 2005;5:161–71.
12. Li KCP, Pandit SD, Guccione S, Bednarski MD. Molecular imaging applications in nanomedicine. Biomed Microdevices. 2004;6(6):113.

13. Narayana A. Applications of nanotechnology in cancer: a literature review of imaging and treatment. J Nucl Med Radiat Ther. 2014;5:1–9.
14. Thakor AS, Gambhir SS. Nanooncology: the future of cancer diagnosis and therapy. CA Cancer J Clin. 2013;63:395–418.
15. Palazzolo S, Bayda S, Hadla M, Caligiuri I, Corona G, Toffoli G, Rizzolio F. The clinical translation of organic nanomaterials for cancer therapy: a focus on polymeric nanoparticles, micelles, liposomes and exosomes. Curr Med Chem. 2017;24:1.
16. Gmeiner WH, Ghosh S. Nanotechnology for cancer treatment. Nanotechnol Rev. 2015;3:111–22.
17. Ajani JA, Bentrem DJ, Besh S, D'Amico TA, Das P, Denlinger C, Fakih MG, Fuchs CS, Gerdes H, Glasgow RE, Hayman JA, Hofstetter WL, Ilson DH, Keswani RN, Kleinberg LR, Korn WM, Lockhart AC, Meredith K, Mulcahy MF, Orringer MB, Posey JA, Sasson AR, Scott WJ, Strong VE, Varghese TK, Warren G, Washington MK, Willett C, Wright CD, McMillian NR, Sundar H, National Comprehensive Cancer Network. Gastric cancer, version 2.2013: featured updates to the NCCN Guidelines. J Natl Compr Cancer Netw. 2013;11:531–46.
18. Yuan M, Yang Y, Lv W, Song Z, Zhong H. Paclitaxel combined with capecitabine as first-line chemotherapy for advanced or recurrent gastric cancer. Oncol Lett. 2014;8:351–4.
19. Schöffski P. New drugs for treatment of gastric cancer. Ann Oncol Off J Eur Soc Med Oncol. 2002;13(Suppl 4):13–22.
20. Li Q, Boyer C, Lee JY, Shepard HM. A novel approach to thymidylate synthase as a target for cancer chemotherapy. Mol Pharmacol. 2001;59:446–52.
21. Meriggi F, Di Biasi B, Caliolo C, Zaniboni A. The potential role of pemetrexed in gastrointestinal cancer. Chemotherapy. 2008;54:1–8.
22. Orditura M, Galizia G, Sforza V, Gambardella V, Fabozzi A, Laterza MM, Andreozzi F, Ventriglia J, Savastano B, Mabilia A, Lieto E, Ciardiello F, De Vita F. Treatment of gastric cancer. World J Gastroenterol. 2014;20:1635–49.
23. Caponigro F, Facchini G, Nasti G, Iaffaioli RV. Gastric cancer. Treatment of advanced disease and new drugs. Front Biosci. 2005;10:3122–6.
24. Johnstone TC, Park GY, Lippard SJ. Understanding and improving platinum anticancer drugs–phenanthriplatin. Anticancer Res. 2014;34:471–6.
25. Minotti G, Menna P, Salvatorelli E, Cairo G, Gianni L. Anthracyclines: molecular advances and pharmacologic developments in antitumor activity and cardiotoxicity. Pharmacol Rev. 2004;56:185–229.
26. Palacio S, Loaiza-Bonilla A, Kittaneh M, Kyriakopoulos C, Ochoa RE, Escobar M, Arango B, Restrepo MH, Merchan JR, Rocha Lima CMSR, Hosein PJ. Successful use of Trastuzumab with anthracycline-based chemotherapy followed by trastuzumab maintenance in patients with advanced HER2-positive gastric cancer. Anticancer Res. 2014;34:301–6.
27. Park S, Woo Y, Kim H, Lee YC, Choi S, Hyung WJ, Noh SH. In vitro adenosine triphosphate based chemotherapy response assay in gastric cancer. J Gastric Cancer. 2010;10:155–61.
28. Pommier Y. Drugging topoisomerases: lessons and challenges. ACS Chem Biol. 2013;8:82–95.
29. Kang BW, Kim JG, Kwon O-K, Chung HY, Yu W. Non-platinum-based chemotherapy for treatment of advanced gastric cancer: 5-fluorouracil, taxanes, and irinotecan. World J Gastroenterol. 2014;20:5396–402.
30. Kang Y-K, Chang H-M, Yook JH, Ryu M-H, Park I, Min YJ, Zang DY, Kim GY, Yang DH, Jang SJ, Park YS, Lee J-L, Kim TW, Oh ST, Park BK, Jung H-Y, Kim BS. Adjuvant chemotherapy for gastric cancer: a randomised phase 3 trial of mitomycin-C plus either short-term doxifluridine or long-term doxifluridine plus cisplatin after curative D2 gastrectomy (AMC0201). Br J Cancer. 2013;108:1245–51.
31. Tsuburaya A, Yoshida K, Kobayashi M, Yoshino S, Takahashi M, Takiguchi N, Tanabe K, Takahashi N, Imamura H, Tatsumoto N, Hara A, Nishikawa K, Fukushima R, Nozaki I, Kojima H, Miyashita Y, Oba K, Buyse M, Morita S, Sakamoto J. Sequential paclitaxel followed by tegafur and uracil (UFT) or S-1 versus UFT or S-1 monotherapy as adjuvant chemotherapy for T4a/b gastric cancer (SAMIT): a phase 3 factorial randomised controlled trial. Lancet Oncol. 2014;15:886–93.
32. Van Cutsem E. The treatment of advanced gastric cancer: new findings on the activity of the taxanes. Oncologist. 2004;9(Suppl 2):9–15.
33. Schulte N, Ebert MP, Härtel N. Gastric cancer: new drugs – new strategies. Gastrointest Tumors. 2014;1:180–94.
34. Carr C, Ng J, Wigmore T. The side effects of chemotherapeutic agents. Curr Anaesth Crit Care. 2008;19:70–9.
35. Kehrer DF, Soepenberg O, Loos WJ, Verweij J, Sparreboom A. Modulation of camptothecin analogs in the treatment of cancer: a review. Anti-Cancer Drugs. 2001;12:89–105.
36. Muggia FM, Burris HA. Clinical development of topoisomerase-interactive drugs. Adv Pharmacol. 1994;29B:1–31.
37. Slichenmyer WJ, Rowinsky EK, Donehower RC, Kaufmann SH. The current status of camptothecin analogues as antitumor agents. J Natl Cancer Inst. 1993;85:271–91.
38. Gaur S, Chen L, Yen T, Wang Y, Zhou B, Davis M, Yen Y. Preclinical study of the cyclodextrin-polymer conjugate of camptothecin CRLX101 for the treatment of gastric cancer. Nanomedicine. 2012;8:721–30.
39. Nabell L, Spencer S. Docetaxel with concurrent radiotherapy in head and neck cancer. Semin Oncol. 2003;30:89–93.
40. Wang S-C, Chen F-L, Lin W-L, Wang P-H, Han C-P. Cytokeratin 8/18 monoclonal antibody was dissimilar to anti-cytokeratin CAM 5.2. Comment

on: A randomized phase III study of adjuvant platinum/docetaxel chemotherapy with or without radiation therapy in patients with gastric cancer. Cancer Chemother Pharmacol. 2011;67:243–4; author reply 245.
41. Sen F, Saglam EK, Toker A, Dilege S, Kizir A, Oral EN, Saip P, Sakallioglu B, Topuz E, Aydiner A. Weekly docetaxel and cisplatin with concomitant radiotherapy in addition to surgery and/or consolidation chemotherapy in stage III non-small cell lung cancer. Cancer Chemother Pharmacol. 2011;68:1497–505.
42. Markman M. Managing taxane toxicities. Support Care Cancer. 2003;11:144–7.
43. Cui F-B, Li R-T, Liu Q, Wu P-Y, Hu W-J, Yue G-F, Ding H, Yu L-X, Qian X-P, Liu B-R. Enhancement of radiotherapy efficacy by docetaxel-loaded gelatinase-stimuli PEG-Pep-PCL nanoparticles in gastric cancer. Cancer Lett. 2014;346:53–62.
44. Fuse N, Kuboki Y, Kuwata T, Nishina T, Kadowaki S, Shinozaki E, Machida N, Yuki S, Ooki A, Kajiura S, Kimura T, Yamanaka T, Shitara K, Nagatsuma AK, Yoshino T, Ochiai A, Ohtsu A. Prognostic impact of HER2, EGFR, and c-MET status on overall survival of advanced gastric cancer patients. Gastric Cancer. 2016;19:183–91.
45. Sakai K, Mori S, Kawamoto T, Taniguchi S, Kobori O, Morioka Y, Kuroki T, Kano K. Expression of epidermal growth factor receptors on normal human gastric epithelia and gastric carcinomas. J Natl Cancer Inst. 1986;77:1047–52.
46. Takehana T, Kunitomo K, Suzuki S, Kono K, Fujii H, Matsumoto Y, Ooi A. Expression of epidermal growth factor receptor in gastric carcinomas. Clin Gastroenterol Hepatol. 2003;1:438–45.
47. Pinto C, Di Fabio F, Siena S, Cascinu S, Rojas Llimpe FL, Ceccarelli C, Mutri V, Giannetta L, Giaquinta S, Funaioli C, Berardi R, Longobardi C, Piana E, Martoni AA. Phase II study of cetuximab in combination with FOLFIRI in patients with untreated advanced gastric or gastroesophageal junction adenocarcinoma (FOLCETUX study). Ann Oncol Off J Eur Soc Med Oncol. 2007;18:510–7.
48. Sreeranganathan M, Uthaman S, Sarmento B, Mohan CG, Park I-K, Jayakumar R. In vivo evaluation of cetuximab-conjugated poly(γ-glutamic acid)-docetaxel nanomedicines in EGFR-overexpressing gastric cancer xenografts. Int J Nanomedicine. 2017;12:7165–82.
49. Gao Z, Li Z, Yan J, Wang P. Irinotecan and 5-fluorouracil-co-loaded, hyaluronic acid-modified layer-by-layer nanoparticles for targeted gastric carcinoma therapy. Drug Des Devel Ther. 2017;11:2595–604.
50. van Rees BP, Saukkonen K, Ristimäki A, Polkowski W, Tytgat GNJ, Drillenburg P, Offerhaus GJA. Cyclooxygenase-2 expression during carcinogenesis in the human stomach. J Pathol. 2002;196:171–9.
51. Shanmugam MK, Ong TH, Kumar AP, Lun CK, Ho PC, Wong PTH, Hui KM, Sethi G. Ursolic acid inhibits the initiation, progression of prostate cancer and prolongs the survival of TRAMP mice by modulating pro-inflammatory pathways. ed G C Jagetia. PLoS One. 2012;**7**:e32476.
52. Limami Y, Pinon A, Leger DY, Mousseau Y, Cook-Moreau J, Beneytout J-L, Delage C, Liagre B, Simon A. HT-29 colorectal cancer cells undergoing apoptosis overexpress COX-2 to delay ursolic acid-induced cell death. Biochimie. 2011;93:749–57.
53. Zhang H, Li X, Ding J, Xu H, Dai X, Hou Z, Zhang K, Sun K, Sun W. Delivery of ursolic acid (UA) in polymeric nanoparticles effectively promotes the apoptosis of gastric cancer cells through enhanced inhibition of cyclooxygenase 2 (COX-2). Int J Pharm. 2013;441:261–8.
54. Salaun B, Coste I, Rissoan M-C, Lebecque SJ, Renno T. TLR3 can directly trigger apoptosis in human cancer cells. J Immunol. 2006;176:4894–901.
55. Paone A, Starace D, Galli R, Padula F, De Cesaris P, Filippini A, Ziparo E, Riccioli A. Toll-like receptor 3 triggers apoptosis of human prostate cancer cells through a PKC-alpha-dependent mechanism. Carcinogenesis. 2008;29:1334–42.
56. Chiron D, Pellat-Deceunynck C, Amiot M, Bataille R, Jego G. TLR3 ligand induces NF-{kappa}B activation and various fates of multiple myeloma cells depending on IFN-{alpha} production. J Immunol. 2009;182:4471–8.
57. Yoneda K, Sugimoto K, Shiraki K, Tanaka J, Beppu T, Fuke H, Yamamoto N, Masuya M, Horie R, Uchida K, Takei Y. Dual topology of functional Toll-like receptor 3 expression in human hepatocellular carcinoma: differential signaling mechanisms of TLR3-induced NF-kappaB activation and apoptosis. Int J Oncol. 2008;33:929–36.
58. Besch R, Poeck H, Hohenauer T, Senft D, Häcker G, Berking C, Hornung V, Endres S, Ruzicka T, Rothenfusser S, Hartmann G. Proapoptotic signaling induced by RIG-I and MDA-5 results in type I interferon-independent apoptosis in human melanoma cells. J Clin Invest. 2009;119:2399–411.
59. Qu J, Hou Z, Han Q, Zhang C, Tian Z, Zhang J. Poly(I:C) exhibits an anti-cancer effect in human gastric adenocarcinoma cells which is dependent on RLRs. Int Immunopharmacol. 2013;17:814–20.
60. Nagini S. Carcinoma of the stomach: A review of epidemiology, pathogenesis, molecular genetics and chemoprevention. World J Gastrointest Oncol. 2012;4:156–69.
61. Wong H, Yau T. Targeted therapy in the management of advanced gastric cancer: are we making progress in the era of personalized medicine? Oncologist. 2012;17:346–58.
62. Che X, Hokita S, Natsugoe S, Tanabe G, Baba M, Takao S, Aikou T. Tumor angiogenesis related to growth pattern and lymph node metastasis in early gastric cancer. Chin Med J. 1998;111:1090–3.

63. Martin-Richard M, Gallego R, Pericay C, Garcia Foncillas J, Queralt B, Casado E, Barriuso J, Iranzo V, Juez I, Visa L, Saigi E, Barnadas A, Garcia-Albeniz X, Maurel J. Multicenter phase II study of oxaliplatin and sorafenib in advanced gastric adenocarcinoma after failure of cisplatin and fluoropyrimidine treatment. A GEMCAD study. Investig New Drugs. 2013;31:1573–9.
64. Mochalin VN, Shenderova O, Ho D, Gogotsi Y. The properties and applications of nanodiamonds. Nat Nanotechnol. 2011;7:11–23.
65. Zhang Z, Niu B, Chen J, He X, Bao X, Zhu J, Yu H, Li Y. The use of lipid-coated nanodiamond to improve bioavailability and efficacy of sorafenib in resisting metastasis of gastric cancer. Biomaterials. 2014;35:4565–72.
66. Ji J-L, Huang X-F, Zhu H-L. Curcumin and its formulations: potential anti-cancer agents. Anti Cancer Agents Med Chem. 2012;12:210–8.
67. Shishodia S, Chaturvedi MM, Aggarwal BB. Role of curcumin in cancer therapy. Curr Probl Cancer. 2007;31:243–305.
68. Hahn Y-B, Ahmad R, Tripathy N. Chemical and biological sensors based on metal oxide nanostructures. Chem Commun (Camb). 2012;48:10369–85.
69. Dhivya R, Ranjani J, Rajendhran J, Mayandi J, Annaraj J. Enhancing the anti-gastric cancer activity of curcumin with biocompatible and pH sensitive PMMA-AA/ZnO nanoparticles. Mater Sci Eng C Mater Biol Appl. 2018;82:182–9.
70. Xiao Y-F, Li J-M, Wang S-M, Yong X, Tang B, Jie M-M, Dong H, Yang X-C, Yang S-M. Cerium oxide nanoparticles inhibit the migration and proliferation of gastric cancer by increasing DHX15 expression. Int J Nanomedicine. 2016;11:3023–34.
71. Mi F-L, Tan Y-C, Liang H-F, Sung H-W. In vivo biocompatibility and degradability of a novel injectable-chitosan-based implant. Biomaterials. 2002;23:181–91.
72. Qi L-F, Xu Z-R, Li Y, Jiang X, Han X-Y. In vitro effects of chitosan nanoparticles on proliferation of human gastric carcinoma cell line MGC803 cells. World J Gastroenterol. 2005;11:5136–41.
73. Dean M, Fojo T, Bates S. Tumour stem cells and drug resistance. Nat Rev Cancer. 2005;5:275–84.
74. Sun M, Zhou W, Zhang Y-Y, Wang D-L, Wu X-L. CD44+gastric cancer cells with stemness properties are chemoradioresistant and highly invasive. Oncol Lett. 2013;5:1793–8.
75. Takaishi S, Okumura T, Tu S, Wang SSW, Shibata W, Vigneshwaran R, Gordon SAK, Shimada Y, Wang TC. Identification of gastric cancer stem cells using the cell surface marker CD44. Stem Cells. 2009;27:1006–20.
76. Zhang C, Li C, He F, Cai Y, Yang H. Identification of CD44+CD24+ gastric cancer stem cells. J Cancer Res Clin Oncol. 2011;137:1679–86.
77. Chen T, Yang K, Yu J, Meng W, Yuan D, Bi F, Liu F, Liu J, Dai B, Chen X, Wang F, Zeng F, Xu H, Hu J, Mo X. Identification and expansion of cancer stem cells in tumor tissues and peripheral blood derived from gastric adenocarcinoma patients. Cell Res. 2012;22:248–58.
78. Platt VM, Szoka FC. Anticancer therapeutics: targeting macromolecules and nanocarriers to hyaluronan or CD44, a hyaluronan receptor. Mol Pharm. 2008;5:474–86.
79. Fuchs D, Daniel V, Sadeghi M, Opelz G, Naujokat C. Salinomycin overcomes ABC transporter-mediated multidrug and apoptosis resistance in human leukemia stem cell-like KG-1a cells. Biochem Biophys Res Commun. 2010;394:1098–104.
80. Kusunoki S, Kato K, Tabu K, Inagaki T, Okabe H, Kaneda H, Suga S, Terao Y, Taga T, Takeda S. The inhibitory effect of salinomycin on the proliferation, migration and invasion of human endometrial cancer stem-like cells. Gynecol Oncol. 2013;129:598–605.
81. Wang Y. Effects of salinomycin on cancer stem cell in human lung adenocarcinoma A549 cells. Med Chem. 2011;7:106–11.
82. Dong T-T, Zhou H-M, Wang L-L, Feng B, Lv B, Zheng M-H. Salinomycin selectively targets "CD133+" cell subpopulations and decreases malignant traits in colorectal cancer lines. Ann Surg Oncol. 2011;18:1797–804.
83. Gupta PB, Onder TT, Jiang G, Tao K, Kuperwasser C, Weinberg RA, Lander ES. Identification of selective inhibitors of cancer stem cells by high-throughput screening. Cell. 2009;138:645–59.
84. Yao H-J, Zhang Y-G, Sun L, Liu Y. The effect of hyaluronic acid functionalized carbon nanotubes loaded with salinomycin on gastric cancer stem cells. Biomaterials. 2014;35:9208–23.
85. Shapira A, Davidson I, Avni N, Assaraf YG, Livney YD. β-Casein nanoparticle-based oral drug delivery system for potential treatment of gastric carcinoma: stability, target-activated release and cytotoxicity. Eur J Pharm Biopharm. 2012;80:298–305.
86. Davis ME, Chen ZG, Shin DM. Nanoparticle therapeutics: an emerging treatment modality for cancer. Nat Rev Drug Discov. 2008;7:771–82.
87. Fang J, Nakamura H, Maeda H. The EPR effect: Unique features of tumor blood vessels for drug delivery, factors involved, and limitations and augmentation of the effect. Adv Drug Deliv Rev. 2011;63:136–51.
88. Farokhzad OC. Using ligands to target cancer cells. Clin Adv Hematol Oncol. 2012;10:543–4.
89. Yoo J-W, Irvine DJ, Discher DE, Mitragotri S. Bio-inspired, bioengineered and biomimetic drug delivery carriers. Nat Rev Drug Discov. 2011;10:521–35.
90. Langer R, Tirrell DA. Designing materials for biology and medicine. Nature. 2004;428:487–92.
91. Irvine DJ, Swartz MA, Szeto GL. Engineering synthetic vaccines using cues from natural immunity. Nat Mater. 2013;12:978–90.
92. Wegst UGK, Bai H, Saiz E, Tomsia AP, Ritchie RO. Bioinspired structural materials. Nat Mater. 2015;14:23–36.

93. Zhang L, Li R, Chen H, Wei J, Qian H, Su S, Shao J, Wang L, Qian X, Liu B. Human cytotoxic T-lymphocyte membrane-camouflaged nanoparticles combined with low-dose irradiation: a new approach to enhance drug targeting in gastric cancer. Int J Nanomedicine. 2017;12:2129–42.
94. Draghiciu O, Walczak M, Hoogeboom BN, Franken KLMC, Melief KJM, Nijman HW, Daemen T. Therapeutic immunization and local low-dose tumor irradiation, a reinforcing combination. Int J Cancer. 2014;134:859–72.
95. Lugade AA, Sorensen EW, Gerber SA, Moran JP, Frelinger JG, Lord EM. Radiation-induced IFN-gamma production within the tumor microenvironment influences antitumor immunity. J Immunol. 2008;180:3132–9.
96. Whitehead KA, Langer R, Anderson DG. Knocking down barriers: advances in siRNA delivery. Nat Rev Drug Discov. 2009;8:129–38.
97. Soutschek J, Akinc A, Bramlage B, Charisse K, Constien R, Donoghue M, Elbashir S, Geick A, Hadwiger P, Harborth J, John M, Kesavan V, Lavine G, Pandey RK, Racie T, Rajeev KG, Röhl I, Toudjarska I, Wang G, Wuschko S, Bumcrot D, Koteliansky V, Limmer S, Manoharan M, Vornlocher H-P. Therapeutic silencing of an endogenous gene by systemic administration of modified siRNAs. Nature. 2004;432:173–8.
98. Jagani H, Rao JV, Palanimuthu VR, Hariharapura RC, Gang S. A nanoformulation of siRNA and its role in cancer therapy: in vitro and in vivo evaluation. Cell Mol Biol Lett. 2013;18:120–36.
99. de Fougerolles A, Vornlocher H-P, Maraganore J, Lieberman J. Interfering with disease: a progress report on siRNA-based therapeutics. Nat Rev Drug Discov. 2007;6:443–53.
100. Ye Q-F, Zhang Y-C, Peng X-Q, Long Z, Ming Y-Z, He L-Y. Silencing Notch-1 induces apoptosis and increases the chemosensitivity of prostate cancer cells to docetaxel through Bcl-2 and Bax. Oncol Lett. 2012;3:879–84.
101. BAI Z, ZHANG Z, QU X, HAN W, MA X. Sensitization of breast cancer cells to taxol by inhibition of taxol resistance gene 1. Oncol Lett. 2012;3:135–40.
102. Miele E, Spinelli GP, Miele E, Di Fabrizio E, Ferretti E, Tomao S, Gulino A. Nanoparticle-based delivery of small interfering RNA: challenges for cancer therapy. Int J Nanomedicine. 2012;7:3637–57.
103. Gravalos C, Jimeno A. HER2 in gastric cancer: a new prognostic factor and a novel therapeutic target. Ann Oncol Off J Eur Soc Med Oncol. 2008;19:1523–9.
104. Hofmann M, Stoss O, Shi D, Büttner R, van de Vijver M, Kim W, Ochiai A, Rüschoff J, Henkel T. Assessment of a HER2 scoring system for gastric cancer: results from a validation study. Histopathology. 2008;52:797–805.
105. Tanner M, Hollmén M, Junttila TT, Kapanen AI, Tommola S, Soini Y, Helin H, Salo J, Joensuu H, Sihvo E, Elenius K, Isola J. Amplification of HER-2 in gastric carcinoma: association with Topoisomerase IIalpha gene amplification, intestinal type, poor prognosis and sensitivity to trastuzumab. Ann Oncol Off J Eur Soc Med Oncol. 2005;16:273–8.
106. Bang Y-J, Van Cutsem E, Feyereislova A, Chung HC, Shen L, Sawaki A, Lordick F, Ohtsu A, Omuro Y, Satoh T, Aprile G, Kulikov E, Hill J, Lehle M, Rüschoff J, Kang Y-K, ToGA Trial Investigators. Trastuzumab in combination with chemotherapy versus chemotherapy alone for treatment of HER2-positive advanced gastric or gastro-oesophageal junction cancer (ToGA): a phase 3, open-label, randomised controlled trial. Lancet (Lond Engl). 2010;376:687–97.
107. Wu F-L, Zhang J, Li W, Bian B-X, Hong Y-D, Song Z-Y, Wang H-Y, Cui F-B, Li R-T, Liu Q, Jiang X-D, Li X-M, Zheng J-N. Enhanced antiproliferative activity of antibody-functionalized polymeric nanoparticles for targeted delivery of anti-miR-21 to HER2 positive gastric cancer. Oncotarget. 2017;8:67189–202.
108. Takahashi T, Saikawa Y, Kitagawa Y. Gastric cancer: current status of diagnosis and treatment. Cancers (Basel). 2013;5:48–63.
109. Dicken BJ, Bigam DL, Cass C, Mackey JR, Joy AA, Hamilton SM. Gastric adenocarcinoma: review and considerations for future directions. Ann Surg. 2005;241:27–39.
110. Kuo C-Y, Chao Y, Li C-P. Update on treatment of gastric cancer. J Chin Med Assoc. 2014;77:345–53.
111. Proserpio I, Rausei S, Barzaghi S, Frattini F, Galli F, Iovino D, Rovera F, Boni L, Dionigi G, Pinotti G. Multimodal treatment of gastric cancer. World J Gastrointest Surg. 2014;6:55–8.
112. Kilic L, Ordu C, Yildiz I, Sen F, Keskin S, Ciftci R, Pilanci KN. Current adjuvant treatment modalities for gastric cancer: from history to the future. World J Gastrointest Oncol. 2016;8:439–49.
113. Cui D, Jin G, Gao T, Sun T, Tian F, Estrada GG, Gao H, Sarai A. Characterization of BRCAA1 and its novel antigen epitope identification. Cancer Epidemiol Biomark Prev. 2004;13:1136–45.
114. Wang K, Ruan J, Qian Q, Song H, Bao C, Zhang X, Kong Y, Zhang C, Hu G, Ni J, Cui D. BRCAA1 monoclonal antibody conjugated fluorescent magnetic nanoparticles for in vivo targeted magnetofluorescent imaging of gastric cancer. J Nanobiotechnol. 2011;9:23.
115. Cui D, Zhang C, Liu B, Shu Y, Du T, Shu D, Wang K, Dai F, Liu Y, Li C, Pan F, Yang Y, Ni J, Li H, Brand-Saberi B, Guo P. Regression of gastric cancer by systemic injection of RNA nanoparticles carrying both ligand and siRNA. Sci Rep. 2015;5:10726.
116. Wu Y, Wang W, Chen Y, Huang K, Shuai X, Chen Q, Li X, Lian G. The investigation of polymer-siRNA nanoparticle for gene therapy of gastric cancer in vitro. Int J Nanomedicine. 2010;5:129–36.
117. Czupryna J, Tsourkas A. Suicide gene delivery by calcium phosphate nanoparticles: a novel method of

targeted therapy for gastric cancer. Cancer Biol Ther. 2006;5:1691–2.
118. Wang JB, Liu LX. Use of photodynamic therapy in malignant lesions of stomach, bile duct, pancreas, colon and rectum. Hepato-Gastroenterology. 2007;54:718–24.
119. Chatterjee DK, Fong LS, Zhang Y. Nanoparticles in photodynamic therapy: an emerging paradigm. Adv Drug Deliv Rev. 2008;60:1627–37.
120. Foote CS. Definition of type I and type II photosensitized oxidation. Photochem Photobiol. 1991;54:659.
121. Hatz S, Lambert JDC, Ogilby PR. Measuring the lifetime of singlet oxygen in a single cell: addressing the issue of cell viability. Photochem Photobiol Sci. 2007;6:1106–16.
122. Babu A, Periasamy J, Gunasekaran A, Kumaresan G, Naicker S, Gunasekaran P, Murugesan R. Polyethylene glycol-modified gelatin/polylactic acid nanoparticles for enhanced photodynamic efficacy of a hypocrellin derivative in vitro. J Biomed Nanotechnol. 2013;9:177–92.
123. Huang P, Wang S, Wang X, Shen G, Lin J, Wang Z, Guo S, Cui D, Yang M, Chen X. Surface functionalization of chemically reduced graphene oxide for targeted photodynamic therapy. J Biomed Nanotechnol. 2015;11:117–25.
124. Lee H-I, Kim Y-J. Enhanced cellular uptake of protoporphyrine IX/linolenic acid-conjugated spherical nanohybrids for photodynamic therapy. Colloids Surf B Biointerfaces. 2016;142:182–91.
125. Shimoyama A, Watase H, Liu Y, Ogura S, Hagiya Y, Takahashi K, Inoue K, Tanaka T, Murayama Y, Otsuji E, Ohkubo A, Yuasa H. Access to a novel near-infrared photodynamic therapy through the combined use of 5-aminolevulinic acid and lanthanide nanoparticles. Photodiagn Photodyn Ther. 2013;10:607–14.
126. Sawamura T, Tanaka T, Ishige H, Iizuka M, Murayama Y, Otsuji E, Ohkubo A, Ogura S-I, Yuasa H. The effect of coatings on the affinity of lanthanide nanoparticles to MKN45 and HeLa cancer cells and improvement in photodynamic therapy efficiency. Int J Mol Sci. 2015;16:22415–24.
127. Li S, Chang K, Sun K, Tang Y, Cui N, Wang Y, Qin W, Xu H, Wu C. Amplified singlet oxygen generation in semiconductor polymer dots for photodynamic cancer therapy. ACS Appl Mater Interfaces. 2016;8:3624–34.
128. Glazer ES, Curley SA. The ongoing history of thermal therapy for cancer. Surg Oncol Clin N Am. 2011;**20**:229–35, vii.
129. Jain PK, Huang X, El-Sayed IH, El-Sayed MA. Noble metals on the nanoscale: optical and photothermal properties and some applications in imaging, sensing, biology, and medicine. Acc Chem Res. 2008;41:1578–86.
130. Yang M, Liu Y, Hou W, Zhi X, Zhang C, Jiang X, Pan F, Yang Y, Ni J, Cui D. Mitomycin C-treated human-induced pluripotent stem cells as a safe delivery system of gold nanorods for targeted photothermal therapy of gastric cancer. Nanoscale. 2017;9:334–40.
131. Singh M, Harris-Birtill DCC, Zhou Y, Gallina ME, Cass AEG, Hanna GB, Elson DS. Application of gold nanorods for photothermal therapy in ex vivo human oesophagogastric adenocarcinoma. J Biomed Nanotechnol. 2016;12:481–90.
132. Wang K, Chen G, Hu Q, Zhen Y, Li H, Chen J, Di B, Hu Y, Sun M, Oupický D. Self-assembled hemoglobin nanoparticles for improved oral photosensitizer delivery and oral photothermal therapy in vivo. Nanomedicine (Lond). 2017;12:1043–55.
133. Li J-L, Hou X-L, Bao H-C, Sun L, Tang B, Wang J-F, Wang X-G, Gu M. Graphene oxide nanoparticles for enhanced photothermal cancer cell therapy under the irradiation of a femtosecond laser beam. J Biomed Mater Res A. 2014;102:2181–8.
134. Imano M, Yasuda A, Itoh T, Satou T, Peng Y-F, Kato H, Shinkai M, Tsubaki M, Chiba Y, Yasuda T, Imamoto H, Nishida S, Takeyama Y, Okuno K, Furukawa H, Shiozaki H. Phase II study of single intraperitoneal chemotherapy followed by systemic chemotherapy for gastric cancer with peritoneal metastasis. J Gastrointest Surg. 2012;16:2190–6.
135. Ishigami H, Kitayama J, Kaisaki S, Hidemura A, Kato M, Otani K, Kamei T, Soma D, Miyato H, Yamashita H, Nagawa H. Phase II study of weekly intravenous and intraperitoneal paclitaxel combined with S-1 for advanced gastric cancer with peritoneal metastasis. Ann Oncol Off J Eur Soc Med Oncol. 2010;21:67–70.
136. Ishigami H, Kitayama J, Kaisaki S, Yamaguchi H, Yamashita H, Emoto S, Nagawa H. Phase I study of biweekly intravenous paclitaxel plus intraperitoneal cisplatin and paclitaxel for gastric cancer with peritoneal metastasis. Oncology. 2010;79:269–72.
137. Zhang L, Zhao D. Applications of nanoparticles for brain cancer imaging and therapy. J Biomed Nanotechnol. 2014;10:1713–31.
138. Baetke SC, Lammers T, Kiessling F. Applications of nanoparticles for diagnosis and therapy of cancer. Br J Radiol. 2015;88:20150207.
139. Ho D. Nanodiamond-based chemotherapy and imaging. Cancer Treat Res. 2015;166:85–102.
140. Ryu JH, Koo H, Sun I-C, Yuk SH, Choi K, Kim K, Kwon IC. Tumor-targeting multi-functional nanoparticles for theragnosis: new paradigm for cancer therapy. Adv Drug Deliv Rev. 2012;64:1447–58.
141. Chen F, Ehlerding EB, Cai W. Theranostic nanoparticles. J Nucl Med. 2014;55:1919–22.
142. Li R, Wu W, Liu Q, Wu P, Xie L, Zhu Z, Yang M, Qian X, Ding Y, Yu L, Jiang X, Guan W, Liu B. Intelligently targeted drug delivery and enhanced antitumor effect by gelatinase-responsive nanoparticles. ed R A de Mello. PLoS One. 2013;8:e69643.
143. Li R, Xie L, Zhu Z, Liu Q, Hu Y, Jiang X, Yu L, Qian X, Guo W, Ding Y, Liu B. Reversion of pH-induced physiological drug resistance: a novel function of copolymeric nanoparticles. ed V Bansal. PLoS One. 2011;6:e24172.

144. Li R, Li X, Xie L, Ding D, Hu Y, Qian X, Yu L, Ding Y, Jiang X, Liu B. Preparation and evaluation of PEG-PCL nanoparticles for local tetradrine delivery. Int J Pharm. 2009;379:158–66.
145. Bakhtiary Z, Saei AA, Hajipour MJ, Raoufi M, Vermesh O, Mahmoudi M. Targeted superparamagnetic iron oxide nanoparticles for early detection of cancer: Possibilities and challenges. Nanomedicine. 2016;12:287–307.
146. Liu W-F, Ji S-R, Sun J-J, Zhang Y, Liu Z-Y, Liang A-B, Zeng H-Z. CD146 expression correlates with epithelial-mesenchymal transition markers and a poor prognosis in gastric cancer. Int J Mol Sci. 2012;13:6399–406.
147. Barzi A, Lenz H-J. Angiogenesis-related agents in esophageal cancer. Expert Opin Biol Ther. 2012;12:1335–45.
148. Wang P, Qu Y, Li C, Yin L, Shen C, Chen W, Yang S, Bian X, Fang D. Bio-functionalized dense-silica nanoparticles for MR/NIRF imaging of CD146 in gastric cancer. Int J Nanomedicine. 2015;10:749–63.
149. Kulhari H, Pooja D, Rompicharla SVK, Sistla R, Adams DJ. Biomedical applications of trastuzumab: as a therapeutic agent and a targeting ligand. Med Res Rev. 2015;35:849–76.
150. Kataoka H, Mori Y, Shimura T, Nishie H, Natsume M, Mochizuki H, Hirata Y, Sobue S, Mizushima T, Sano H, Mizuno Y, Nakamura M, Hirano A, Tsuchida K, Adachi K, Seno K, Kitagawa M, Kawai T, Joh T. A phase II prospective study of the trastuzumab combined with 5-weekly S-1 and CDDP therapy for HER2-positive advanced gastric cancer. Cancer Chemother Pharmacol. 2016;77:957–62.
151. Fornaro L, Lucchesi M, Caparello C, Vasile E, Caponi S, Ginocchi L, Masi G, Falcone A. Anti-HER agents in gastric cancer: from bench to bedside. Nat Rev Gastroenterol Hepatol. 2011;8:369–83.
152. Chen T-J, Cheng T-H, Chen C-Y, Hsu SCN, Cheng T-L, Liu G-C, Wang Y-M. Targeted Herceptin-dextran iron oxide nanoparticles for noninvasive imaging of HER2/neu receptors using MRI. J Biol Inorg Chem. 2009;14:253–60.
153. Jang M, Yoon YI, Kwon YS, Yoon T-J, Lee HJ, Hwang SI, Yun BL, Kim SM. Trastuzumab-conjugated liposome-coated fluorescent magnetic nanoparticles to target breast cancer. Korean J Radiol. 2014;15:411–22.
154. Rajagopal I, Niveditha SR, Sahadev R, Nagappa PK, Rajendra SG. HER 2 expression in gastric and gastro-esophageal junction (GEJ) adenocarcinomas. J Clin Diagn Res. 2015;9:EC06–10.
155. De Carli DM, da Rocha MP, Antunes LCM, Fagundes RB. Immunohistochemical expression of HER2 in adenocarcinoma of the stomach. Arq Gastroenterol. 2015;52:152–5.
156. Zhou Z, Zhang C, Qian Q, Ma J, Huang P, Zhang X, Pan L, Gao G, Fu H, Fu S, Song H, Zhi X, Ni J, Cui D. Folic acid-conjugated silica capped gold nanoclusters for targeted fluorescence/X-ray computed tomography imaging. J Nanobiotechnol. 2013;11:17.
157. Cheng C-C, Huang C-F, Ho A-S, Peng C-L, Chang C-C, Mai F-D, Chen L-Y, Luo T-Y, Chang J. Novel targeted nuclear imaging agent for gastric cancer diagnosis: glucose-regulated protein 78 binding peptide-guided 111In-labeled polymeric micelles. Int J Nanomedicine. 2013;8:1385–91.
158. Jian-Hui C, Shi-Rong C, Hui W, Si-le C, Jian-Bo X, Er-Tao Z, Chuang-Qi C, Yu-Long H. Prognostic value of three different lymph node staging systems in the survival of patients with gastric cancer following D2 lymphadenectomy. Tumour Biol. 2016;37:11105–13.
159. Kang W-M, Meng Q-B, Yu J-C, Ma Z-Q, Li Z-T. Factors associated with early recurrence after curative surgery for gastric cancer. World J Gastroenterol. 2015;21:5934–40.
160. Qiao R, Liu CC, Liu M, Hu H, Liu CC, Hou Y, Wu K, Lin Y, Liang J, Gao M. Ultrasensitive in vivo detection of primary gastric tumor and lymphatic metastasis using upconversion nanoparticles. ACS Nano. 2015;9:2120–9.
161. Tatsumi Y, Tanigawa N, Nishimura H, Nomura E, Mabuchi H, Matsuki M, Narabayashi I. Preoperative diagnosis of lymph node metastases in gastric cancer by magnetic resonance imaging with ferumoxtran-10. Gastric Cancer. 2006;9:120–8.
162. Wang M, Abbineni G, Clevenger A, Mao C, Xu S. Upconversion nanoparticles: synthesis, surface modification and biological applications. Nanomedicine. 2011;7:710–29.
163. Tummers QRJG, Boogerd LSF, de Steur WO, Verbeek FPR, Boonstra MC, Handgraaf HJM, Frangioni JV, van de Velde CJH, Hartgrink HH, Vahrmeijer AL. Near-infrared fluorescence sentinel lymph node detection in gastric cancer: a pilot study. World J Gastroenterol. 2016;22:3644–51.
164. Hoshino I, Maruyama T, Fujito H, Tamura Y, Suganami A, Hayashi H, Toyota T, Akutsu Y, Murakami K, Isozaki Y, Akanuma N, Takeshita N, Toyozumi T, Komatsu A, Matsubara H. Detection of peritoneal dissemination with near-infrared fluorescence laparoscopic imaging using a liposomal formulation of a synthesized indocyanine green liposomal derivative. Anticancer Res. 2015;35:1353–9.
165. Lozano N, Al-Ahmady ZS, Beziere NS, Ntziachristos V, Kostarelos K. Monoclonal antibody-targeted PEGylated liposome-ICG encapsulating doxorubicin as a potential theranostic agent. Int J Pharm. 2015;482:2–10.
166. Hill TK, Mohs AM. Image-guided tumor surgery: will there be a role for fluorescent nanoparticles? Wiley Interdiscip Rev Nanomed Nanobiotechnol. 2016;8:498–511.
167. Yaseen MA, Yu J, Jung B, Wong MS, Anvari B. Biodistribution of encapsulated indocyanine green in healthy mice. Mol Pharm. 2009;6:1321–32.
168. Hill TK, Abdulahad A, Kelkar SS, Marini FC, Long TE, Provenzale JM, Mohs AM. Indocyanine green-

loaded nanoparticles for image-guided tumor surgery. Bioconjug Chem. 2015;26:294–303.
169. Ma Y, Tong S, Bao G, Gao C, Dai Z. Indocyanine green loaded SPIO nanoparticles with phospholipid-PEG coating for dual-modal imaging and photothermal therapy. Biomaterials. 2013;34:7706–14.
170. Tsujimoto H, Morimoto Y, Takahata R, Nomura S, Yoshida K, Horiguchi H, Hiraki S, Ono S, Miyazaki H, Saito D, Hara I, Ozeki E, Yamamoto J, Hase K. Photodynamic therapy using nanoparticle loaded with indocyanine green for experimental peritoneal dissemination of gastric cancer. Cancer Sci. 2014;105:1626–30.
171. Hara E, Makino A, Kurihara K, Sugai M, Shimizu A, Hara I, Ozeki E, Kimura S. Evasion from accelerated blood clearance of nanocarrier named as 'Lactosome' induced by excessive administration of Lactosome. Biochim Biophys Acta. 2013;1830:4046–52.
172. Fan X, Wang L, Guo Y, Tong H, Li L, Ding J, Huang H. Experimental investigation of the penetration of ultrasound nanobubbles in a gastric cancer xenograft. Nanotechnology. 2013;24:325102.
173. Zavaleta CL, Garai E, Liu JTC, Sensarn S, Mandella MJ, Van de Sompel D, Friedland S, Van Dam J, Contag CH, Gambhir SS. A Raman-based endoscopic strategy for multiplexed molecular imaging. Proc Natl Acad Sci U S A. 2013;110:E2288–97.
174. Aroca RF. Surface-enhanced infrared spectroscopy surface-enhanced vibrational spectroscopy. Chichester: Wiley; 2007. p. 185–222.
175. Daniel M-C, Astruc D. Gold nanoparticles: assembly, supramolecular chemistry, quantum-size-related properties, and applications toward biology, catalysis, and nanotechnology. Chem Rev. 2004;104:293–346.
176. Aroca RF. Plasmon enhanced spectroscopy. Phys Chem Chem Phys. 2013;15:5355–63.
177. Mody VV, Siwale R, Singh A, Mody HR. Introduction to metallic nanoparticles. J Pharm Bioallied Sci. 2010;2:282–9.
178. Pieczonka NPW, Aroca RF. Single molecule analysis by surfaced-enhanced Raman scattering. Chem Soc Rev. 2008;37:946–54.
179. Wang Y, Irudayaraj J. Surface-enhanced Raman spectroscopy at single-molecule scale and its implications in biology. Philos Trans R Soc Lond Ser B Biol Sci. 2013;368:20120026.
180. Liu H, Zhang L, Lang X, Yamaguchi Y, Iwasaki H, Inouye Y, Xue Q, Chen M. Single molecule detection from a large-scale SERS-active $Au_{79}Ag_{21}$ substrate. Sci Rep. 2011;1:112.
181. Chen Y, Chen G, Zheng X, He C, Feng S, Chen Y, Lin X, Chen R, Zeng H. Discrimination of gastric cancer from normal by serum RNA based on surface-enhanced Raman spectroscopy (SERS) and multivariate analysis. Med Phys. 2012;39:5664–8.
182. Feng S, Chen R, Lin J, Pan J, Wu Y, Li Y, Chen J, Zeng H. Gastric cancer detection based on blood plasma surface-enhanced Raman spectroscopy excited by polarized laser light. Biosens Bioelectron. 2011;26:3167–74.
183. Feng S, Pan J, Wu Y, Lin D, Chen Y, Xi G, Lin J, Chen R. Study on gastric cancer blood plasma based on surface-enhanced Raman spectroscopy combined with multivariate analysis. Sci China Life Sci. 2011;54:828–34.
184. Qian X, Peng X-H, Ansari DO, Yin-Goen Q, Chen GZ, Shin DM, Yang L, Young AN, Wang MD, Nie S. In vivo tumor targeting and spectroscopic detection with surface-enhanced Raman nanoparticle tags. Nat Biotechnol. 2008;26:83–90.
185. Nguyen AH, Sim SJ. Nanoplasmonic biosensor: detection and amplification of dual bio-signatures of circulating tumor DNA. Biosens Bioelectron. 2015;67:443–9.
186. Wang YW, Kang S, Khan A, Bao PQ, Liu JTC. In vivo multiplexed molecular imaging of esophageal cancer via spectral endoscopy of topically applied SERS nanoparticles. Biomed Opt Express. 2015;6:3714–23.
187. Wang YW, Khan A, Leigh SY, Wang D, Chen Y, Meza D, Liu JTC. Comprehensive spectral endoscopy of topically applied SERS nanoparticles in the rat esophagus. Biomed Opt Express. 2014;5:2883–95.
188. Perfézou M, Turner A, Merkoçi A. Cancer detection using nanoparticle-based sensors. Chem Soc Rev. 2012;41:2606–22.
189. Vilela D, González MC, Escarpa A. Sensing colorimetric approaches based on gold and silver nanoparticles aggregation: Chemical creativity behind the assay. A review. Anal Chim Acta. 2012;751:24–43.
190. Baker GA, Moore DS. Progress in plasmonic engineering of surface-enhanced Raman-scattering substrates toward ultra-trace analysis. Anal Bioanal Chem. 2005;382:1751–70.
191. Salvati E, Stellacci F, Krol S. Nanosensors for early cancer detection and for therapeutic drug monitoring. Nanomedicine. 2015;10:3495–512.
192. Tothill IE. Biosensors for cancer markers diagnosis. Semin Cell Dev Biol. 2009;20:55–62.
193. Hayat A, Catanante G, Marty J. Current trends in nanomaterial-based amperometric biosensors. Sensors. 2014;14:23439–61.
194. Swierczewska M, Liu G, Lee S, Chen X. High-sensitivity nanosensors for biomarker detection. Chem Soc Rev. 2012;41:2641–55.
195. Shiddiky MJA, Rauf S, Kithva PH, Trau M. Graphene/quantum dot bionanoconjugates as signal amplifiers in stripping voltammetric detection of EpCAM biomarkers. Biosens Bioelectron. 2012;35:251–7.
196. Huang S, Zhu F, Qiu H, Xiao Q, Zhou Q, Su W, Hu B. A sensitive quantum dots-based "OFF-ON" fluorescent sensor for ruthenium anticancer drugs and ctDNA. Colloids Surf B Biointerfaces. 2014;117:240–7.
197. Wittrup A, Zhang S-H, Svensson KJ, Kucharzewska P, Johansson MC, Morgelin M, Belting M. Magnetic

nanoparticle-based isolation of endocytic vesicles reveals a role of the heat shock protein GRP75 in macromolecular delivery. Proc Natl Acad Sci. 2010;107:13342–7.
198. Shao H, Chung J, Lee K, Balaj L, Min C, Carter BS, Hochberg FH, Breakefield XO, Lee H, Weissleder R. Chip-based analysis of exosomal mRNA mediating drug resistance in glioblastoma. Nat Commun. 2015;6:6999.
199. Muluneh M, Issadore D. Microchip-based detection of magnetically labeled cancer biomarkers. Adv Drug Deliv Rev. 2014;66:101–9.
200. Ravalli A, Marrazza G. Gold and magnetic nanoparticles-based electrochemical biosensors for cancer biomarker determination. J Nanosci Nanotechnol. 2015;15:3307–19.
201. Nie L, Liu F, Ma P, Xiao X. Applications of gold nanoparticles in optical biosensors. J Biomed Nanotechnol. 2014;10:2700–21.
202. Jena BK, Ghosh S, Bera R, Dey RS, Das AK, Raj CR. Bioanalytical applications of au nanoparticles. Recent Pat Nanotechnol. 2010;4:41–52.
203. Viswambari Devi R, Doble M, Verma RS. Nanomaterials for early detection of cancer biomarker with special emphasis on gold nanoparticles in immunoassays/sensors. Biosens Bioelectron. 2015;68:688–98.
204. Chan WCW, Maxwell DJ, Gao X, Bailey RE, Han M, Nie S. Luminescent quantum dots for multiplexed biological detection and imaging. Curr Opin Biotechnol. 2002;13:40–6.
205. Kim S, Bawendi MG. Oligomeric ligands for luminescent and stable nanocrystal quantum dots. J Am Chem Soc. 2003;125:14652–3.
206. Zhang Y, Zhou D. Magnetic particle-based ultrasensitive biosensors for diagnostics. Expert Rev Mol Diagn. 2012;12:565–71.
207. Zhong Z, Wu W, Wang D, Wang D, Shan J, Qing Y, Zhang Z. Nanogold-enwrapped graphene nanocomposites as trace labels for sensitivity enhancement of electrochemical immunosensors in clinical immunoassays: carcinoembryonic antigen as a model. Biosens Bioelectron. 2010;25:2379–83.
208. Hou L, Wu X, Chen G, Yang H, Lu M, Tang D. HCR-stimulated formation of DNAzyme concatamers on gold nanoparticle for ultrasensitive impedimetric immunoassay. Biosens Bioelectron. 2015;68:487–93.
209. Chen H, Tang D, Zhang B, Liu B, Cui Y, Chen G. Electrochemical immunosensor for carcinoembryonic antigen based on nanosilver-coated magnetic beads and gold-graphene nanolabels. Talanta. 2012;91:95–102.
210. Ling S, Yuan R, Chai Y, Zhang T. Study on immunosensor based on gold nanoparticles/chitosan and MnO2 nanoparticles composite membrane/Prussian blue modified gold electrode. Bioprocess Biosyst Eng. 2009;32:407–14.
211. Das J, Kelley SO. Protein detection using arrayed microsensor chips: tuning sensor footprint to achieve ultrasensitive readout of CA-125 in serum and whole blood. Anal Chem. 2011;83:1167–72.
212. Tang D, Su B, Tang J, Ren J, Chen G. Nanoparticle-based sandwich electrochemical immunoassay for carbohydrate antigen 125 with signal enhancement using enzyme-coated nanometer-sized enzyme-doped silica beads. Anal Chem. 2010;82:1527–34.
213. Wu D, Guo Z, Liu Y, Guo A, Lou W, Fan D, Wei Q. Sandwich-type electrochemical immunosensor using dumbbell-like nanoparticles for the determination of gastric cancer biomarker CA72-4. Talanta. 2015;134:305–9.
214. Chun L, Kim S-E, Cho M, Choe W, Nam J, Lee DW, Lee Y. Electrochemical detection of HER2 using single stranded DNA aptamer modified gold nanoparticles electrode. Sensors Actuators B Chem. 2013;186:446–50.
215. Căinap C, Nagy V, Gherman A, Cetean S, Laszlo I, Constantin A-M, Căinap S. Classic tumor markers in gastric cancer. Current standards and limitations. Clujul Med. 2015;88:111.
216. Jokerst JV, Raamanathan A, Christodoulides N, Floriano PN, Pollard AA, Simmons GW, Wong J, Gage C, Furmaga WB, Redding SW, McDevitt JT. Nano-bio-chips for high performance multiplexed protein detection: determinations of cancer biomarkers in serum and saliva using quantum dot bioconjugate labels. Biosens Bioelectron. 2009;24:3622–9.
217. Khazanov E, Yavin E, Pascal A, Nissan A, Kohl Y, Reimann-Zawadzki M, Rubinstein A. Detecting a secreted gastric cancer biomarker molecule by targeted nanoparticles for real-time diagnostics. Pharm Res. 2012;29:983–93.
218. Daneshpour M, Omidfar K, Ghanbarian H. A novel electrochemical nanobiosensor for the ultrasensitive and specific detection of femtomolar-level gastric cancer biomarker miRNA-106a. Beilstein J Nanotechnol. 2016;7:2023–36.
219. Lin M, Chen J-F, Lu Y-T, Zhang Y, Song J, Hou S, Ke Z, Tseng H-R. Nanostructure embedded microchips for detection, isolation, and characterization of circulating tumor cells. Acc Chem Res. 2014;47:2941–50.
220. Myung JH, Tam KA, Park S, Cha A, Hong S. Recent advances in nanotechnology-based detection and separation of circulating tumor cells. Wiley Interdiscip Rev Nanomed Nanobiotechnol. 2016;8:223–39.
221. Wang H-Y, Wei J, Zou Z-Y, Qian X-P, Liu B-R. Circulating tumour cells predict survival in gastric cancer patients: a meta-analysis. Współczesna Onkol. 2015;6:451–7.
222. Yoon HJ, Kozminsky M, Nagrath S. Emerging role of nanomaterials in circulating tumor cell isolation and analysis. ACS Nano. 2014;8:1995–2017.
223. Bhana S, Wang Y, Huang X. Nanotechnology for enrichment and detection of circulating tumor cells. Nanomedicine. 2015;10:1973–90.
224. Chen Z, Hong G, Wang H, Welsher K, Tabakman SM, Sherlock SP, Robinson JT, Liang Y, Dai

H. Graphite-coated magnetic nanoparticle microarray for few-cells enrichment and detection. ACS Nano. 2012;6:1094–101.
225. Hou S, Zhao L, Shen Q, Yu J, Ng C, Kong X, Wu D, Song M, Shi X, Xu X, OuYang W-H, He R, Zhao X-Z, Lee T, Brunicardi FC, Garcia MA, Ribas A, Lo RS, Tseng H-R. Polymer nanofiber-embedded microchips for detection, isolation, and molecular analysis of single circulating melanoma cells. Angew Chem Int Ed. 2013;52:3379–83.
226. Lee HJ, Cho H-Y, Oh JH, Namkoong K, Lee JG, Park J-M, Lee SS, Huh N, Choi J-W. Simultaneous capture and in situ analysis of circulating tumor cells using multiple hybrid nanoparticles. Biosens Bioelectron. 2013;47:508–14.
227. Galanzha EI, Shashkov EV, Kelly T, Kim J-W, Yang L, Zharov VP. In vivo magnetic enrichment and multiplex photoacoustic detection of circulating tumour cells. Nat Nanotechnol. 2009;4:855–60.
228. Xu H, Aguilar ZP, Yang L, Kuang M, Duan H, Xiong Y, Wei H, Wang A. Antibody conjugated magnetic iron oxide nanoparticles for cancer cell separation in fresh whole blood. Biomaterials. 2011;32:9758–65.
229. Song E-Q, Hu J, Wen C-Y, Tian Z-Q, Yu X, Zhang Z-L, Shi Y-B, Pang D-W. Fluorescent-magnetic-biotargeting multifunctional nanobioprobes for detecting and isolating multiple types of tumor cells. ACS Nano. 2011;5:761–70.
230. He R, Zhao L, Liu Y, Zhang N, Cheng B, He Z, Cai B, Li S, Liu W, Guo S, Chen Y, Xiong B, Zhao X-Z. Biocompatible TiO2 nanoparticle-based cell immunoassay for circulating tumor cells capture and identification from cancer patients. Biomed Microdevices. 2013;15:617–26.
231. Chou C-P, Chen Y-W, Liou G-G, Pan H-B, Tseng H-H, Hung Y-T. Specific detection of CD133-positive tumor cells with iron oxide nanoparticles labeling using noninvasive molecular magnetic resonance imaging. Int J Nanomed. 2015;10:6997.
232. Chen Y, Lian G, Liao C, Wang W, Zeng L, Qian C, Huang K, Shuai X. Characterization of polyethylene glycol-grafted polyethylenimine and superparamagnetic iron oxide nanoparticles (PEG-g-PEI-SPION) as an MRI-visible vector for siRNA delivery in gastric cancer in vitro and in vivo. J Gastroenterol. 2013;48:809–21.
233. Sumer B, Gao J. Theranostic nanomedicine for cancer. Nanomedicine. 2008;3:137–40.
234. Janib SM, Moses AS, MacKay JA. Imaging and drug delivery using theranostic nanoparticles. Adv Drug Deliv Rev. 2010;62:1052–63.
235. Muthu MS, Feng S-S. Theranostic liposomes for cancer diagnosis and treatment: current development and pre-clinical success. Expert Opin Drug Deliv. 2013;10:151–5.
236. Muthu MS, Singh S. Targeted nanomedicines: effective treatment modalities for cancer, AIDS and brain disorders. Nanomedicine. 2009;4:105–18.
237. Muthu MS, Rajesh CV, Mishra A, Singh S. Stimulus-responsive targeted nanomicelles for effective cancer therapy. Nanomedicine. 2009;4:657–67.
238. Muthu MS, Leong DT, Mei L, Feng S-S. Nanotheranostics – application and further development of nanomedicine strategies for advanced theranostics. Theranostics. 2014;4:660–77.
239. Mei L, Zhang Z, Zhao L, Huang L, Yang X-L, Tang J, Feng S-S. Pharmaceutical nanotechnology for oral delivery of anticancer drugs. Adv Drug Deliv Rev. 2013;65:880–90.
240. Xie J, Lee S, Chen X. Nanoparticle-based theranostic agents. Adv Drug Deliv Rev. 2010;62:1064–79.
241. Ye Y, Chen X. Integrin targeting for tumor optical imaging. Theranostics. 2011;1:102–26.
242. Xu C, Zhao W. Nanoparticle-based monitoring of stem cell therapy. Theranostics. 2013;3:616–7.
243. Anbarasu M, Anandan M, Chinnasamy E, Gopinath V, Balamurugan K. Synthesis and characterization of polyethylene glycol (PEG) coated Fe3O4 nanoparticles by chemical co-precipitation method for biomedical applications. Spectrochim Acta A Mol Biomol Spectrosc. 2015;135:536–9.
244. Zhao J, Mi Y, Feng S-S. siRNA-based nanomedicine. Nanomedicine. 2013;8:859–62.
245. Huang K, Yinting Chen W, wei-wei Wang G, Guoda Lian C, Chenchen Qian L, Lingyun Wang L, Linjuan Zeng C, Chengde Liao B, Biling Liang B, Bing Huang K, Shuai X-T. Development of an MRI-visible nonviral vector for siRNA delivery targeting gastric cancer. Int J Nanomedicine. 2012;7:359.
246. Luo X, Peng X, Hou J, Wu S, Shen J, Wang L. Folic acid-functionalized polyethylenimine superparamagnetic iron oxide nanoparticles as theranostic agents for magnetic resonance imaging and PD-L1 siRNA delivery for gastric cancer. Int J Nanomedicine. 2017;12:5331–43.
247. Sun Z, Song X, Li X, Su T, Qi S, Qiao R, Wang F, Huan Y, Yang W, Wang J, Nie Y, Wu K, Gao M, Cao F. In vivo multimodality imaging of miRNA-16 iron nanoparticle reversing drug resistance to chemotherapy in a mouse gastric cancer model. Nanoscale. 2014;6:14343–53.
248. Wang F-Q, Li P, Zhang J-P, Wang A-Q, Wei Q. A novel pH-sensitive magnetic alginate–chitosan beads for albendazole delivery. Drug Dev Ind Pharm. 2010;36:867–77.
249. Ma H, Liu Y, Shi M, Shao X, Zhong W, Liao W, Xing MMQ. Theranostic, pH-responsive, doxorubicin-loaded nanoparticles inducing active targeting and apoptosis for advanced gastric cancer. Biomacromolecules. 2015;16:4022–31.
250. Wu J, Shen Y, Jiang W, Jiang W, Shen Y. Magnetic targeted drug delivery carriers encapsulated with pH-sensitive polymer: synthesis, characterization and *in vitro* doxorubicin release studies. J Biomater Sci Polym Ed. 2016;27:1303–16.
251. Huang P, Lin J, Wang X, Wang Z, Zhang C, He M, Wang K, Chen F, Li Z, Shen G, Cui D, Chen X. Light-triggered theranostics based on photosensitizer-conjugated carbon dots for simultaneous enhanced-fluorescence imaging and photodynamic therapy. Adv Mater. 2012;24:5104–10.

252. Huang P, Li Z, Lin J, Yang D, Gao G, Xu C, Bao L, Zhang C, Wang K, Song H, Hu H, Cui D. Photosensitizer-conjugated magnetic nanoparticles for in vivo simultaneous magnetofluorescent imaging and targeting therapy. Biomaterials. 2011;32:3447–58.
253. Tsujimoto H, Morimoto Y, Takahata R, Nomura S, Yoshida K, Hiraki S, Horiguchi H, Miyazaki H, Ono S, Saito D, Hara I, Ozeki E, Yamamoto J, Hase K. Theranostic photosensitive nanoparticles for lymph node metastasis of gastric cancer. Ann Surg Oncol. 2015;22:923–8.
254. Lotfi-Attari J, Pilehvar-Soltanahmadi Y, Dadashpour M, Alipour S, Farajzadeh R, Javidfar S, Zarghami N. Co-delivery of curcumin and chrysin by polymeric nanoparticles inhibit synergistically growth and hTERT gene expression in human colorectal cancer cells. Nutr Cancer. 2017;69:1290–9.
255. Mariano RN, Alberti D, Cutrin JC, Geninatti Crich S, Aime S. Design of PLGA based nanoparticles for imaging guided applications. Mol Pharm. 2014;11:4100–6.
256. Chang Y-N, Zhang M, Xia L, Zhang J, Xing G. The toxic effects and mechanisms of CuO and ZnO nanoparticles. Materials (Basel). 2012;5:2850–71.
257. Sharma A, Madhunapantula SV, Robertson GP. Toxicological considerations when creating nanoparticle-based drugs and drug delivery systems. Expert Opin Drug Metab Toxicol. 2012;8:47–69.
258. Bergin IL, Witzmann FA. Nanoparticle toxicity by the gastrointestinal route: evidence and knowledge gaps. Int J Biomed Nanosci Nanotechnol. 2013;3:163.
259. Liu L, Ye Q, Lu M, Lo Y-C, Hsu Y-H, Wei M-C, Chen Y-H, Lo S-C, Wang S-J, Bain DJ, Ho C. A new approach to reduce toxicities and to improve bioavailabilities of platinum-containing anti-cancer nanodrugs. Sci Rep. 2015;5:10881.
260. Chapman S, Dobrovolskaia M, Farahani K, Goodwin A, Joshi A, Lee H, Meade T, Pomper M, Ptak K, Rao J, Singh R, Sridhar S, Stern S, Wang A, Weaver JB, Woloschak G, Yang L. Nanoparticles for cancer imaging: the good, the bad, and the promise. Nano Today. 2013;8:454–60.
261. Blanco E, Shen H, Ferrari M. Principles of nanoparticle design for overcoming biological barriers to drug delivery. Nat Biotechnol. 2015;33:941–51.

Index

© Springer Nature Switzerland AG 2019

V. Canzonieri, A. Giordano (eds.), *Gastric Cancer In The Precision Medicine Era*, Current Clinical Pathology, https://doi.org/10.1007/978-3-030-04861-7

D

E

F

G

H

I

J

K

L

M

N

Printed by Printforce, the Netherlands